The Vaccine Guide is a highly informative discussion of key issues necessary for making informed decisions about vaccination. Chapters address adverse reactions, chemical preservatives, and legal exemptions, as well as bioterrorism and adult vaccinations.

—Mothering Magazine

The Vaccine Guide is surprisingly readable and despite the vastness of this field and the potentially turgid and macabre nature of this catalogue of woes, it is gripping.

—Homeopathic Links

The Vaccine Guide is a thorough, well-researched introduction to a complicated, explosive subject. For any parent who believes in informed choice, this book makes all the sense in the world.

—Natural Health Magazine

I have discussed [this] book virtually every day my practice. I couldn't get away from it even if I want to—which I do not.

—Jay Gordon MD, pediatrician

This well organized, user-friendly guide.... [It] will prove an indispensable aid for those trying to make educated decisions about this controversial topic.

—Janet Levatin MD, pediatrician

This book is an invaluable guide to help p rents make an informed choice about this vital health issue.

—Kenneth P. Stoller MD, pediatrician

The first edition of *The Vaccine Guide* was published in 1972 and the recently published revised edition specifically addresses the threat of bioterrorism.... With a vaccine reference guide and the CDC's published information, you can start to connect the dots on your own. Dying for your country over a lousy shot is not something the government should recommend for millions of Americans.

—Jennie Rose at Blogcritics.org

Vaccine Facts

Compulsory vaccination laws exist in every state.

All vaccines carry risks of adverse reactions.

Every parent has the legal right to exempt children from vaccination.

The vaccination campaign has traded infectious diseases of childhood for chronic autoimmune diseases that afflict both children and adults.

THE VACCINE GUIDE
Risks and Benefits for Children and Adults

Randall Neustaedter, OMD

REVISED EDITION

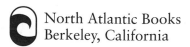

North Atlantic Books
Berkeley, California

Homeopathic Educational Services, Berkeley, California

Published by

North Atlantic Books
P.O. Box 12327
Berkeley, California 94712

Homeopathic Educational Services
2124 Kittredge Street
Berkeley, California 94704

Cover design © Ayelet Maida, A/M Studios

Book design and production by Jan Camp, JCamp Studio

Printed in the United States of America

The Vaccine Guide is sponsored by the Society for the Study of Native Arts and Sciences, a nonprofit educational corporation whose goals are to develop an educational and crosscultural perspective linking various scientific, social, and artistic fields; to nurture a holistic view of arts, sciences, humanities, and healing; and to publish and distribute literature on the relationship of mind, body, and nature.

This book has been written as an information resource. It is not intended as medical advice. As with any medical procedure, consumers should base their decisions about vaccines on careful research. Consultation with professionals, including health care providers and attorneys with expertise in the area of vaccination, will also help to clarify the issues involved in this important decision.

Library of Congress Cataloging-in-Publication Data

Neustaedter, Randall, 1949–
    The vaccine guide: risks and benefits for children and adults / by Randall Neustaedter.
      p. ; cm.
    Includes bibliographical references and index.
      1. Vaccination—Popular works. 2. Immunization of children—Popular works.
    3. Vaccines—Popular works. 4. Risk Assessment—Popular Works.
QW806 N496v 2002] I. Title.
    RA638 .N485 2002
    614.4'7—dc21   2002012036
                                                                        CIP

4 5 6 7 8 9 DATA 06

Dedicated to my wife, Michele

Acknowledgments

I would like to thank the parents, child advocates, clinicians, crusaders, and scientific researchers who have been in the forefront as pioneers challenging the vaccine campaigns.

Harris Coulter (author and historian)

Barbara Loe Fisher and Kathi Williams (cofounders of the NVIC)

Congressman Dan Burton

Researchers and clinicians Bernard Rimland, Andrew Wakefield, Vijendra Singh, F. Edward Yazbak, Meryl Nass, Harold Buttram, Bart Classen, and John Martin

Outspoken parents Ray Gallup, Cindy Goldenberg, Michael Belkin, Danielle Burton Sarkine

Organizers Dawn Richardson, Dawn Winkler, Meryl Dorey

And all the valiant children who have been injured by vaccines.

Contents

Part II: The Vaccines

Preface to the New Edition

The Vaccine Guide now includes issues that relate to vaccination of adults as well as children. Smallpox and anthrax vaccines have emerged as urgent topics as a result of terrorist attacks on America. Since publication of the first edition, adult readers have repeatedly asked about flu vaccines and vaccination for international travel, and I have included chapters on these topics as well. Reports of new conditions associated with vaccine reactions have also appeared in research studies since the previous version of the book. Autism, asthma, diabetes, and the Gulf War Syndrome have each been directly linked to adverse vaccine reactions. A new edition seemed essential.

The accumulated evidence of devastating disease caused by vaccines is shocking and scandalous. These drugs that supposedly protect our population from deadly illness have been shown in recent years to wreak their own brand of havoc. The damage that vaccines cause on immune functions is now undeniable, but the repeated denial of serious adverse events and deaths by vaccine manufacturers is reminiscent of the tobacco industry's stonewalling. The power of drug companies and their influence in government has created a system where vaccine reactions are ignored and dismissed. Since 1986, drug companies have enjoyed immunity from liability for children's vaccine reactions.

In this protected environment, vaccine manufacturers continue to develop and dispense a growing number of increasingly expensive and dangerous vaccines. These vaccines are rushed into the market, where they undergo extensive testing on America's children. The tragic deaths caused by the rotavirus vaccine for diarrhea in children serve as a reminder of the dangers inherent in this vaccine industry process.

Within six months of being approved and recommended for all children, the rotavirus vaccine was withdrawn. Later investigations revealed that government committees ignored studies that warned of the vaccine's deadly side effects. In recent years, vaccine critics and outraged parents have demanded and won congressional hearings to investigate the newer childhood vaccines, their approval process, and the conflicts of interest inherent in a system where members of government committees are also paid representatives of drug companies.

Vaccine decisions are made in four circumstances.

1. Parents confront the issue of vaccines beginning with the birth of a child, and subsequent doctor visits focus on the ritual of vaccination.

2. Adults must decide whether to maintain the vaccinations begun during childhood.

3. When contemplating international travel, adults and children are advised to get vaccinated against exotic diseases.

4. The recent threat of bioterrorism has triggered an emergency interest in smallpox and anthrax vaccines.

Most parents are surprised to learn that they have a choice about vaccination. Usually, pediatricians do not give parents any information about potential adverse reactions. They assure parents that babies need vaccines and the ritual begins, first at their child's birth and then again at the two-month office visit. Parents may have made conscious choices about natural childbirth, circumcision, and breastfeeding, but never considered the issues surrounding vaccines. Adults, especially the elderly, are expected to get their flu shots every year. And now the issue of mandatory smallpox has once again made headlines, just as it did during protests against compulsory vaccination in the early twentieth century.

Who decided that our citizens require all of these vaccines? Why have we adopted a policy of universal immunization for every childhood ailment? Why is the public left out of a process considered too technical for their understanding? Who do we trust?

It is only in recent years that large numbers of people have begun to question routine medical procedures. People are voicing their own choices in health care. Questions have been raised about the overuse of antibiotics, the many unnecessary surgeries performed on breast cancer patients, and the useless procedure of infant circumcision. Even amidst criticisms of the medical establishment, however, very few assail the venerable institution of vaccines. We have been conditioned and convinced to accept vaccination as a savior of children and a miracle that freed us from deadly infectious disease. That refrain, repeated so often, has become a watchword of our culture. Politicians concerned about their ratings in the polls pick up a baby and announce their support for more immunizations to safeguard our children, an ever-popular position. In recent memory, President Ford energetically supported the swine flu vaccine catastrophe. President Carter sponsored an immunization campaign that increased Congress's allocated funding from 7 million to 47 million dollars within the first two years after his election. President Reagan passed the National Childhood Vaccine Injury Act of 1986 to ensure adequate vaccine production. And President Clinton passed the Comprehensive Child Immunization Act of 1993.

Unfortunately, complete information about vaccines is not generally available. Parents feel poorly informed. Like most decisions about health care, the choice of which vaccines to give, the timing of vaccines, and their child's safety rest in the hands of the doctor. But doctors receive recommendations from vaccine advisory committees, and the committees rely upon studies conducted by drug manufacturers. Parents who do not make an informed choice place their child's health in the hands of drug companies with a profit motive.

Parents have the responsibility to provide the best health care possible for their own children. They must decide whether it is better for their child's health to give the vaccines or not. If parents question the validity or wisdom of administering vaccines to their child, they receive little support in their efforts to make an informed choice. Even adults who are advised to receive the vaccine for hepatitis, tetanus, typhoid, or flu have difficulty foraging through information on the Internet to make an informed decision.

This book is intended to help parents investigate the subject of vaccination, and to guide readers to an informed choice about each vaccine. *The Vaccine Guide* provides consumers with information about the diseases, the vaccines, their risks and their benefits. Parents, especially, need to know the issues and the controversies surrounding these drugs, since the potential adverse effects of vaccines are usually cloaked in secrecy. Medical professionals have often stated that broadcasting adverse effects of vaccines to the public would cause unnecessary concern and hinder vaccine campaigns. Dr. Paul Meier summarized this position quite clearly in a panel discussion on the efficacy of the polio vaccine campaign of the 1950s:

> It is hard to convince the public that something is good. Consequently, the best way to push forward a new program is to decide on what you think the best decision is and not question it thereafter, and further, not to raise questions before the public or expose the public to open discussion of the issues (Intensive Immunization Programs, Hearings, 1962).

Similar sentiments were published later in a more recent dialogue concerning the release of information from a study that suggested the measles vaccine could cause chronic intestinal disease. The Chief Medical Officer of England's Department of Health wrote, "It would be most unfortunate if the publication of this controversial work led to public anxiety over the safety of measles vaccine" (Calman, 1995). The authors of that study responded, "We reported the measles vaccination study for discussion by the scientific community, not only with many qualifications . . . but also with great care not to excite media over-reaction. . . . We realized that the measles vaccination programme is of great importance to the community and the public health of the nation, but it would have been unethical to suppress this result because its preliminary conclusions were uncomfortable or inconvenient" (Thompson *et al.*, 1995a). I would commend the ethical stance of these authors. Unfortunately, information about vaccine reactions is constantly suppressed because such findings run contrary to policy decisions about vaccination.

The passage by Congress of the National Childhood Vaccine Injury

Act has required more disclosure about vaccines and encouraged informed consent, but parents still have little information about the vaccines, and suppression of information remains a goal of many pharmacies and pediatrician organizations. For example, when the American Academy of Pediatrics' former president, Dr. Martin Smith, reviewed information brochures for parents prepared by the US Department of Health and Human Services, he recommended that they be simplified. He said, "The length and complexity of the materials . . . would confuse many parents and could even needlessly alarm them" (AAP News, 1989).

Parents are hungry for information about the vaccines, especially their adverse effects. They are unwilling to blindly accept the opinions of doctors concerning medical care. This book seeks to provide information that is usually unavailable to parents.

The Vaccine Guide also places the issues surrounding vaccines within the context of a health care philosophy. Natural medical care and alternative medicine support the body's own healing mechanisms, and the result is a stronger, more resilient immune system. Modern technological medicine manipulates the immune system with drugs, a process that sometimes goes awry, resulting in a self-destructive immune reaction. When consumers view vaccinations as part of an overall medical philosophy it places vaccine choices within a more familiar perspective, one they have given a lot of thought.

The subject of vaccines can be confusing and overwhelming. In *The Vaccine Guide* I have simplified the issues without sacrificing the detail that consumers need to make an informed choice. I present the ideas and facts here as I do with patients in my office. I state the facts about each disease and vaccine, summarize the information, and present the options regarding individual vaccines as a personal strategy. Ultimately, each individual and parent must decide what is best based on their philosophy, comfort level, and understanding of the real issues that surround vaccinations. Only then will your choice be based upon intelligent reasoning and not blind faith.

I recommend that you read at least the first chapter, "Making an Informed Choice," and the Conclusion of this book, to understand the philosophical issues involved in making a choice about vaccination. The second chapter, "Adverse Vaccine Reactions," presents a sobering view of the damage caused by vaccines, effects that have led many observers to note that our program of eliminating infectious disease through vaccination has resulted in an epidemic of devastating chronic illness. The other chapters about legal requirements and the individual diseases can be studied individually as reference materials when you are confronted with a new vaccine.

A note on conventions used throughout the book is warranted here. The words "vaccinate" and "vaccination" are used to denote the process in preference to "immunize" and "immunization" because vaccines do not always induce immunity. In fact, vaccines very clearly suppress the immune system. Although vaccine research is conducted throughout the world, legal issues and statistics discussed in the book usually refer to the United States. Other issues relating to vaccine effectiveness, reactions, and options should be applicable in all developed nations.

Part I: Choices

MAKING AN INFORMED CHOICE

Childhood Vaccines

The experience of childhood vaccination is not pleasant. Babies scream and develop fevers with the first illness of their lives in reaction to the vaccine. Preschoolers learn to fear the doctor because they are jabbed with needles whenever they go for well-child check-ups. Older children run around the doctor's office refusing to be poked, or cling to their mothers in abject terror awaiting the dreaded needle. Parents are informed that vaccines may damage their child's nervous system. This causes understandable apprehension in everyone. Parents are convinced that all of this is worthwhile. Or are they? Most have doubts, but little information. They have been told that vaccines are the greatest achievement of modern preventive medicine. The polio epidemic of the 1950s, the March of Dimes, and the eradication of smallpox are historical events of the recent past. We are assured that one more generation of vaccines will eliminate whooping cough, measles, and mumps as threats to our children, just as polio and diphtheria have disappeared into memory. This is a reassuring and convincing argument: Risk a few cases of rare adverse effects to eliminate these serious and life-threatening diseases. But lingering doubts remain.

Parents must accommodate themselves to the vaccines' adverse effects. They must steel themselves against their children's inevitable anxiety about the doctor visit and dread of the shot. They wonder about the publicized cases of vaccine-damaged children. Measles, mumps, and chickenpox were simple childhood diseases. Why all the excitement about them now? Parents are upset when their child develops a fever after a shot, though it usually is not serious. Parents are devastated if their child develops polio, seizures, or retardation after a vaccination, but these reactions are relatively uncommon. We are told that this is the price we pay for eliminating these diseases from our population. We are reassured that the incidence of these problems would be higher from the natural diseases if the vaccines were not given routinely.

What is the truth about the vaccine campaign? Isn't someone making a lot of money from these billions of shots? Most parents put these doubts aside and rationalize: My pediatrician would not be influenced by a drug company's desire for profit. Doctors would not recommend these vaccines unless they were convinced of their necessity. I have to leave the decision to the doctor. I just don't know enough to make a judgment about such a complex issue.

As a parent you are faced with many decisions soon after your baby is born. Most of these are retractable. You can decide to use cloth diapers after four months of plastic ones. If you say the wrong thing to your child, you can recant. If you decide that giving ice cream to Jennifer for breakfast so she gets at least a little protein is not such a great idea after all, you can change your mind tomorrow. Even medical decisions are usually reversible. The decongestant makes Jesse too groggy; let's try a humidifier tonight. But some medical decisions are momentous. Circumcision, vaccination—these are weighty issues with permanent effects.

Parents have a responsibility to avoid toxic exposure and toxic hazards. Locking up the cupboards and childproofing hazardous areas of the kitchen can prevent poisoning from household chemicals. Avoiding chemicals in foods takes extra effort. Parents can shop at health-food stores to sidestep the antibiotics and growth hormones in milk, the pesticides on fruits and vegetables, the preservatives in packaged foods. Some toxic exposure cannot be prevented so easily—pollution, ozone depletion, pesticides used on lawns and trees in public parks and playgrounds. Escaping city life may be the only possible solution for these problems. But the toxicity of vaccines, the injection of virulent neurotoxins and heavy metals into an infant's bloodstream, can be avoided by simply saying *no* to the pediatrician.

You must rely on various advisors to give you their opinions. Family, friends, and health professionals can all be helpful and informative, but you must ultimately take responsibility for the choices. The issues of medical decisions are not out of your reach. Except for emergency situations that require immediate action, you can weigh the pros and cons of a medical decision. Some of these may be obvious and simple, others may be agonizing. Any decision will be easier if you have support and reassurance that you are doing the right thing. Unfortunately, the subject of vaccinations often involves heated emotions and recriminations.

I encourage parents to gather information from professionals with differing views about vaccination. The medical issues are controversial, and you need to be aware of these controversies when making a truly informed decision about your child's health care. Individuals with differing perspectives will examine the same data and arrive at different conclusions. For that reason I have included here reviews of the medical literature for parents to examine themselves. I also recommend that parents obtain and read those materials listed at the end of this book that seem most interesting (see Resources). These publications are generally critical of vaccinations for children. Pediatricians and most books on child health care are good alternative sources for pro-vaccination information.

I recommend that parents take a careful look at the vaccine question in general and each vaccine individually before making a decision for their child. In the following sections of this book, I outline a practical approach that should help guide you through the maze of the vaccine question.

Four steps are necessary for parents who want to make an informed decision.

1. Understand the philosophical issues surrounding vaccines.

2. Get information about the vaccines.

3. Decide which vaccines you do or don't want.

4. If you decide to vaccinate, then choose the right time.

Adult Vaccines

Childhood vaccination has resulted in a shift of some formerly childhood diseases to the adult population. The percentage of adults who contract whooping cough, measles, and mumps compared to children has increased. The protective effect of childhood vaccines decreases over time, and eventually after ten or twenty years, adults become susceptible once again to these infectious diseases. The same will be true for chickenpox when this generation grows up. Some diseases, such as whooping cough, are typically milder in adults than in children. In fact, many thousands of cases of whooping cough in adults go undiagnosed every year because the cough is minimal. Other diseases, like chickenpox, are typically much more severe in adulthood. Chickenpox in children lasts for about a week. In adults symptoms persist for a month. Adults are now faced with the decision of whether to continue these childhood vaccines on a regular booster schedule, just as they have always done with tetanus.

Adults are presented with many vaccine decisions in addition to those vaccines begun in childhood. Hepatitis is a potential threat inherent to various adult lifestyles. Hepatitis B is primarily a sexually transmitted disease, and adults with multiple sexual partners are encouraged to have the vaccine. Since hepatitis B is also transmitted by exposure to the blood of infected patients, hepatitis vaccination is required for health care workers. Hepatitis A is a disease contracted by drinking contaminated water, and the vaccine is encouraged for people in areas where the disease is endemic. Flu vaccine is recommended for all adults every year, but especially encouraged for those who suffer from chronic respiratory disease and the elderly, who could suffer more than others from the effects of a severe viral illness. A vaccine for pneumococcal pneumonia is usually recommended for elderly people. College students are required to receive measles and meningitis vaccines. Women who do not have antibodies to the rubella virus in their bloodstream are expected to obtain the rubella vaccine to protect their unborn children in case of exposure during pregnancy. Immigrants are required to obtain vaccines when applying for citizenship or work permits and extended visas. Multiple vaccinations are required for induction into the military. And now the threat of terrorism has opened the possibility for compulsory vaccination against smallpox and anthrax. Finally, the recommendations for international travel often include vaccination against typhoid, yellow fever, and hepatitis A.

Adverse effects of vaccines are not limited to infants whose immune systems and nervous systems are especially vulnerable. Some of the most dramatic and debilitating reactions to vaccines have occurred in adults following the hepatitis, flu, and rubella vaccines. Many adults make careful health care decisions for their children, but conform to expectations for their own vaccination program.

Philosophy and Medical Care

Modern (allopathic) medicine is based upon several underlying assumptions. The first is the concept of reduction. The body can be reduced to its parts—the organs, the tissues, and the "systems." This allows for the manipulation of one part—the immune system for example—without any regard for the effect this will have on the integrity of the person as a whole. The second assumption is that diseases are bad and need to be combated. This leads to the concept of chemical warfare conducted against the kingdom of diseases. If some innocent civilians lose their lives as a result of the weapons employed, then that is the unfortunate cost of war. This has certainly been the stated position of leaders in the vaccine campaign. The third assumption is that diseases should be prevented by chemicals. This takes the form of lifelong medication with drugs, for example fluoridation of water systems to prevent tooth decay, estrogen replacement in post-menopausal women to prevent bone loss, and periodic vaccine administration beginning in infancy to prevent infectious diseases.

It is important for parents, and all health care consumers, to examine their beliefs about these assumptions because the administration of vaccines implies tacit approval of the allopathic medical philosophy. We do have a choice about our medical treatment. The United States

Constitution is based upon the principle of freedom of choice. The widespread belief that vaccination of an entire population is necessary, however, has threatened our basic rights and our ability to legally make an informed decision.

The history of mandatory vaccinations reads like the story of martial law in an occupied country. The freedom to choose is suspended in an all-out effort to eradicate an enemy. This is the mentality of war.

The problem with warfare lies in its basically destructive principles. The casualties are usually heavy. In the vaccine war, the casualties have been devastatingly damaged children with resultant lifelong retardation, asthma, autism, and fatalities directly caused by the vaccines.

The crime and the shame of the vaccine industry and the medical establishment have been the routine and blatant denial of these casualties in public testimony and in daily practice. In their view, the good fight has been staged, and these supposed casualties represent merely the deluded suspicions of parents with a sick child who are all too eager to point at vaccines as the cause of their problems. The Vaccine Injury Act was instituted not because the vaccine industry admitted its culpability in these tragedies, but simply because the drug companies refused to continue production of these substances that resulted in multimillion-dollar lawsuits. The government chose to subsidize vaccine production by paying awards out of tax dollars and limiting the amount to an administrative budget. Litigation against drug companies was eliminated, and parents were left seeking recompense from a government bureaucracy. This protection of the drug companies ensured continuing profits. Vaccine production was re-established. Parents' claims were deflected and continued to be denied, and no further recourse was left to the victims. The war against disease could continue unabated.

The drug companies' production of vaccines and the government's requirements for their administration has been a very successful partnership. When a consumer evaluates medical pronouncements about drug prescriptions for the entire world's population, one should never lose sight of the fact that drug companies reap tremendous profits. The same companies that make and sell these drugs fund their research.

In fact, research and marketing go hand-in-hand. The next simple step is for the drug companies to assist in legislative efforts to make drug prescribing mandatory for all citizens. The desire for profits has shaped the law.

The war on disease represents the driving force behind vaccine use. The basic assumptions of our culture fuel the policies adopted for our citizens in the areas of medicine and defense. Waging war provides a simple black-and-white perspective: Identify an enemy and declare war. In medicine the concept of disease provides us with the unwitting, elusive, and destructive enemy. The lowly virus and bacterium become the identified targets, the carriers, the weapons, and the tangible troops of the invading army. The analogy is striking. It has become so integrated into our personal belief systems that it seems ludicrous to question it. Who would call disease an ally?

Yet the analogy upon which allopathic medicine is based has no logical foundation. The body is not a battleground. Hostile enemy forces are not threatening our way of life, and biochemical war is not the only solution to illness. There is another philosophy of medicine, which has been ignored in the assumptions of the allopathic worldview. In our population and in our lifetime a shift in consciousness has already occurred. This awareness encompasses the notion that the body itself has an innate intelligence and healing ability.

In this view, the body needs to be nurtured, not attacked with chemicals. The body does have a fundamental order and integrity. This ordered and harmonious function benefits from life-promoting activities, and suffers under the stressful influence of hostile interventions. A philosophy of healing that respects the natural order inherent within the body and the body's innate healing abilities may provide us with an approach to prevention that avoids chemical warfare. When the organism is seen as a whole, when we view nutritional factors, lifestyle, the body's natural integrity, and their overall effect on healing, then we can view vaccines from a different perspective.

All actions have the ability to influence the inherent order of the organism. The body seeks to maintain a healthy balance or homeostasis. Some actions will promote order and others will disorder the internal balance that the body has created. For example, when a child makes a transition from one environment to another, like going to a new preschool, this has the potential to create disorder. The transition may be interpreted by the child as threatening, and the resulting internal disorder might manifest as a tantrum. The parent can then take actions that reassure the child and re-establish balance and homeostasis. Other actions may have a more disordering effect.

To continue the analogy in the emotional realm, the death of a pet or a family member will provoke a deeper injury and greater imbalance. The emotional reactions of fear and grief may cause symptoms. When managed appropriately, with respect for the child's feelings and emotional maturity, these stresses can result in a stronger, more resilient personality. Similarly, different physical stresses on the system will cause varying degrees of imbalance and disorder. When we view the body as an organism in balance, we see everything that occurs as potentially ordering or disordering. An apparent stress can result in order. A continued stress can upset the balance, and a toxic stress can cause damage that throws the body into a tailspin.

Drugs have the potential to cause a significant degree of imbalance because of their inherent toxicity. Vaccines can provoke toxic reactions, and they are also capable of causing these same types of imbalances. They can be just as devastating as other severe shocks to the system. The degree of the imbalance and disorder will depend upon the toxic potential of the vaccine and the susceptibility of the organism. By contrast, when an infectious disease causes stress on the body, a vital healing response is mounted as a defense. Marshalling this response can result in a stronger immune system. Illness can thus be seen as a strengthening process, due to its dynamic effect on the body as opposed to the specific antigen-antibody stimulating mechanism of vaccination.

An acute illness can cause a remission of a chronic disease precisely because the acute illness mobilizes healing forces within the body. For example, a report in the British medical journal *Lancet* described two patients with multiple sclerosis who experienced remission of their neurologic symptoms after they contracted chickenpox.

Both patients had been severely disabled prior to the chickenpox infection. A year later both were participating in normal activities, and one was jogging. Follow-up after two years and six years in the respective cases revealed no further relapse (Ross, 1991). The principle that a similar acute illness can cure a chronic disease was elucidated during the early nineteenth century by Samuel Hahnemann, the founder of homeopathic medicine. Multiple sclerosis and the chickenpox herpes zoster virus both affect the nerves. Hahnemann showed that such an acute infectious disease often cures a chronic problem. In his *Organon of Medicine,* first published in 1810, he wrote the following:

> Two diseases, different in nature but very similar in their manifestations and effects, their respective suffering and symptoms, always and infallibly destroy each other as soon as they meet in the organism. . . . Smallpox . . . has removed and cured a host of ills that have similar symptoms. . . . When measles meets a disease that is similar to it in its main symptom—the eruption— it will undeniably destroy and cure it (Hahnemann, 1982).

The decision about the use of vaccines involves weighing these considerations and viewing them in the context of an underlying philosophy of health and disease.

Looking at the body as a whole, as an integrated organism, encompasses a philosophy in contrast to the allopathic reduction of the body to a set of parts. Modern technological medicine views only short-term reactions and the localized effects of its interventions. There is little attention paid to long-term effects because there is no model for viewing or evaluating these. The double-blind study looks at limited effects on distinct physiological systems in the body. Vaccines stimulate specific antibody responses in the immune system. That is the desired effect, and the ultimate goal is prevention of a specific disease in the tested population. These tests run for a few years at the most. The issue of long-term detrimental effects of vaccines never arises in these study designs because that concept defies the objective of those tests.

Politically, it would not be useful to look for these effects because studies are conducted by vaccine manufacturers and the government, both of whom have a vested interest in the product and a long-term political and monetary commitment to the promotion of the vaccine campaign. They have no interest in revealing vaccine toxicity. This intentionally myopic view encourages the limited perspective of allopathic medicine, but parents and other consumers of medical services are questioning this limited view. They increasingly seek the perspectives of alternative medical systems that do view the body as a whole.

The systems of Traditional Chinese Medicine (TCM), homeopathy, naturopathy, and Ayurvedic medicine all share the belief that interventions have global, long-term effects in the body. The goal of these systems is to bring the body into a higher state of order and balance. Their interventions create harmony. Within these systems, diet, drug use, herbs, medicines, exercise, emotions, thoughts, beliefs, and relationships all play a role in the overall health of each person. The physical body and the mind are linked in the sense that an imbalance in one realm will affect other realms. Physical illness can cause emotional stress, and emotional turmoil can cause physical reactions. When the natural energetic balance and harmony of body systems is upset, then the resulting disorder may manifest in symptoms and destructive physiological processes. A persistent unremitting stress may cause chronic problems. For example, repressed anger can result in physical changes within the body, causing high blood pressure or a depressed immune system and consequent cancer growth.

Vaccine critics have postulated that the constant stress caused by manipulating and altering the immune system with vaccines could also result in these types of imbalances and disease processes. Healing systems that address these imbalances intend the opposite effect—to create harmony and re-establish balance in the body. The goal is a healthy life and prevention of illness. The crisis-oriented approach of allopathic medicine and its attention to isolated, disjointed reactions exist in sharp distinction to the curative and preventive healing approaches of these other medical systems.

A shift has occurred in the West, from a fear of isolated diseases towards a focus on the organism as a whole and the strength of its immune response. Fear of disease has fueled the fire of allopathic medicine throughout its history and caused a preoccupation with infection. Perhaps this was appropriate during medieval and early industrial historical periods, when infectious disease ran rampant. In the era of waste-disposal technology systems, the frequency and severity of these diseases have steadily declined. Perhaps shifting the focus away from fear and toxic assaults on the immune system through antibiotics and vaccines is now appropriate for our culture.

The subject of immune system deficiencies has occupied a great deal of attention in the health care industry, especially the health-foods arena. Many products now exist that purport to strengthen the immune system including herbs, mushrooms, and algae, as well as meditation and movement techniques. This interest stems from the widespread rise in immune system disorders and in new diseases that never existed prior to the modern chemical era of industrial pollution and drugs (AIDS, cancer, lupus, chronic fatigue syndrome, hypothyroidism, and a whole array of autoimmune disorders). Opportunistic viruses may also play a role in the declining health of the population, but concern over the fundamental immune system failure lies at the core of the efforts to develop immune enhancement.

The possible role of vaccines in causing these immune system deficiencies has been the subject of much speculation and controversy. Many health care providers and consumer advocates have pointed to vaccines as a cause of immune failure. The coincident emergence of these diseases and the mass vaccination of populations has led to suspicions that an entire generation has suffered immune system crippling from the vaccines that should be protecting us from illness.

The vaccines may also impact other body systems. The nervous system seems to be particularly sensitive to the toxic properties of vaccines. Subtle nervous system damage caused by vaccines has been identified as a possible source of the recently observed epidemic problems of attention disorders, criminal behavior in children, and the emergence of autism as a new disease since the advent of mass vaccination (Coulter, 1990). More immediate and dramatic nervous system reactions can occur soon after vaccine administration, often after the third or fourth dose. These include convulsions sometimes resulting in lifelong epilepsy, persistent high-pitched screaming, bizarre grimacing, and sudden unexplainable death (SIDS). Of course, these types of reactions are continuously denied by the vaccine industry (Institute of Medicine, 1994).

Another significant shift in consciousness that affects the way parents make health care decisions includes the evolving view of the doctor. Some parents have discovered that the exalted position of the medical doctor who dictates all treatment decisions may involve misplaced trust. Doctors are trained by drug companies, both in medical schools and later in their offices and clinics. Medical textbooks teach drug prescribing, clinical training involves learning the proper way to prescribe drugs, and seminars for doctors in practice teach the latest advances in drug development. All of this information is derived from research conducted by the pharmaceutical industry, whose only goal is to sell drugs. Increasingly, drug companies own the health care delivery institutions themselves. In this way they can supervise and design the delivery of their products.

This phenomenon has not escaped the consumer's awareness. If an individual citizen in the role of patient wants something other than drugs, then he or she must turn to sources outside the medical establishment simply because the world of physicians represents the position of the drug-manufacturing industry. Many parents have realized that accepting the opinion of their physician about vaccines is similar to believing the car salesman's pitch. Both have a product to push. Vaccines represent consumer goods—and we should research this product far more carefully than other purchases because our lives could be at stake.

The doctor-as-God philosophy is gradually losing ground. Consumers want information. The scandals and tragedies associated with drug company products have created a more wary public. Thalidomide, the IUD, silicone breast implants, and unnecessary mutilations in the form of mastectomies and hysterectomies have resulted in widespread mistrust. People have discovered that drug companies may not have our best interests at heart. Doctors do what they are told. The consumer who does not beware is the unwitting participant and potential victim.

Personal Choice, Politics, and Profits

What constitutes personal choice in health care decisions? The first parameter involves the freedom to choose. When some group or authority dictates policies, there can be no personal decision. Parents are especially at risk of legal action if they refuse vaccines. The freedom to make health care decisions is a fundamental right, and yet parents in many states have been denied the right to choose whether their children are injected with chemicals recommended by the vaccine industry. The requirement to vaccinate makes parents criminals if they refuse to comply. Religious and medical exemptions to vaccination merely place the decision in the hands of another authority, the church or the doctor. This well-guarded authority has been upheld by courts in some states, which require that parents prove their membership in a recognized church that proscribes vaccines before they qualify for a religious exemption. If parents who live in those states do make a personal decision that a particular vaccine is too toxic for their child, they cannot exercise their right to choose avoidance of vaccines. The remaining states that do provide parents with the option of a personal belief or philosophical exemption to vaccination at least allow parents to choose for themselves.

Adults are required to obtain vaccines for themselves in the following situations: for attendance at a college or university, to work in the health care industry, for immigration, to join the armed services, and for international travel.

The second parameter in a personal decision requires that you assess your own needs. This involves getting information, weighing your choices, and evaluating the pros and cons of an issue. The reasoning for a family may differ from the reasoning for an entire population. You may find that your needs are significantly different than those of someone else. For example, is your child at a higher risk than the general population due to overcrowding, poor nutrition, and inadequate sanitation? These are factors that could make an individual child more susceptible and more likely to come in contact with infectious diseases.

A public health official may have a completely different agenda for the nation than you do for your own family. The strategy for eliminating diseases from a population usually includes universal measures for everyone, regardless of risk of exposure or consequences for the individual. The population takes precedence over the individual. The following quote taken from an article in the British medical journal, *Lancet,* makes this abundantly clear.

> There is still much to be learned about how best to use vaccines for maximum benefit to the community as well as to the individual. For a pathogenic microbe to persist within a population, the density of susceptible individuals needs to exceed a critical value such that, on average, each primary case of infection generates at least one secondary. Thus, it may be to the benefit of society as a whole for an individual to be immunised but in that individual's interest not to be! As with other matters bearing on altruism in society, the promotion of vaccination to secure herd immunity raises complex issues (Moxon, 1990).

The "complex issue" to an epidemiologist amounts to this for an individual parent: Are you willing to sacrifice your child to satisfy a public health official's objectives? Some children will inevitably be sacrificed to achieve certain goals for the community. Are you prepared to take that risk with your child? In answering that question, consider whether you agree with the philosophy that underlies the methods. Is it necessary or even wise to wipe out diseases, to prevent the body's management of childhood illnesses, to manipulate the immune system, beginning at birth, with toxic chemicals? What is the risk from these diseases? What are the dangers of vaccines? Why have parents not been told about the devastating reactions that can occur? This massive marketing scheme has been heralded as the greatest preventive health measure of modern times, brought to us by the pharmaceutical industry and their vaccine researchers. It is time that vaccines and their promotion campaign are viewed with a critical eye. Are you ready to inject these powerful and toxic drugs into your child, on the advice of drug manufacturers, at the insistence of doctors who are paid by these drug companies, delivered to you by doctors trained by those same companies? Look at the facts, and reach your own conclusions.

Organizations of parents have been formed to fight the policy of mandatory vaccines for children. These parents represent their vaccine-injured children. They have learned about vaccines because their toxic effects destroyed their child's health. Listen to their experience and see their side before you meekly rest assured in the word of your doctor, who tells you exactly what he was told by the drug company. Question the effects of drugs used on your child. These are not difficult issues to understand. You can take control of these decisions. Make sure that you feel comfortable in your choices. Do not become the naive victim of wholesale drug policies. This is an area of your life and your family's health that you can control.

With such powerful combined forces at work—the vaccine manufacturers, medical associations, government committees, legislature, and media—it is not surprising that vaccine acceptance pervades our culture. Public health policies support this vast industry. Considering the range of organizations and forces involved in this field, a multitude of motives emerges that drives the vaccine campaign.

First and foremost is modern medicine. The medical world has very little to offer in the treatment of infectious disease. This impotence in the face of illness leads to a strong desire to prevent these untreatable problems, even at a high cost in the form of adverse effects. Viruses and whooping cough are not responsive to antibiotics. That covers measles, mumps, rubella, polio, chickenpox, hepatitis, and pertussis. But more and more bacteria have become resistant to antibiotics. That threatens the effectiveness of the few drugs that treat the remaining microbes in question, Haemophilus, diphtheria, and tetanus.

The ineffectiveness of allopathic medicine creates a compelling desire to develop vaccines, which shifts the research arm of the industry into hyperdrive. The fact that other forms of treatment could be utilized to manage infectious diseases is ignored. Allopathic medicine denies the effectiveness of any treatment besides its own drugs. The model does not allow for recognition of other healing systems. This occurs even when another healing modality proves effective. Generally, this merely encourages the harshness of the medical world's opposition. For example, when homeopathic medicine proved clinically effective in treating yellow-fever epidemics and severe influenza outbreaks, the allopathic medical establishment redoubled its efforts to discredit and destroy the competition (Coulter, 1973). Modern medicine has bet its money on vaccines to such an extent that the belief in their goodness pervades all discussions. The universally accepted credo that the benefits derived from vaccines outweigh their risks fuels the research, adoption, and dissemination of vaccines despite any evidence that they may be harmful.

The nearly compulsive desire to wipe out diseases governs public health policies. In this great battle we lose lives to vaccine injuries. Even this unfortunate fact is vehemently denied. The obvious self-justification that more lives would be lost to the disease is a specious and convenient argument that ends discussion. The medical world first blinds itself to the possibility of treating these illnesses with anything beyond its own meager methods, then justifies its use of toxic drugs to wipe out the offenders. The concept of mutual existence between humans and these microbes has never been considered. The possibility that the body can be encouraged to manage these diseases has never entered the worldview of modern medicine. This results in a simple, self-perpetuating philosophy: Vaccines are good, diseases are bad. And this war cry is echoed throughout the modern world.

Drug manufacturers realized that the allopathic goal of wiping out diseases held the promise of vast fortunes. They were quick to combine forces and supply physicians with the armaments for their massive campaign. Vaccine researchers have provided the vaccine manufacturers with a guaranteed world market for their product. Their alliance in this effort is apparent at all public hearings, government committee meetings, and court cases involving vaccine toxicity and injuries to children. The vaccine producers have one goal—profits. They will produce a vaccine for anything if they are guaranteed a market, especially if they are protected from lawsuits. They are not motivated by improving world health. They are not willing to lose money on vaccines. If vaccines stop producing a profit, they stop producing vaccines, a simple equation.

Government provides the seal of approval for the vaccine campaign. Politicians get into the vaccine business because of their own personal beliefs, their alliance with the medical establishment viewpoint, and their need to adopt popular causes. Protecting children and improving the health status of disadvantaged populations represent non-controversial political positions. If the pharmaceutical industry profits from such government decisions, so much the better. They mount a tremendous lobbying effort, and mandatory vaccine policies translate to lucrative gold mines. Testifying at government hearings, providing expert paid researchers for government committees, advising politicians about vaccine campaign plans—all represent solid marketing strategies. After all, the government is a vaccine company's biggest single customer. There is no mystery in the motives of vaccine manufacturers' efforts to sponsor and lobby for state legislation that requires vaccination for school entry. Every new vaccine's marketing strategy includes vast sums from the manufacturer, SmithKline, Merck, or Lederle, to get it mandated for the entire population of children in every state.

The vaccine business also provides jobs for physicians. Positions for vaccine experts occur in the form of pharmaceutical researchers, academic researchers, and membership on professional organization and government committees. This medical wing of the vaccine industry supports itself through promotion of vaccines. Their promotion of vaccines ensures self-employment, continuation of research funds, and academic positions.

Conflict of interest abounds in the vaccine business. It starts with a government committee. The Centers for Disease Control appoints members to the Advisory Committee on Immunization Practices (ACIP), which makes recommendations to the FDA. These recommendations are tremendously influential because state legislatures rely on them to draft immunization requirements for their citizens. Members of the Advisory Committee are often employed by or funded by vaccine manufacturers. Dr. John Modlin was simultaneously Chairman of the Advisory Committee, served on the Merck Immunization Advisory Board, and was a Merck shareholder. Merck is one of the world's largest vaccine manufacturers. Committee members typically receive multiple contracts of $200,000 or more per year per contract from vaccine companies (Committee on Government Reform, 2000).

In June 2000 the US House of Representatives Committee on Government Reform concluded its investigation of conflicts of interest in vaccine policy making with the publication of their report, a veritable indictment of the CDC Advisory Committee. This congressional committee found that the CDC routinely grants waivers from conflict of interest rules to every member of its Advisory Committee. Committee members with admitted conflict of interest are nonetheless allowed to participate in committee deliberations and advocate specific positions. Committee members often fill out incomplete financial disclosure statements, and are not required to provide the missing information. Finally, the investigation revealed that an overwhelming majority of committee members commonly vote to approve guidelines for specific vaccines despite their own substantial financial ties to pharmaceutical companies developing versions of these vaccines.

The recommendation/approval process for vaccines takes place in a closed club with few checks on the members. No wonder more and more vaccines are rushed to market. Those scientists and physicians who dare to question the sacrosanct act of vaccination risk their careers and livelihood. When Dr. Andrew Wakefield persisted in defending his research findings on the link between autism and vaccines, he was fired from his position at the Royal Free Hospital of London where he had conducted his clinical studies. When Dr. John Martin persisted in investigating the transmission of dangerous stealth viruses from monkeys to humans through vaccines, funding for his research dried up.

Let's consider an example of how drug-company recommendations can influence your doctor and government policy about vaccines. The following facts represent just one drama in the vaccine world, where billions of dollars in revenues and vaccine-injury claims are at stake. In 1990, Marie Griffin and her associates at Vanderbilt University School of Medicine in Nashville, Tennessee, published a study on the risk of seizures and other neurologic events following the DTP (Diphtheria-Tetanus-Pertussis) vaccine. This study appeared in the *Journal of the American Medical Association (JAMA)*. The study was big in scope, including more than 38,000 children who received 107,000 doses of DTP. Their conclusion? "No child who was previously normal without a prior history of seizures had a seizure in the 0 to 3 days following vaccination that marked the onset of either epilepsy or other neurological or developmental abnormality." This seems to provide the final word about the supposed neurotoxicity of the pertussis vaccine and brain damage (encephalopathy). Accompanying the article, an editorial titled "'Pertussis vaccine encephalopathy': It is time to recognize it as the myth that it is" by James Cherry proclaimed the end of the long debate about pertussis vaccine and nervous system damage (Cherry, 1990).

Later that year, Vincent Fulginiti published another editorial titled "A pertussis vaccine myth dies" in another AMA-sponsored journal, *The American Journal of Diseases of Children (AJDC)* (Fulginiti, 1990). Similar editorials occurred across the nation (California Department of Health Services, 1994).

Several problems, however, taint the purity of these clinical studies and their interpretation. First, Marie Griffin was reported to be financially supported by Burroughs Wellcome, one of the world's largest pertussis (whooping cough) vaccine manufacturers. James Cherry, MD, of UCLA, was a paid consultant for Lederle Laboratories, the largest American manufacturer of pertussis vaccine (Conflict . . . , 1990). Cherry was paid by the vaccine-production companies and also headed the 1988 American Academy of Pediatrics task force on pertussis and pertussis immunization, whose report also denied any major problems with the vaccine. In 1988 Cherry admitted receiving $50,000 per year for testifying in lawsuits on behalf of vaccine manufacturers in vaccine-damage cases, obtained $400,000 in grant funds for UCLA, partly covering his expenses and salary, and his department at UCLA received $450,000 in "gifts" from Lederle Laboratories (Coulter and Fisher, 1991). Vincent Fulginiti, as editor of *AJDC*, chose to publish a disclaimer about his own drug-company affiliations. "Many years ago he received support from a variety of pharmaceutical firms to undertake studies of many vaccines, including pertussis vaccine. He has also, in the past but not in recent years, testified as an expert witness for physicians and pharmaceutical firms, for which he received compensation, in trials concerning the alleged side effects of pertussis vaccine" (Fulginiti, 1990).

James Cherry also headed a task force of pediatricians that dismissed the findings of a British study that did show a significant association between the vaccine and serious neurologic disorders. That task force delivered a bizarre rationalization. "The data can be interpreted as demonstrating a temporal association in which DTP calls attention to or brings out something that is to occur anyway but is just moved forward in time because of the immunization" (Cherry *et al.*, 1988). The drug manufacturers blame the parents for seeking retribution against them, and claim that vaccine-injured children would have acquired these problems anyway. Then the government steps in to protect the drug companies. Who is in control here?

All of the denial and self-congratulation in this particular drama were based on the findings of the Griffin study. But the quality and methods of that study itself were called into question. For example, the identified cases included only those vaccine recipients who experienced a "first nonneonatal seizure or episode of encephalopathy that resulted in Medicaid reimbursement for a medical encounter between the first DTP immunization and the end of study follow-up." Coulter, in his critique of this study, asks, "How about the children who did not apply for a Medicaid reimbursement? Not every parent rushes to the Medicaid office for medicines just because the child has seizures or 'spells'" (Coulter, 1990a).

The study also looked at deaths following the vaccine. They found that in a period of 15 to 30 days after vaccination, there was a 20 percent increase in deaths compared to the control group. Yet in their summary they say only that they found no increased risk of SIDS (Sudden Infant Death Syndrome) in the 0- to 14-day interval after DTP vaccination. This exclusion of possible late effects allows them to "conclude that in this large population of children there was no increase in the risk of SIDS after immunization with the DTP vaccine" (Coulter, 1990b).

Another reviewer also questioned the methods and conclusions of the Griffin study, noting that office neurological examinations and

Medicaid mothers' reporting of seizures did not represent a reliable system of measurement for detecting mild to moderate pertussis vaccine encephalopathies (Lewis, 1990).

Since the Griffin article appeared and the vaccine industry so readily dismissed any association between the pertussis vaccine and neurologic sequelae, other studies have continued to reveal the vaccine's problems. Apparently, other researchers did not believe that the "myth" had been put to rest. A follow-up survey was conducted of the children identified as suffering "severe acute neurological events within seven days of pertussis immunisation" in the famous British study conducted ten years prior. This survey showed that after ten years, "significantly more children with such illnesses die or suffer subsequent educational, behavioural, or neurological deficits than expected by comparison with controls" (Miller et al., 1993).

Another study published the same year as the Griffin study showed a positive association between severe acute neurologic illnesses and recent administration of DTP vaccine (Gale et al., 1990). Either these studies have continued to perpetuate the "myth" of vaccine damage to the nervous system, or the vaccine defenders were suspiciously premature in their verdicts. A summary of the evidence, including the Griffin article, published by the American Academy of Pediatrics, confirmed that the vaccine was associated with nervous system disorders. The authors conclude with two points: "1. There is an association between DTP vaccine and serious acute neurologic illness. . . . 2. We do not know whether pertussis vaccine causes permanent brain damage" (Wentz & Marcuse, 1991). Nonetheless, the vaccine defenders made their point, which was echoed in the popular press. The drama merely reflects the high stakes involved in the form of salaries, profits, and the defense of a personal belief. Ironically, within a few years the whole-cell pertussis vaccine was removed from the recommended list of vaccines for children and replaced with a new acellular form of the vaccine because of the severe, toxic reactions to the DTP vaccine so vehemently denied by Griffin, Cherry, and Fulginiti.

The scandal surrounding the rotavirus vaccine fiasco provides another dramatic example of vaccine industry corruption. In August 1998 the rotavirus vaccine was licensed for use in children to combat viral diarrhea. Less than one year later the vaccine was withdrawn from the market because of reports that as many as 99 infants developed a life-threatening bowel obstruction after receiving the vaccine, and two of these babies died. The withdrawal of this vaccine represented a serious blow to the vaccine industry's reputation for safety, but subsequent news was even worse. Data revealed that during clinical trials prior to vaccine approval this bowel problem occurred at a level 30 times the expected rate in a normal population. A study conducted ten years previously in China also found an exceptionally high incidence of the same bowel obstruction in vaccine recipients, but this study was ignored by the US approval committees (Harris, 1999). It also came to light during congressional investigations into the rotavirus vaccine approval process that four out of eight CDC advisory committee members who voted to approve guidelines for the vaccine in June 1998 had financial ties to pharmaceutical companies that were developing different versions of the vaccine. Additionally, three out of five FDA advisory committee members who voted to approve the rotavirus vaccine in December 1997 had financial ties to pharmaceutical companies that were developing different versions of the vaccine (Committee on Government Reform, 2000).

For many reasons, the factors that influence a government to adopt vaccine requirements may differ considerably from the individual parent's personal goals for a family. Politicians, vaccine companies, and medical organizations have their own concerted agenda for their immunization campaign. This agenda may coincide with your choices as a consumer of medical services, or it may not. Since administering the vaccines involves significant health risks, it makes sense to base your choice on health considerations for the individual and not on a public policy determined by drug companies.

When a vaccine proves less profitable than planned, vaccine manufacturers stop production. Increased consumer demand for safer vaccines has led to greater quality control of manufacturing practices and increased production costs. In October 2000 the FDA leveled a record $30 million fine against Wyeth-Ayerst Laboratories because of quality-control problems. Two months later Wyeth-Ayerst stopped producing tetanus and DtaP vaccines (Russell, 2002). A second company, Baxter Hyland, also quit DtaP production The 1999 regulation to remove mercury from all drugs including vaccines has also increased manufacturing costs. Vaccine companies are simply dropping out of the market. This has created shortages of many vaccines, including DtaP, MMR, and hepatitis vaccine, requiring doctors to ration shots. If vaccines do not produce a profit, drug companies will turn to other drugs that do. These are business decisions. Vaccine companies are not in the business of public health.

Nonetheless, the vaccine campaign continues. Vaccine promoters make the claim that everyone must continue to comply with government recommendations or the diseases will return; but they have no proof that this will occur. The much-touted success of vaccine campaigns is debatable in any case. The incidence of many infectious diseases such as diphtheria and tetanus has consistently declined over the past hundred years. Many diseases disappeared long ago without the benefit of vaccines (typhoid, yellow fever). Vaccines in current use have only been widely used since the 1940s, and some are much more recent. The pressure to vaccinate is founded upon vaccine company claims, and a commitment to a belief system that runs deeply in economic and philosophical veins. Consumers should remain wary of the motives and methods involved in these public health measures.

Options for Parents: Choosing and Timing Vaccines

When it comes to making a choice about whether or not to vaccinate, parents usually have two simultaneous voices vying for their attention. If they have come this far in their thinking, if they are questioning whether it is actually wise to give their child these shots, then doubts have crept into the equation. They are not absolutely sure that the pediatrician is telling them the whole story. They are not altogether convinced. The doubts speak through an instinctual, protective, parental voice. They have heard about adverse vaccine effects through friends, or articles and books. They want information, but their pediatrician is not forthcoming. All they get from that side is calm reassurance that the vaccines are safe, that the diseases represent a far greater risk. It is a comforting paternalistic tone that lulls their distracting doubts and intimidates them through a subtle coercion. Belief systems cannot really be questioned; too much time is usually spent attempting to prove that they are correct.

Some parents, however, continue to question the accepted wisdom despite the heresy this entails. They want to be responsible and make the right decision. An internal voice says, maybe giving all these vaccines is not the best thing to do right now. My baby seems so vulnerable and delicate. Maybe we could wait.

Confronted with this, the pediatrician usually becomes furious and accusatory. Parents remain in a quandary. If they have little information, they usually succumb. With no support for their doubts, they capitulate. Only the most stalwart parents continue to pursue their questions. In most cases, the second voice raises its competing song. This voice doubts the doubting voice. How could all of these people be wrong about vaccines? We must be crazy to question what is so accepted by everyone around us. Lulled thus into submission, the first voice often turns tail and slips off gain. It returns fleetingly when the mother watches the syringe enter her baby's skin, sees her baby scream, and dreads the possible reactions she has acknowledged when signing off her informed consent.

Anxiety is the keynote of this internal fugue. Emotions run high when confronting time-honored beliefs. Ultimately, a parent's choice comes down to one question: Are we more anxious about the diseases or the vaccines? The fear of diseases runs deep in our culture. Anxiety on this score already tops the charts. It is fueled by vivid stories recounting the horrors of infectious diseases of bygone eras, deaths from diphtheria, and iron-lung hospital wards during the great polio wars. High drama in the fight against disease provides the backdrop for the savior legends of modern medicine, glorifying the inventors of vaccines, Pasteur, Salk, and Sabin. Anxiety about diseases stirs easily in the parental breast.

Anxiety about vaccines runs along more nebulous lines. Parents have few resources to inform them about problems with vaccines.

Their fear of vaccines stems from their own childhood experiences with needles. They have personally felt the initial pain and the subsequent illness caused by vaccines. Inflicting this on their children is not a pleasant prospect. Of course, this anxiety is consciously repressed because of its illogical nature.

Other anxieties stem from hearsay and second-hand information that sporadically leaks into mainstream culture. Reports of the dangers associated with vaccines are vehemently denied by the vast industry that controls the media. In 1982, when NBC-TV released a vaccine exposé that revealed the devastating damage to children caused by the pertussis vaccine, the Centers for Disease Control (CDC), the American Medical Association (AMA), and the American Association of Pediatrics (AAP) called it biased, histrionic, amoral, and psychopathic. The producer of the show said the American press did not pick up the story "because doctors have squelched it" (Coulter, 1991).

There is little support for parents' doubts. Their anxieties are labeled hysterical, and then repudiated. Parents wonder if their concerns are exaggerated. Given their doubts about vaccine safety and the doubts about these doubts, it is no wonder that parents are confused. In fact, parents have anxiety about vaccines because they sense and know the physical stress on the system that vaccines do cause. They have experienced this in their own bodies, and in the reactions of their children. In some children this reaction presents more obvious symptoms than in others. Parents who have seen dramatic changes in their child's behavior following a vaccine will be more anxious about the next one in the schedule. If their children make it through the vaccine reaction without developing severe symptoms, then they breathe a sigh of relief and think, "there, it wasn't so bad after all."

Going against the grain, rejecting an almost universally held belief that vaccines have saved us from disease, and refusing them causes painful experiences for parents. Self-doubt creeps in and parents wonder, have I done the right thing? Grandparents, friends, and medical providers become accusatory. Standing firm in the choice can be difficult. Parents often need support and continual reinforcement that they have made the right choice. Overcoming the anxiety instilled by such deep cultural expectations may require time, patience, and repeated exposure to views that question the authoritative statements of the vaccine industry that continually bombard parents.

One thing that vaccines surely accomplish is the relief of parental guilt. When parents consent to the vaccines, they rest assured in the belief that they have done everything humanly possible in modern medicine. If the disease strikes, then it was an unfortunate case of vaccine failure, a not uncommon event. (Ninety percent or more of measles cases in some epidemics occur in those previously vaccinated.) If a crippling reaction to a vaccine occurs, at least parents do not feel guilty, because they did what they were told. They may be angry and distraught, but they reassure themselves that it was not their fault. The less thinking that occurs prior to giving the vaccine, the less guilt. This places all the authority and all the responsibility on the shoulders of vaccine experts who dictate the path that parents must follow. If their motives are not always in the best interest of the individual child, well, parents will never discover it.

What options are available to parents in their choice about vaccines? First, parents may decide they want less than the total range of recommended vaccines. It comes as a surprise to some parents that they can choose to have one or some vaccines and refuse others. You are responsible for your child's health. You are in control. If a child suffers a dramatic and tragic reaction to a vaccine, it is the parents who must cope with it. The doctors may be sympathetic, but they are personally uninvolved. They view it merely as a casualty in the war against disease, if they admit any culpability at all.

When would a parent choose to give some vaccines and not others? Simply stated, some vaccines apparently represent a more dangerous threat to the body than others. This is inferred from the types of immediate, short-term reactions that we can observe. We assume that those vaccines with the most dramatic short-term toxicity also pose a more dangerous risk for long-term reactions, though this has not been proven because no one has studied the long-term effects of vaccines.

Given that the long-term risks are unknown, parents usually make choices about individual vaccines based on the history of short-term reactions they have caused. The pertussis, measles, and rubella vaccines tend to cause more significant observable reactions than others, though hepatitis and polio vaccines can also cause serious illness. The most commonly avoided vaccine is pertussis because by now, after more than sixty years of medical reports of horrific reactions (deaths, epilepsy, and retardation) from the whole-cell pertussis vaccine, public fear of the vaccine has mounted. The fact that many other countries have abandoned the pertussis vaccine has strengthened the resolve of many parents to also refuse the vaccine. These parents have held their ground, and many physicians, though they may not take the same position, admit that a parent's concern about possible reactions may be justified, despite the consistent denial of the American vaccine industry.

Parents can pick and choose from the list of vaccines based on their own individual family's needs and their own research. They may decide that some diseases pose enough danger to their child to risk the adverse effects of the vaccine. Even a parent who has rejected most vaccines because of their potential adverse effects may choose to give one or a few individual vaccines. Typically, tetanus is a disease that concerns many parents. Since the vaccine causes less immediate severe reactions than others, because the vaccine always works to prevent tetanus, and because tetanus represents a life-threatening situation when it does occur, parents who refuse other vaccines sometimes opt to get the tetanus shots for their child. A parent's concern may be greater for a very active child, especially around horses, since both these factors increase the risk of wounds and exposure to tetanus. Other families may be considering travel to areas of the world (Asia or Africa) where polio still exists, and they will consider giving that vaccine even if they realize that polio does not occur in their own part of the world.

Typically, parents will avoid and refuse specific vaccines for two reasons. Either they fear serious vaccine reactions because of a vaccine's history, or the disease causes so little concern that the vaccine does not seem necessary to them. Other diseases represent a greater threat, and parents may feel more secure giving the vaccine than risking the disease in their child.

Vaccines That Parents Commonly Refuse

HIGH VACCINE TOXICITY	LOW DISEASE INCIDENCE OR SEVERITY
Pertussis	Chickenpox
Measles	Hepatitis
Mumps	Diphtheria
Rubella	Polio

Diseases That Commonly Concern Parents the Most

Tetanus
Meningitis
Polio
Diphtheria

The most difficult aspect of rejecting or refusing vaccines may be finding a cooperative pediatrician or family physician. The decision itself can be complicated and agonizing. Parents must consider conflicting opinions and resources, including unsolicited advice, and then search their own hearts and minds for the answers that make sense to them. Through this process their child also may require a medical provider as a resource for health problems, concerns, or for general advice. It may be difficult to find a compassionate and understanding doctor who will respect and accept parents' decisions about vaccine use for their child. When interviewing a potential doctor, the question of his or her position about the issue of parental choice concerning vaccines may be crucial to their search.

Increasingly, parents may not have a choice about their child's doctor. They must take what they get from their health care plan. Parents may need to steel themselves for a fight. The pressure exerted by doctors to give vaccines is enormous. Many pediatricians in private practice will refuse to care for children whose parents reject vaccinations. Doctors will often bully and harass parents who question them or who refuse to follow standard vaccination recommendations. It takes a strong parent to confront this kind of blatant persecution.

Since the medical establishment's certainty about vaccines constitutes a belief system, any other view is considered heresy. The more zealous defenders of vaccine policies and promoters of the mass vaccine campaign will sometimes vehemently confront parents, and have even proposed seeking out these recalcitrant citizens. Parents should be on their guard when discussing vaccines with medical professionals, schools, or government administrators. Doctors have accused parents of neglect and even contacted Child Protective Services upon discovering that a child was not fully vaccinated. So far, federal legislation that proposed tracking children's vaccine status in a computerized database has failed to be enacted due to the efforts of parent advocacy groups. This would allow state governments to seek and find families who refuse vaccines.

An understanding doctor will provide support and comfort to families who confront the *status quo* of vaccine laws. A caring family doctor or pediatrician should respect parents enough to accept their well-considered decisions about vaccine use for their own family. He or she may even be willing to write a medical exemption for admittance to schools.

The second option that parents can consider concerns the timing of vaccines. It is not necessary to begin giving vaccines at birth or two months of age. Delaying vaccines will at least give you time to make your choices. It will also give your baby's body a chance to develop a less vulnerable immune system and nervous system, which are so susceptible to the vaccines' toxic effects. Delay of DTP vaccination until two years of age in Japan resulted in a dramatic decrease in adverse vaccine effects. During the period 1970 through 1974, when DTP vaccine was begun at 3 to 5 months of age, the Japanese national compensation system paid claims for 57 permanent severe vaccine reactions and 37 deaths. During the following six-year period, 1975 through 1980, when DTP vaccine was begun at 24 months of age, severe reactions were reduced to a total of eight with three deaths (Noble *et al.*, 1987). This is an 85 to 90 percent reduction in severe reactions and deaths calculated according to total doses of vaccine administered during these years. Dr. James Cherry and colleagues, reporting the American Academy of Pediatrics Task Force on Pertussis findings, conclude, "It is clear that delaying the initial vaccination until a child is 24 months . . . reduces most of the temporally associated severe adverse events" (Cherry *et al.,* 1988).

Delaying the initiation of vaccines in a child will not reduce the effectiveness of the vaccine. In fact, the early administration of vaccines has created problems with effective antibody production in response to the vaccine itself. For example, measles, mumps, and rubella vaccines do not produce persistent antibody responses if they are administered prior to 15 months of age. The effort to manufacture more effective vaccines has focused on the issue of how soon a vaccine can be used and still maintain persistent effects over time. So if you delay giving vaccines to your child, then the length of effectiveness will probably be enhanced.

Only two diseases that have corresponding vaccines cause any significant problems within the first year of life in countries with modern sanitation systems. These two are whooping cough (pertussis) and Haemophilus meningitis. The pertussis vaccine caused so many dangerous reactions that Western European countries eliminated it from the roster of routinely administered vaccines. If you decide not to give the pertussis vaccine for the same reasons, then the remaining vaccines to consider are those for meningitis (Haemophilus, pneumococcal, and meningococcal vaccines). These are relatively new and experimental vaccines. The latter two have barely been tested and remain controversial. The risk of exposure to Haemophilus for infants under one year increases in large day-care settings, so this may be a consideration. Breastfeeding exerts a continuing protective effect against Haemophilus meningitis, so parents may want to factor this into their decision (Silfverdal, 1997). Parents should carefully read the discussion in the meningitis chapter.

Certain other diseases—diphtheria, tetanus, polio, hepatitis, and chickenpox—do not threaten babies. Diphtheria and polio do not exist in the United States. The possibility of exposure to tetanus is extremely unlikely in a child under two years old, since tetanus can only be acquired from an injury to the skin such as a puncture wound. Hepatitis is primarily a sexually transmitted disease, and chickenpox causes minimal problems if acquired during childhood at any age. Delaying vaccination causes minimal risk of disease and can result in a dramatically reduced risk of toxic reactions. After infancy your child has developed his or her own antibody production mechanisms and a more resilient defense system for coping with toxic substances. Even if you do nothing else outside the recommended or state-required vaccine onslaught on the body, you might consider the delay of this attack on the system until your child is beyond infancy and less vulnerable to vaccine reactions.

Vaccines are usually recommended for use during infancy, as opposed to some later age, for two reasons. First, the incidence of diseases that do pose a health risk to infants can be reduced in this way. This assumes that the individual vaccine is effective, which may or may not be true.

The second, and much more important, reason is that doctors have access to babies during the first year of life. Parents bring their babies for well-child check-ups every two or three months during infancy. This provides the perfect opportunity to give several doses of vaccines. The recommended vaccine schedule has been devised to conform to this spacing of check-ups. After two years of age, children would not normally visit their doctor every few months for any reason other than shots if the vaccines were begun at that age.

The timing of this medical intervention has evolved out of convenience and the strategies of a mass-coverage plan, rather than considering the needs and safety of the individual child. Timing of vaccines may represent another instance where your family's needs do not coincide with those of the vaccine industry. You do have a choice about the age at which your child receives shots, because the vaccine laws are linked to school admission, which may be at five or six years of age (except for those infants who attend day-care programs or preschoolers). Delaying vaccination could be a significant step in your efforts to minimize the risk of adverse effects from vaccines given to your child.

A number of vaccines are commonly given simultaneously. This may create more of a burden on the system and cause a greater likelihood of adverse reactions than giving the vaccines individually. No studies have evaluated the effect on the immune system of single versus combined vaccines, but since vaccines have been shown to temporarily suppress various immune system functions, it is conceivable that combination vaccines could compound this effect (Jaber *et al.,* 1988; Hirsch *et al.,* 1981; Nicholson *et al.,* 1992).

There is also some concern that combining vaccines could reduce the effectiveness of individual vaccines contained within the shot. For example, young children receiving the HIB vaccine may develop lower antibody response titers to the other childhood vaccinations when they are all given at once (Clemens *et al.,* 1992). If you feel that the administration of four to seven vaccines at one time could constitute a greater risk than giving less at each doctor visit, then this option might be one for you to consider. The problem with this option is that a doctor or clinic may not have the vaccines in isolated preparations, since giving combination vaccines spares the child more doctor visits and more shots, at the same time reducing the cost of medical care.

As the number of vaccines given to children continues to increase, the number in each shot continues to rise as well. Pharmacies have plans for the development of a "supervaccine" that will contain all of the recommended shots (ten or more) in one syringe. Their ultimate goal is to have this shot available at birth.

SUMMARY OF OPTIONS FOR YOUR CHILD

- Using some vaccines and not others
- Delaying vaccines until after one year of age or later
- Administering individual vaccines separately rather than giving them in combination

Individual Disease Incidence and Severity

The concept of consumers choosing individual vaccines implies that they understand the issues surrounding the individual diseases. They must decide whether a specific disease poses a significant threat. The factors that affect this decision process include the possibility of exposure to a disease, the severity of a disease if it occurs, and comparison of these risks to the possible risks of the specific vaccine. For some diseases this equation is simple, and for others it is much more complicated.

Chickenpox, for example, poses no health risks for a generally healthy child. The illness lasts longer and involves much more suffering in adults who may be susceptible when the effectiveness of the childhood vaccine wanes. It confers lifelong immunity, however, after children acquire the illness naturally. And the vaccine has potential adverse effects. Most parents will conclude that the risks from the chickenpox vaccine are greater than the risks from the disease. Other diseases, like Hepatitis B and C, involve different issues for children and adults. Since these forms of hepatitis are primarily sexually transmitted diseases, children have minimal risk of infection, but adults in high-risk situations, such as those with multiple sexual partners or health workers exposed to the blood of patients, may want to consider the vaccines for their use.

Risking a serious vaccine reaction in order to prevent a mild childhood disease may not be the best alternative for your child. On the other hand, you may decide that preventing a potentially life-threatening disease may be worth the risk of the vaccine if you or your child have a significant chance of exposure.

Following three simple steps will enable consumers to form an educated opinion about each of the diseases and their vaccines. Extensive information about the diseases in question and the individual vaccines comprises the entire second part of this book. Using these chapters, readers can evaluate each disease and the adverse effects of each vaccine. At the end of each chapter, a summary of the information serves as a reference for quick review. Additionally, the information contained in the following general discussion of vaccine adverse effects can serve as background considerations to weigh in the balance when a choice is not perfectly clear about an individual vaccine. Your own philosophy about health care, your perception of the medical profession's reporting of vaccine reactions, your intuition, and a lot of information will establish a context to help you make these choices.

FACTORS TO CONSIDER ABOUT INDIVIDUAL DISEASES

1. Disease incidence and the likelihood of exposure

2. Severity and possible complications of the disease

3. Comparing the risks from the disease with the risks from the vaccine.

ADVERSE VACCINE REACTIONS

All of the vaccines have significant adverse effects. These can be separated into two groups: (a) immediate or short-term reactions that occur soon after giving a vaccine, and (b) delayed or long-term reactions. Immediate reactions include fevers, allergic responses, deafness, convulsions, paralysis, central nervous system disease resulting in temporary or permanent disabilities, and death. Delayed reactions may be more insidious and less obvious. They can also result in persistent conditions that include epilepsy, mental retardation, learning disabilities, and behavior disorders.

Adverse events resulting from vaccines may be due to the bacterial toxin or virus component of the vaccine, or to the chemicals used in the preparation and preserving of the solution. These chemicals include mercury, formaldehyde, aluminum, and a variety of other known toxic materials.

These adverse vaccine reactions are notoriously under-reported. A 1994 survey of 159 doctors' offices by the National Vaccine Information Center (NVIC) revealed that only 18 percent of doctors said they make a report to the government when a child suffers a serious health problem following vaccination. Many factors contribute to the reluctance of physicians to report a vaccine reaction, not the least of which is outright denial. Self-protection and self-reassurance are other psychological motives. Physicians do not want to admit that they have caused a problem. They like to think that their interventions are helpful, not harmful. They have also been assured and instructed by the vaccine industry that certain reactions that parents regularly observe, such as brain damage and death, cannot be attributed to the vaccines. A whole range of bizarre and pathological behaviors that infants display after they receive vaccines must have another cause, they argue. It would have occurred anyway, regardless of the shot.

This type of denial and obtuse reasoning runs rampant in the medical literature. Case reports of severe vaccine reactions, whether published in the medical literature or reported to VAERS (the Vaccine Adverse Event Reporting System), are ignored and dismissed. The generally casual, cynical, and paternalistic stance of the medical profession results in constant denial of claims for compensation for vaccine reactions, and absolute refusal to report adverse reactions.

Short-term Reactions

Immediate or short-term reactions following vaccine administration have been consistently reported in the medical literature since vaccines have been in common use. Reports of these reactions have caused rebellion within the populations of various countries, and governments have responded in various ways.

In 1975, Japanese parents refused to give their children the pertussis vaccine after widespread publication of two deaths following vaccination. The Japanese government changed its policy in response to this protest, and delayed the recommended age for vaccination until two years. During the late nineteenth century, individuals in the United States protested that mandatory smallpox vaccination infringed upon their constitutional right of personal liberty. The issue was brought to trial and, in 1905, the Supreme Court upheld the rule that state police power included the need to protect its citizens from diseases. All cases since then have resulted in the same conclusion based on this precedent. When European countries began suspecting that the pertussis vaccine was dangerous, they eliminated it from the recommended schedule of childhood vaccinations. When parents in the United States have refused to administer this vaccine to their children, however, their children have been taken into protective custody by the state.

When vaccine companies began losing million-dollar lawsuits to parents with vaccine-damaged children, the United States government intervened and removed all vaccine manufacturer liability, assuming and limiting damage claims, and removing the possibility of any other compensation. This was the origin of the National Childhood Vaccine Injury Act of 1986 and the Vaccine Compensation Amendments of 1987. This legislation mandated that the Institute of Medicine conduct a scientific review of possible adverse consequences of vaccines. The Vaccine Safety Committee was established, and published several voluminous reports, including *Adverse Effects of Pertussis and Rubella Vaccines* in 1991 and *Adverse Events Associated with Childhood Vaccine: Evidence Bearing on Causality* in 1994 (Institute of Medicine, 1991; 1994).

The Vaccine Safety Committee searched the literature, culling every report of a possible vaccine reaction. They found thousands of vaccine-reaction case reports and studies of adverse effects of vaccines in the medical literature. They reviewed the cases of vaccine-injury claims reported to the Vaccine Adverse Event Reporting System (VAERS), which receives approximately 1,000 reports of vaccine reactions per month. All of these reactions were catalogued by type of event and then evaluated by the committee. A judgment was made about each type of reaction associated with each vaccine, placing them within one of five categories. These five categories refer to the likelihood that a vaccine can cause a particular reaction. Their conclusions about vaccine reactions dictate medical opinion, official positions, and compensation rewards. The weight of these judgments warrants some discussion of their methods and criteria for determining the relationship between adverse events and vaccines.

CATEGORIES OF CAUSAL RELATIONS FOR ADVERSE VACCINE EFFECTS

Institute of Medicine, Vaccine Safety Committee

1. No evidence bearing on a causal relation.

2. The evidence is inadequate to accept or reject a causal relation.

3. The evidence favors rejection of a causal relation.

4. The evidence favors acceptance of a causal relation.

5. The evidence establishes a causal relation.

The Vaccine Safety Committee did an exhaustive job, citing every report available. They applied stringent criteria to these reports and studies, and determined that most conditions fit into category two—inadequate evidence to accept or reject a causal relation. The only conditions that earned a category-five rating, establishment of a causal relation, were:

- anaphylaxis (a sudden, potentially life-threatening systemic allergic response) caused by several vaccines

- polio and death caused by the polio vaccine

- thrombocytopenia (a decrease in the number of platelets, the cells involved in blood clotting) caused by the measles vaccine

- death caused by the measles vaccine

- acute arthritis caused by the rubella vaccine

The only conditions that earned a category-four rating, evidence favors a causal relation, were:

- acute encephalopathy after DTP

- shock and unusual shock-like states after DTP

- chronic arthritis after rubella vaccine

- Guillain-Barré syndrome after DT and polio vaccines

All of the other thousands of reports from countries around the world—from distraught parents whose children died within hours of a shot to physicians convinced that a vaccine resulted in meningitis, or deafness, or sudden onset of central nervous system disorders—proved inadequate to convince the committee that any causal relation exists between these events and the recently administered vaccines. Most types of adverse reactions reported in the medical literature and through the adverse event reporting systems were not recognized by the Vaccine Safety Committee as having a causal relationship to the vaccines. The list of conditions that fit category two, "inadequate evidence to accept or reject a causal relation," is embarrassingly long. That list includes

44 reported conditions and reactions that occurred following the 8 vaccines considered by the Institute of Medicine Committees. The list includes conditions with literally hundreds of reported cases—conditions such as meningitis and diabetes following mumps vaccine, and subacute sclerosing panencephalitis (SSPE) after measles vaccine. Other types of reactions, such as deaths from the pertussis vaccines, are denied. These conclusions are now used as guidelines in the award of compensations for vaccine-injured children.

Is there a problem with the Vaccine Safety Committee's findings? The charge of this committee was "the evaluation of the weight of scientific and medical evidence bearing on the question of whether a causal relation exists between certain vaccines and specific serious adverse events." The principle of proving causality occupied the majority of their deliberations. Simply put, they wanted to know if a specific vaccine *can* cause a specific adverse reaction, and whether it *did* cause adverse reactions in individual case reports.

This determination depended upon the concept of relative risk—the ratio of the rate of occurrence of the adverse event in vaccinated persons to the rate in otherwise comparable unvaccinated persons. The question of whether a vaccine can cause a specific reaction could only be answered affirmatively if the relative risk ratio were greater than 1:1. In other words, a greater number of people suffered a specific disease or reaction soon after a vaccine compared to those people not vaccinated. The greater the relative risk, the more likely the committee would attribute a causal relation to the vaccine. Therefore, the only way to establish a causal relation was to examine studies that observed the rate of occurrence compared to a control group.

They admit the problem: no such control group exists for most vaccines. "In controlled cohort studies, a defined group of individuals exposed to a given vaccine are followed longitudinally for the occurrence of one or more adverse events of interest, and the rate of such occurrence is compared with the rate in an otherwise similar group of nonexposed individuals. . . . In many populations, however, exposure to vaccines is virtually universal." They overcome this by establishing an arbitrary time period during which the reaction must occur: "Exposure can then be defined within a rather narrow time window; that is, the rate of occurrence of an adverse event within 2 weeks of vaccine administration can be compared with the rate of occurrence of an adverse event several weeks or months thereafter."

Who says that delayed reactions do not occur? The committee. Most clinical studies accept reactions within an even shorter time window than that. The vaccine injury table contained within Public Law 99-660, upon which compensation awards are based, allows only a 3-day window for development of encephalopathy (impairment of brain function) or residual seizure disorder following the DTP vaccine. However, numerous studies have consistently shown that nervous system reactions to DTP vaccine occur after a latent period of up to two weeks following vaccination (Gorter, 1933; Munoz, 1984).

The strict rules governing the analysis of causation result in the rejection of most clinical case reports. If your child developed sudden seizures and extreme sleepiness within hours of receiving a measles vaccine and then experienced persistent problems with speech and walking, you would attribute the disease to the vaccine. You would have no doubt about it. The Vaccine Safety Committee, however, would view this report with skepticism because your child was not entered in a controlled study of adverse reactions. They have received dozens of such reports. Their conclusion reads, "Although there are a number of reports of encephalitis or encephalopathy following vaccination with measles vaccines of various strains, the rates quoted are impossible to distinguish from background rates. Good case-control or controlled cohort studies of these conditions in similar unvaccinated populations . . . are lacking. . . . The evidence is inadequate to accept or reject a causal relation between measles or mumps vaccine and encephalitis or encephalopathy" (Institute of Medicine, 1994).

When evaluating case reports of vaccine adverse events, the committee examined the following factors (and a few others) in assessing causality.

- *Previous general experience with the vaccine*—How often have vaccine recipients experienced similar events? How often does the event occur in the absence of vaccine exposure?

- *Alternative etiologic candidates*—Can a pre-existing or new illness explain the sudden appearance of the adverse event?

- *Timing of events*—Does the adverse event occur with the timing that would be expected if the vaccine were the cause?

- *Characteristics of the adverse event*—Are there any available laboratory tests that either support or undermine the hypothesis of vaccine causation?

In evaluating the available case reports, the committee adopted an analytical approach to calculate the probability of vaccine causation based on "likelihood ratios" for each element of the observed case. The likelihood ratio is calculated by comparing the vaccine as the probable cause to the probability of the same occurrence given non-vaccine causation. "The main elements of the case reports used in the committee's assessments included the individual's medical history, the timing of onset of the adverse event following vaccine administration, specific characteristics of the adverse event, and follow-up information concerning its evolution" (Institute of Medicine, 1994). Each case report was systematically reviewed, and very few could measure up to this strict protocol for determining causation.

The guidelines themselves predetermined that the committee would seldom find a causal relation between the vaccine and the disease, death, or disability that followed the receipt of a vaccine, no matter how many similar reports existed and no matter how quickly the reactions occurred. The reason for this is that an adverse effect would occur at the same rate after a vaccine as it does in the general population when the entire population has received the vaccines. This very complex analytical model falls apart because vaccinated children are being compared to the background population of vaccinated children. The frequency of vaccine reactions will be the same in these two equivalent groups, and the committee or any other vaccine researchers will call them "spontaneous events."

The other essential criterion for acceptance of a reaction involves the principle of biological plausibility. Simply put, this principle amounts to the idea that if science can't explain it, then we won't admit it. In the words of the Vaccine Safety Committee, "The vaccine-adverse event association should be plausible and coherent with current knowledge about the biology of the vaccine and the adverse event" (Institute of Medicine, 1994). If there is a biological model that makes sense, then that reinforces an association between the event and the vaccine. Lack of a biological explanation, however, may only show the limited knowledge we have of immune system mechanisms; not understanding it doesn't mean it isn't real.

Long-term Reactions

Deep controversy surrounds the issue of delayed or long-term reactions, because these do not have a clear causal link to vaccines. In vaccine-industry jargon, they are not "temporally related"—that is the definition of a delayed reaction. For example, how do we know that the increased number of ear infections in a population of vaccinated children, or in any individual child, was caused by the vaccine? No one has studied this question. How do we know that the rise in attention disorders in school-age children has a relationship to vaccines? It would seem to be a logical conclusion given the other forms of neurologic damage linked to vaccine reactions, but no one has studied ADD in vaccinated versus unvaccinated children. Parents must make judgments in this area based on the experience of other parents and practitioners whose children and patients have not been vaccinated. Lawmakers are concerned with the lack of interest among drug researchers in studies on long-term adverse effects of vaccines. In May 2001 Congressman Dan Burton observed that "there is a paucity of research looking at long-term safety of any vaccine" (Burton, 2001).

Three types of long-term sequelae are associated with vaccination: autoimmune reactions, depression of immune function, and injury to the nervous system. All of these consequences may involve similar neuroimmune mechanisms, and several theories have been proposed explaining how vaccines trigger these disease processes. For the world's populations, however, the toll exacted by vaccines in the form of chronic disease may be an exorbitant price to pay for our attempt to wipe out these infectious diseases. The list of chronic disease associated with vaccines is now long. Immune system problems resulting from vaccines include asthma and allergies. Several autoimmune disorders seem to have their onset after vaccines—diabetes, arthritis, and multiple sclerosis. And neurologic injury caused by vaccines has resulted in autism, epilepsy, retardation, and attention deficits.

Parents have established Internet networks and membership organizations to track and treat those problems obviously caused by vaccines, particularly autism and other forms of brain injury, conditions whose treatment eludes the skills of modern medicine. Asthma and diabetes are treated according to standard protocols, and the causative relationship to vaccines is ignored. It is primarily the drastic increase in childhood asthma, diabetes, autism, and attention deficits that has drawn worldwide attention to these conditions, but the medical establishment remains perplexed about the reasons for the exponential rise in the numbers of children with these disorders. Continual denial of these effects is standard policy, even when angry parents confront drug companies at congressional hearings on vaccine safety.

Autism

Three important events stimulated intense interest in the association between autism and vaccination. First, disturbing reports of a wildly escalating incidence of autism has parents and researchers searching for the cause. Second, in 1998 Dr. Andrew Wakefield published a research study that showed an association between the MMR vaccine, intestinal disease, and autism. And third, Congressman Dan Burton's grandson developed autism within a week of receiving nine vaccines, thereby joining the legions of autistic children whose symptoms have been attributed to vaccine reactions. These parents are angry, and not inclined to accept denials by drug company magnates.

In 1999, a report released by the California Department of Developmental Services (DDS) revealed the phenomenal statistic that the number of children with autism increased by 273 percent between 1987 and 1998. In 2001 an all-time one-year record number of cases were added to California's system, a 20 percent increase over the previous year. Autism in 2001 became the number-one disability entering California's system.

Similar increases have been noted throughout the country. In Maryland the number of autistic children increased by 513 percent between 1993 and 1998 according to Maryland Special Education Census Data. The number of children with autism served under the Individuals with Disabilities Education Act showed an increase of 300 percent between 1992 and 1997 in more than 25 states. The incidence of autism in Brick Township, New Jersey, in 1998 was 1 in 150 children. In Granite Bay, California, the incidence is 1 in 132 children. Most of these autistic cases are children. Of the nearly 17,000 autistic individuals treated in California during 2001, 80 percent were born after 1980, and 66 percent are children between the age of 0 and 13 years old.

Dr. Andrew Wakefield along with 13 colleagues gained a great deal of attention and scientific criticism when they dared to publish their findings associating autism with measles vaccine exposure (Wakefield, 1998). Since their original work with 12 children who simultaneously developed intestinal disease and autism, Dr. Wakefield has studied over 150 children with autism and intestinal disease. A significant number of these children have elevated levels of IgG measles antibodies compared to controls, and measles-specific antigens in cells of the colon (Wakefield, 2000). The onset of autism in these cases occurred after administration of the MMR vaccine, and Dr. Wakefield has speculated that the compound effect of three live viruses could initiate brain injury, just as the simultaneous occurrence of more than one natural viral infection has been known to increase the risk of encephalitis. Wakefield's findings were later verified and replicated by other researchers. Both Dr. John O'Leary and Dr. H. Kawashima identified measles virus in the intestinal lining of the same children (O'Leary, 2000; Kawashima et al., 2000). A follow-up study conducted by Wakefield, O'Leary, and others also showed the presence of persistent measles virus and inflammatory bowel disease in children with developmental disorder. In that study, 91 children with developmental disorder and bowel disease were compared to 70 developmentally normal controls, some of whom also had inflammatory bowel disease, Crohn's disease, or ulcerative colitis. Among the children with developmental disorder 75 of 91 (82 percent) had persistent measles virus, presumably from the MMR vaccine, compared to 5 of 70 (7 percent) developmentally normal children (Uhlmann *et al.*, 2002).

The mechanism for production of autism by measles vaccine has been presented by Dr. Vijendra Singh's research. He has identified specific antibodies that produce an autoimmune attack on brain tissue in response to measles vaccine (Singh, 1996; Singh, 1998). Brain injury from the measles vaccine has long been suspected, and a recent report has verified the causal relationship between permanent brain injury and the vaccine (Weibel *et al.*, 1998). It should come as no surprise that measles vaccine could also cause an insult to the brain resulting in autism.

A questionnaire administered to mothers of autistic children revealed another alarming connection to vaccines. This time the effects were apparently passed from mother to infant. Of the 240 mothers surveyed, 25 had received a rubella vaccine or MMR vaccine during the postpartum period, and 20 of these women (80 percent) had children with autism. Nine of these children were born just prior to the vaccination, and it is presumed that transmission occurred through the mother's breast milk. The rubella vaccine insert states that "lactating postpartum women immunized with rubella live attenuated vaccine may secrete the virus in breast milk and transmit it to breast fed infants." The author states that "caution should be exercised when the vaccine is administered to a nursing mother." In ten of the cases the subsequent child developed autism, suggesting a placental or genetic transmission of factors that could cause the disease (Yazbak, 1999). Seven women in this survey received a rubella, measles, hepatitis B, or MMR during pregnancy. "Six out of the seven children (85%) who resulted from these pregnancies were diagnosed with autism, and the seventh whose mother received a measles vaccine, exhibits symptoms which suggest autistic spectrum. This child's twin brother was stillborn" (Yazbak, 1999a).

In the fall of 2000, the National Institutes of Health (NIH) established a committee to investigate the relation between MMR vaccine and autism. Despite the findings of clinical studies showing the association, the committee's report concluded that "the evidence favors rejection of a causal relationship at the population level between MMR vaccine and autistic spectrum disorders (ASD)" (Institute of Medicine, 2001). Immediately upon release of the report in April 2001, Chairman Dan Burton of the House Committee on Government Reform blasted the analysis as a "disservice to the American people." Burton also accused two of the report's reviewers of having ties to the pharmaceutical industry, and raised concerns that some of the information clearing the vaccine came from Merck, the vaccine's manufacturer. The following month Burton testified that he believed his grandson became autistic one week after he received nine vaccines in one day, and that the vaccines were responsible (Burton, 2001).

Other researchers have associated the dramatic rise in autism cases with the toxic exposure to the mercury preservative contained in vaccines. In 1998 the FDA banned the use of mercury in all drugs because of its recognized neurotoxicity and lack of safety. In 1999 the US Public Health Service and the American Academy of Pediatrics supported the FDA directive to remove mercury from all vaccines. In May of 2001 Congressman Burton noted that many vaccines still contained mercury, and he demanded that mercury be removed from all vaccines (Burton, 2001).

Mercury poisoning produces parallel symptoms to those of autism, including seizures, lack of coordination, retardation, and unresponsive behaviors. During the first six months of life, an infant who receives all recommended vaccines will accumulate 187 micrograms of mercury, a cumulative level of exposure higher than that recommended by the Environmental Protection Agency (Committee on Infectious Disease, 1999). Parent advocacy groups have concluded that this level of mercury exposure is responsible for the onset of autism. As a result of this concern, a consortium of ten law firms led by the firm of Waters & Kraus has filed lawsuits alleging that the mercury preservative in vaccines caused neurological damage resulting in autism in clients' children. These lawsuits are based on a confidential study conducted by Centers for Disease Control scientists who studied autism as a potential neurological injury caused by mercury in vaccines. The attorneys contend that a different version of the study was made public and cited by the Institutes of Medicine report as inconclusive on the role of mercury in initiating autism symptoms. The confidential version of the study demonstrates that an exposure of 62.5 micrograms of mercury in the first three months of life significantly increased a child's risk of autism. The currently recommended course of vaccines would expose an infant to 75 micrograms of mercury in the first three months of life. Children exposed to this level of mercury were more than twice as likely to develop autism as children not exposed (Waters & Krause, 2001).

Several mechanisms have been proposed to explain the onset of mercury-induced autism. In a study of 503 autism patients, 499 (99 percent) showed a defect in metal metabolism that impairs the development of the brain and can result in hypersensitivity to toxic substances. This defect was reported by William Walsh, Ph.D., and Anjum Usman, M.D., of the Pfeiffer Center, Naperville, IL *(www.hriptc.org)*. Their findings were presented at the annual meeting of the American Psychiatric Association in May 2001. The authors suggest that the primary cause of autism may be a genetic defect in metal metabolism (metallothionein dysfunction) or an environmental insult which disables the metallothionein protein (MT). These MT proteins regulate blood levels of metals, detoxify mercury and other heavy metals, and assist in neuronal development.

Immune System Disorders

Critics of vaccinations have asserted that vaccines are capable of causing recurrent infections in children because they weaken the immune system. They say that the dramatic rise in ear infections, allergies, and asthma in children can be attributed (at least in part) to the damaging effects of vaccines. The incidence of asthma, the most serious and life-threatening of these conditions, has steadily increased in the modern era since the introduction of vaccines. During the period 1980 through 1989 the prevalence rate of self-reported asthma in the United States increased 38 percent, and the death rate for asthma increased 46 percent (Centers for Disease Control, 1992). In the five years from 1985 through 1990, projected estimates for asthma's medical costs increased 53 percent. The total estimated cost of asthma rose from $4.5 billion to $6.2 billion, or 1 percent of all US health-care costs (Weiss *et al.*, 1992). In other parts of the world as many as 30 percent of children suffer from asthma, and the rate of asthma increases by 50 percent every decade. This dramatic increase has been attributed to increased exposure to environmental pollutants, and to the toxic effect of asthma medications themselves, but the increasing burden on the immune system caused by vaccines cannot be ignored.

Several clinical studies have confirmed an association between vaccination and asthma. A team of New Zealand researchers followed 1,265 children born in 1977. Of the children who were vaccinated 23 percent had asthma episodes. A total of 23 children did not receive the DTP vaccines, and none of them developed asthma (Kemp *et al.*, 1997). A study in Great Britain produced similar findings that associated asthma with the pertussis vaccine. In that study 243 children received the vaccine and 26 of them later developed asthma (10.7 percent), compared to only 4 of the 203 children who had never received the pertussis vaccine (2 percent). The relative risk of developing asthma from the pertussis vaccine was 5.4. Additionally, of the 91 children who received no vaccines at all, only one had asthma. Therefore the risk of developing asthma was about one percent in children receiving no vaccines and 11 percent for those children who received vaccines including pertussis (Odent *et al.*, 1994). A third study was conducted in the US from data in the National Health and Nutrition Examination Survey of infants through adolescents aged 16. Data showed that children vaccinated with DTP or tetanus were twice as likely to develop asthma compared to unvaccinated children (Hurwitz and Morgenstern, 2000).

One study revealed that the MMR vaccine can cause human white blood cells to develop IgE antibodies, which is the primary characteristic of asthma (Imani & Kehoe, 2001). This induction of an allergic reactivity may explain the increased incidence of asthma in vaccinated children.

Several studies have examined the effect of vaccines on subsequent illness patterns in children to investigate whether vaccines can suppress immune system functions. The studies were stimulated in part by previous reports of an increased risk of acquiring serious invasive infections within the three weeks following receipt of the older capsular *Haemophilus influenzae* (Hib) vaccine (Black *et al.*, 1987) and the deaths of four children from invasive bacterial disease in Sweden after receiving acellular pertussis vaccines (Storsaeter *et al.*, 1988).

One study examined the incidence of acute illnesses in the 30-day period following vaccine compared to the incidence in the same children for the 30-day period prior to a vaccine. This study showed a significant and dramatic increase in nonbacterial fevers, diarrhea, and cough in the month following DTP vaccine (Jaber *et al.*, 1988). Children had a higher incidence of illness after DTP compared to their health before the shot.

The ability of pertussis and DTP vaccines to stimulate the onset of paralytic polio provides further evidence that vaccines can promote serious disease processes and immune system dysfunction. Paralytic polio has occurred frequently following vaccination. This phenomenon was first reported in 1909. Scattered cases were reported over the next 40 years. Then, during the polio epidemics of the 1950s, series of cases of polio following pertussis-vaccine injections were reported around the world: in Australia (McCloskey, 1950; McCloskey, 1952), the United Kingdom (Hill & Knowelden, 1949; Medical Research Council, 1956), and the United States (Korn *et al.*, 1952; Greenberg *et al.*, 1952).

During a polio epidemic in Oman, the problem of paralytic polio infection's onset soon after DTP vaccination occurred again. In this epidemic, 70 children 5 to 24 months old contracted paralytic polio during the period 1988–1989. When compared to a control group of children without polio, it was found that a significantly higher percentage of these children had received a DTP shot within 30 days of the onset of polio (43 percent of polio victims compared to 28 percent of controls) (Sutter *et al.*, 1992). The mechanism of this provoking effect of vaccination on polio onset has never been adequately explained, but it seems clear that an immune-suppressing effect of vaccines must be responsible.

Many clinical studies have also shown immune-suppressive effects of vaccines. For example, mice showed an increased susceptibility to infection following pertussis vaccine (Abernathy & Spink, 1956). Laboratory studies in humans have revealed evidence of immune system suppression as well. After measles vaccination certain lymphocyte functions essential in fighting pathogenic organisms are depressed (Hirsch *et al.*, 1981), and the number of lymphocytes, a type of white blood cell that fights disease, decreases (Nicholson *et al.*, 1992; Hussey *et al.*, 1996). Similarly, measles-mumps-rubella (MMR) vaccine has been reported to have a temporary suppressive effect on the function of neutrophils, another white blood cell (Toraldo *et al.*, 1992). Immune suppression caused by the measles vaccine was also observed in human recipients who then developed an increased susceptibility to other infections (Auwaerter *et al.*, 1996).

The *Haemophilus influenzae* (Hib) meningitis vaccine causes a decrease in measured antibody concentrations to Hib. This is true for both the older capsular vaccine and the new conjugate vaccine (Daum *et al.*, 1989). This depression of antibody levels is responsible for the early onset of Hib infection in the 7 days following Hib vaccine. Four case-control studies showed an increased risk of children developing Hib after receiving the capsular vaccine to prevent Hib (Black *et al.*, 1988; Harrison *et al.*, 1988; Shapiro *et al.*, 1988; Osterholm *et al.*, 1988).

The use of this vaccine was abandoned with the development of the new conjugated Hib vaccines. However, ten cases of Hib disease that occurred within 5 days after the Hib conjugate vaccine were reported through the Vaccine Adverse Event Reporting System (VAERS) between 1990 and 1992. Case-controlled studies have failed to show a significant increase in early-onset Hib disease after the conjugate vaccine compared to the prevaccine era incidence rate (Institute of Medicine, 1994). The Vaccine Safety Committee therefore rejected a causal relation between vaccination with Hib conjugate vaccines and early-onset Hib disease. Despite these individual studies, the weight of evidence in a large body of studies, cases, and laboratory findings indicates that vaccines can suppress immune system function.

Other researchers have shown that vaccines stimulate the body's production of naturally occurring interferon gamma (Pabst, 1997). One function of interferon gamma is to increase tissue permeability, thus allowing activated B-cells and T-cells of the human immune system to infiltrate the brain and nerves, where they can destroy tissue in an autoimmune process (Benveniste, 1992; Matyszak, 1998).

Our understanding of these processes is very limited, and the long-term effects of persistent circulating antigen in the body are unknown. It may cause a continual immune suppression, which disables the body's ability to react normally to disease. Or the autoimmune reaction may be due to "molecular mimicry, when a structural similarity exists between some viral antigen (or other component of the vaccine) and a self-antigen. This similarity may be the trigger to the autoimmune reaction" (Shoenfeld and Aron-Maor, 2000). Certainly the continual reports of autoimmune phenomena that occur as reactions to vaccines provide us with incontrovertible evidence that tampering with the immune system through vaccination practices has led to immune system dysfunction.

The Institute of Medicine Vaccine Safety Committee identifies various autoimmune phenomena as well-documented adverse effects of vaccines. Many of these autoimmune responses to vaccines result in permanent, chronic disease conditions. The committee's report acknowledges the repeated incidence of specific autoimmune diseases triggered by vaccines that attack nerves and cause destruction of the nerve sheath (myelin). These demyelinating diseases, such as multiple sclerosis and Guillain-Barré syndrome (GBS), have plagued the vaccine industry. Reports of their occurrence following vaccination continue to pour in from around the world. In their attempt to explain the demyelinating autoimmune diseases that repeatedly occur as reactions to vaccines, the committee members admit that,

It is biologically plausible that injection of an inactivated virus, bacterium, or live attenuated virus might induce in the susceptible host an autoimmune response by deregulation of the immune response, by nonspecific activation of the T-cells directed against myelin proteins, or by autoimmunity triggered by sequence similarities of proteins in the vaccine to host proteins such as those of myelin (Institute of Medicine, 1994).

Multiple Sclerosis

The repeated reports of multiple sclerosis (MS) and other demyelinating nervous system diseases occurring subsequent to vaccinations have not gone unnoticed. In October 1998, France became the first country to stop hepatitis B vaccination requirements for schoolchildren after reports of chronic arthritis, symptoms resembling multiple sclerosis, and other serious health problems following hepatitis B vaccination became so numerous that the Health Minister of France suspended the school requirement. Health Minister Bernard Kouchner said inoculations were stopped because of fears that the vaccine could cause neurological disorders, in particular multiple sclerosis. Hundreds of case reports have been filed that associate the hepatitis B vaccine with nervous system disorders, and a French court ruled that there was sufficient evidence to conclude there was a connection between a vaccine produced by British drug maker SmithKline Beecham and multiple sclerosis symptoms. The French government compensated three recipients of hepatitis B vaccine for their development of MS.

The first clinical report of demyelination after the hepatitis B vaccination was noted in 1983 (Ribera and Dutka, 1983). The complication was transient. A second clinician observed seven cases of a neurologic picture resembling multiple sclerosis after hepatitis B vaccination (Waisbren, 1992). In 1993, an 11-year-old girl developed transverse myelitis following a recombinant hepatitis vaccination (Trevisani, 1993). The same year another report appeared of a classic MS case following ten days after a recombinant vaccination (Nadler *et al.*, 1993).

Following the news reports and resulting concerns among the population, SmithKline published a report that attributed the association between the hepatitis vaccine and MS to pure coincidence

(Monteyne and Andre, 2001). Other studies of nurses who developed MS (Ascherio *et al.*, 2001) and MS patients who experienced relapses (Confavreux *et al.*, 2001) could not find an association between the onset of symptoms and a recent hepatitis vaccination. Nonetheless, concerns remain about this severe autoimmune phenomenon.

Diabetes

A dramatic increase in the incidence of diabetes has clinicians puzzling over possible causes. The US population has approximately doubled since the 1940s, but the number of diabetics has risen more than twenty-fold (Coulter, 1997). In 1947 there were an estimated 600,000 cases of diabetes in the US, and by 1997 there were an estimated 13 million diabetics (Libman, 1997). Like autism, asthma, and other autoimmune diseases, many researchers have pinpointed vaccines as a primary cause of this increased incidence.

The onset of diabetes has been associated with the mumps, Haemophilus, and hepatitis B vaccines. Finland has the highest rate of type-1 (juvenile onset, insulin-dependent) diabetes in the world. The incidence of diabetes in children aged 0–4 rose 62 percent between the years 1980–82 and 1990–92 following a widespread *Haemophilus influenzae* vaccine campaign begun in 1986 (Tuomilehto *et al.*, 1995; Classen and Classen, 1997). A later study in Finland compared the effect of 4 doses of Haemophilus vaccine to 0 doses and noted a relative risk of 1.26 for the onset of diabetes in the vaccinated group compared to those not vaccinated (Classen, 1999; Karvonen *et al.*, 1999). A similar phenomenon occurred in the US. In Allegheny County, Pennsylvania, the Haemophilus vaccine was introduced in 1985. This county has the oldest type-1 diabetes registry in the US. An epidemic of diabetes occurred in the 0–4 age group during the years 1985–1993, following introduction of the vaccine. The annual incidence of diabetes in these children rose 60 percent during the postvaccine years (1985–1989), compared to the prevaccine years (1980–1984) (Dokheel, 1993). This temporal association does not prove causation, but it is certainly suspicious, especially when considering an identical rise in diabetes following the hepatitis vaccine.

Christchurch, New Zealand, has the only existing diabetes registry in the country. A massive hepatitis B vaccination program began in 1988, and over 70 percent of children in Christchurch were vaccinated (Classen, 1996). The annual incidence of type-1 diabetes in persons 0–19 years of age rose from 11.2 cases/100,000 in 1982–1987 (preceding the vaccine) to 18.1 cases in 1989–1991, an increase of 60 percent (Classen, 1996; Classen 1997). Dr. Bart Classen has postulated that the most likely mechanism for the onset of diabetes after vaccination is the release of interferons, since vaccines can cause the release of interferons that produce autoimmune reactions including diabetes (Huang *et al.*, 1995; Stewart *et al.*, 1993).

Since the publication of these findings, a follow-up study failed to show any association between vaccination and diabetes (DeStefano *et al.*, 2001); however, the fact that the onset of diabetes may occur several years after vaccination could explain the lack of a clear correlation. Long-term reactions and delayed reactions are difficult to study for this very reason. Classen has suggested that it may take up to four years to develop diabetes following the insult of vaccination. A vaccine assault will destroy some percentage of pancreatic islet cells, and it may take several such assaults by vaccines or other agents to deplete the ability of the pancreas to produce insulin (Classen, 1996a).

CONTAMINATED VACCINES

Vaccines are prepared from viruses and bacteria grown in cultures and media of animal cells and animal meat extracts. Therefore, the finished product contains many contaminants in the form of animal proteins. If those animals were infected with viruses, then viral contaminants can be present in the vaccine. Most vaccines have chemicals added that kill the live viruses, and the vaccines are screened for known viruses and bacteria. However, the oral polio vaccine depends upon transmission of a live virus, and killing other viruses would result in an inactive vaccine. Additionally, manufacturers can only find what they are looking for, and any currently unknown viruses can escape detection.

At least one vaccine researcher has agreed to talk about his experience with contamination and safety of vaccines. He worked for more than ten years in the labs of major pharmaceutical houses and the US government's National Institutes of Health, and agreed to a printed interview with Jon Rappaport only on condition of complete anonymity. "I was 'part of the inner circle.' If now I began to name names and make specific accusations against researchers, I could be in a world of trouble." He relates stories of other researchers with critical views who were "harassed" and "put under surveillance" by the FBI and the IRS. When asked about vaccine safety, he scoffs. "If the FDA were run by honorable people, these vaccines would not be granted licenses. They would be investigated to within an inch of their lives." Focusing on the contaminants he found in vaccines he states, "If you try to calculate what damage these contaminants can cause, well, we don't really know, because no testing has been done, or very little testing. It's a game of roulette. You take your chances." Some contaminants have been identified. "Who knows how many others there are? Others we don't find because we don't think to look for them. If tissue from, say, a bird is used to make a vaccine, how many possible germs can be in that tissue? We have no idea. We have no idea what they might be, or what effects they could have on humans."

Would he agree to get vaccinated? "If I had a child now, the last thing I would allow is vaccination. I would move out of the state if I had to. I would change the family name. I would disappear. With my family, I'm not saying it would come to that. There are ways to side-step the system with grace, if you know how to act. There are exemptions you can declare, in every state, based on religious and/or philosophic views. But if push came to shove, I would go on the move" (Rappaport at *www.whale.to/v/rapp.html*).

Extensive research has been conducted on three viral contaminants suspected of causing disease in recipients—SV40 (a monkey virus that causes cancer), HIV (the virus associated with AIDS), and a stealth virus associated with chronic fatigue syndrome and autism.

Monkey Virus and Cancer

Polio vaccine has traditionally been prepared in monkey cell cultures. A virus harbored by monkeys could grow in the vaccine culture and infect humans. In the early days of polio vaccine research, everyone assumed that monkey viruses caused no problems in humans, and regulations of the 1950s referred only to the exclusion of "viable" microbial agents, not monkey viruses (Papers, 1959). However, monkey B viruses, first identified by Albert Sabin, the inventor of the oral polio vaccine, were later shown to infect humans and to cause illness and death.

Since that time, many different monkey viruses have been transmitted from monkeys to humans. One particular monkey virus, SV40, contaminated the IPV (killed polio) vaccine during the period 1954 to 1963. The term SV40 refers to Simian virus 40, so named because it was the 40th virus identified in monkeys. An estimated 98 million

Americans were exposed to SV40 through IPV injections, and hundreds of millions of people worldwide received the contaminated vaccine (Fisher *et al.*, 1999). Prior to 1961, vaccine manufacturers did not give monkeys a blood test for SV40 before using their kidneys for vaccine production. No one knows whether the contaminated vaccine caused any form of illness or symptoms because adverse effects of the vaccine were never studied comprehensively. However, an increased incidence of brain tumors was found among persons who had received the contaminated vaccine (Geissler, 1990). A study of more than 58,000 women who had received IPV during the years that SV40 contaminated the vaccine (1959–1965) showed a thirteenfold increased risk of brain tumors in their children (Rosa *et al.*, 1988).

Later research confirmed the association between the SV40 virus transmitted through polio vaccine and cancers. SV40 does cause cancer when injected into laboratory animals. Now, more than 60 scientific studies have found SV40 in human brain, bone, and lung-related cancers, the same kinds of tumors the virus causes in laboratory animals. Researchers also determined that SV40 viral stains can infect humans, and that the authentic SV40 present in monkeys is associated with brain tumors in early childhood (Butel *et al.*, 1998). A study conducted in China confirmed that SV40 was present in a majority of brain tumors tested, and that the SV40 involved was actively expressing proteins and stimulating tumor production (Zhen *et al.*, 1999). In a study of 154 patients with lymphoma, 64 (42 percent) contained DNA sequences of SV40 virus. The data from that study also suggest that SV40 caused the cancers (Vilchez *et al.*, 2002). A second study found SV40 in 29 (43 percent) of 68 lymphomas tested (Shivapurkar *et al.*, 2002). There is no doubt that the SV40 virus can cause lymphoma. When hamsters are injected with SV40, 72 percent of the animals develop lymphomas (Diamandopoulos, 1972).

Skeptics still questioned whether the SV40 found in tumors was the same virus as that transmitted through the polio vaccine of the 1950s and 60s, especially since many of the SV40-containing tumors were discovered in children born three decades later. To solve this question, Michele Carbone, one of the primary researchers of SV40 cancers, sought out the original polio vaccine. He found an unopened case of vaccine from 1955 in a Chicago doctor's office. When he tested the vials he found that they contained SV40 genetically identical to the strains found in human bone and brain tumors and in monkeys. "This proves that the SV40 that was present in the polio vaccine is identical to the SV40 we are finding in these human tumors," Carbone says (Bookchin and Schumacher, 2000). Researchers attribute the transmission of virus to blood transfusions, breastfeeding, and sexual contact. In other words, a virus transmitted from monkeys to humans through the polio vaccine in the 1950s is still being passed among the population and causing cancer.

For more information and updates on the most recent studies linking SV40 and cancer, see the website at *www.SV40cancer.com.*

HIV and AIDS

Did early oral polio vaccine experiments in Africa transmit an AIDS-related monkey virus to humans and begin the AIDS epidemic? In 1980, Robert Gallo of the National Cancer Institute identified the first retroviruses that infected humans, the two human T-lymphotropic viruses, HTLV-I and HTLV-II. These viruses cause leukemia and cancer of lymph nodes in people. Two years later a virus with remarkably similar effects was discovered in monkeys, designated the simian T-lymphotropic virus, STLV. In a search for the origins of HTLV in humans, researchers began looking for monkeys in the wild that harbored the STLV virus. Genetic studies of monkey STLVs showed that human HTLV was closely related to the simian virus seen in the African green monkey (Kanki *et al.*, 1985). Gallo proposed that HTLV originated in Africa, infecting humans and primates, and was spread to the Americas by the slave trade.

A similar search for a monkey virus related to HIV (the human immunodeficiency virus) began in 1984. At this time the human AIDS-related virus was called HTLV-III, and later renamed HIV. A new virus was soon discovered in monkeys that caused simian acquired immune deficiency, simian AIDS. Researchers who isolated this virus named it SIV. Genetic studies have shown that SIV is approximately 50 percent related to HIV (Essex & Kanki, 1988).

Later studies of high-risk populations in West Africa revealed that 10 percent of their blood samples had antibodies that reacted with both HIV and SIV. This West African virus was found to be more closely related to SIV than to HIV, and it was named HTLV-IV and later renamed HIV-2. The reactions of the human blood samples were indistinguishable from the antibody reactions of infected African green monkeys. According to retrovirus researcher Robert Gallo, SIV is "virtually indistinguishable from some human variants of HIV-2" associated with West African AIDS (Curtis, 1992). According to viral researchers, "people infected with HIV-2 have antibodies entirely cross-reactive with SIV antigens; in fact, it is impossible to distinguish between SIV and HIV-2 on the basis of serological criteria." They go on to confirm, "All of this suggests at least that the primate and human viruses share evolutionary roots and at most that there may have been interspecies infection—that SIV-infected monkeys transmitted the virus to humans or vice versa" (Essex & Kanki, 1988).

Later researchers also proposed that HIV-2 was probably spread to humans from the SIV-infected monkeys through scratches, bites, or blood exposures while humans hunted and butchered the West African mangabey monkeys in the wild (Nowak, 1992). Another simian virus, this time SIV from chimpanzees, proved to be remarkably similar to several HIV-1 viral strains, thus connecting AIDS in both the United States (HIV-1) and Africa (HIV-2) with primates (Huet et al., 1990). Some researchers referred to this connection between SIV in chimpanzees with HIV as the missing link to the origins of HIV-1 in humans (Desrosiers, 1990). Similarly, HIV can infect macaque (Agy et al., 1992) and African green monkeys (Lecatsas & Alexander, 1992). Researchers continually discover these connecting links between SIV and HIV strains, HIV in monkeys, and SIV infections in humans. SIV was found in the cancer cells of an AIDS patient (Bohannon et al., 1991), and SIV infections have been discovered in laboratory workers, agricultural workers, and urban dwellers (Khabbaz et al., 1992; Gao et al., 1992).

Although the SIV virus causes AIDS in captive macaque monkeys, infected African green monkeys remain symptom-free. Researchers found that a surprisingly high number of African green monkeys carried the SIV virus—30–70 percent of monkeys in the wild (Essex & Kanki, 1988). These were the same green monkeys used in polio vaccine production, and these carrier monkeys were never excluded from vaccine production because they appeared healthy. US government tests in 1976–1977 detected retroviruses in polio vaccines, but authorities approved them for release if the vaccine contained fewer than 100 organisms per dose (Kyle, 1992).

In 1976, however, researchers at the US Bureau of Biologics recorded that three samples of Lederle polio vaccine contained between 1,000 and 100,000 simian viruses per ml. of vaccine, a much higher concentration than later safety regulations allowed (Kyle, 1992). Vaccine manufacturers were so concerned about monkey virus contamination of live polio vaccines that some pharmaceutical companies (e.g. Merck and Co.) refused to participate in vaccine production (Developments . . . , 1961).

Several investigators have speculated that the contamination of oral polio vaccine with monkey viruses may have been the origin of AIDS. They have criticized the "cut hunter" hypothesis in which African hunters were supposedly infected by contaminated monkey blood as taking too long to spread AIDS compared to the rapid epidemic that actually occurred. They have searched for a more massive population exposure of humans to infected monkeys. What better way to spread a lethal virus and ignite mass epidemics than giving live monkey viruses to humans in a vaccine campaign?

Such a massive vaccine campaign in the Belgian Congo (now Zaire, Rwanda, and Burundi) using an oral polio vaccine contaminated with monkey SIV virus may have started AIDS outbreaks in Africa (Elswood & Stricker, 1993; Curtis, 1992). An experimental oral polio vaccine campaign during 1957 to 1959 included 320,000 infants and children in that area of Africa, which then became the center of the radiating African AIDS epidemics. That vaccine was prepared in monkey kidney cells that were known to be contaminated with at least 18 different simian viruses (Hayflick *et al.,* 1962). The polio vaccine used in the Congo experiments was never approved for human use and never used after 1960 (Elswood & Stricker, 1994). This connection between the contaminated polio vaccine, the Congo polio experiments, and the first outbreaks of AIDS in Africa has led several independent investigators to suspect the vaccine as the origin of AIDS (Pascal, 1991). One reviewer stated it boldly and simply: "It is difficult to believe that the outbreak of HIV infection in Africa at the same time and location as this mass polio vaccine trial is a coincidence" (Elswood & Stricker, 1994).

Oral polio vaccine was used in repeated monthly doses beginning in 1974 to treat recurrent genital herpes (Tager, 1974). This treatment could have seeded the homosexual population with these simian retroviruses, producing the first United States AIDS epidemics (Kyle, 1992).

Investigators called for the testing of polio vaccines for the presence of simian viruses (SIV). A panel was convened to assess the credibility of the polio vaccine hypothesis as the origin of AIDS. The Wistar Institute, producers of the polio vaccine used in the Congo experiments, financed this in response to accusations about contaminated vaccines. Not surprisingly, this panel found the argument that AIDS arose from the polio vaccine extremely unlikely: "The panel found flaws in every step of the hypothetical pathway of transmission. It points out that neither SIV nor HIV is known to infect or multiply in . . . cells from monkey kidneys."

They acknowledged that cell cultures could contain white blood cells infected with HIV, but they argued that the freezing and thawing cycles would have "greatly reduced concentration and infectivity of any contaminating retrovirus" (Poliovaccine, 1992). They neglected to explain, however, how the live polio vaccine could survive processing that destroyed other viruses. As a matter of fact, it could not. According to Tom Folkes, chief virologist of the retrovirus laboratory at the Centers for Disease Control, vaccine manufacturers could not kill one virus and have other viruses survive. He said in reference to the oral polio vaccine, "The fact that it's a live vaccine would indicate that they had not gone through any inactivation procedures to denature the AIDS virus, because it would probably denature the polio virus. So the polio virus is kept alive, and the SIV virus would just travel with it. The theory, the possibility is real" (Curtis, 1992). Finally, the panel could not refute the possibility of transmission, and suggested that relevant samples of vaccine stock be tested for HIV/SIV viruses (Poliovaccine, 1992).

This is exactly what a group of researchers at the National Institute for Biological Standards in England proceeded to do. They conducted a laboratory examination of oral polio vaccine preparations from 4 manufacturers used between 1975 and 1984, the era prior to testing for SIV contamination. They found no evidence of HIV or SIV gene sequences in these samples—but these were not the same cultures as those used in the period 1957 to 1960 in the Congo. A vaccine used 20 years later, in 1975, would not necessarily have the same problems of contamination as those used in the African vaccine campaign. They tested the wrong vaccines.

These researchers also studied the ability of monkey kidney cell cultures to grow HIV. Cell cultures from uninfected monkeys failed to support the growth of HIV when it was added to the culture. They claimed that HIV could not survive and multiply in the conditions required for the growth of poliovirus.

They conducted a third experiment as well. They infected monkeys with SIV and examined cells derived from their kidneys. No SIV virus or SIV antigens could be found in the kidney cell cultures after 10 days. As a result of those studies the authors concluded that "there is no evidence for HIV or SIV contamination in the polio vaccines we examined and that SIV from infected monkeys would be unlikely to survive the procedures involved in the production of [vaccine] or to replicate under the conditions required for the growth of poliovirus" (Garrett *et al.*, 1993). However, they did not examine specimens of vaccine used in the original African experiments, nor did they prove that SIV could not contaminate the vaccine. Furthermore, John Garrett, the researcher who conducted these experiments "conceded that there were many ways in which his experiments might not, in practice, reflect what had actually gone on during the early days of OPV production.

It was not easy, he explained, to reproduce tissue cultures like those of forty years earlier . . ." (Hooper, 1999, p. 662). Until HIV is found in polio vaccine, the theories about transmission of AIDS from monkeys to humans through the vaccine will remain speculative.

For a complete history of the polio vaccine transmission theory of AIDS, readers are referred to the scholarly and exhaustive book by Edward Hooper, *The River: A Journey to the Source of HIV and AIDS* (Little, Brown and Co., 1999).

A new discovery has created another link between monkey viruses, polio vaccine, and mysterious debilitating illnesses. This time the detection of a virus in patients with chronic fatigue syndrome (CFS) led to the monkey again.

Stealth Virus

Dr. John Martin discovered an unusual virus in cultures isolated from at least two patients with chronic fatigue syndrome, a cytomegalovirus-like stealth virus. These viruses are termed "stealth" because they fail to evoke an inflammatory reaction in the patients from whom they were isolated because the viruses lack target antigens for recognition by the body's cellular immune system. Comparison of DNA sequences with other known viruses showed that this stealth virus was closely related to a strain of simian cytomegalovirus found in African green monkeys (Martin *et al.*, 1995). The most likely source for infection by an African green monkey virus is the live polio vaccine. This study provides further evidence that the polio vaccine or other vaccines produced in monkey cell cultures or monkey tissues could harbor unrecognized simian viruses capable of causing chronic infections in humans.

Dr. Martin has identified stealth viral infection in all of the following conditions: chronic fatigue syndrome, autism (Martin, 1995), fibromyalgia, Gulf War Syndrome, depression and dementia in adults, and attention deficit and behavioral disorders in children. Stealth viral infection can also cause severe encephalopathy (Martin, 1996).

For a complete discussion of stealth viruses see *www.ccid.org*.

Other Viruses

Viruses can only be detected in vaccines if researchers know what they are trying to find. Monkey viruses have been transferred from monkeys to humans through the live polio vaccine because manufacturers did not know about their existence. It is possible that still other unidentified viruses that cause disease in humans could be contained in vaccines, their discovery awaiting further research findings. Infants exposed to these monkey viruses could develop infections transmitted from monkeys to humans, the same type of infections suspected in the spread of AIDS, chronic fatigue syndrome, autism, and cancer.

Laboratory analysis of vaccines has identified dozens of foreign protein contaminants in vaccines, including a long list of pathogens. According to one scientist who has come forward, the list is forbidding. "In polio vaccine, we found acanthamoeba, which is a so-called 'brain-eating' amoeba. Simian cytomegalovirus in polio vaccine. Simian foamy virus in the rotavirus vaccine. Bird-cancer viruses in the MMR vaccine. Various micro-organisms in the anthrax vaccine. I've found potentially dangerous enzyme inhibitors in several vaccines. Duck, dog, and rabbit viruses in the rubella vaccine. Avian leucosis virus in the flu vaccine. Pestivirus in the MMR vaccine."

Flu vaccine and MMR vaccine are prepared in chick embryo cells, which are commonly contaminated with avian leukosis viruses (ALV). These leukosis viruses cause many kinds of cancers in chickens, and they are transmissible, but humans are not considered susceptible to the virus. No attempt has been made to eliminate the use of avian leukosis-containing hens' eggs in the large-scale production of these vaccines because there is no perceived safety issue.

Here is a typical statement. "There is currently no evidence that exposure to ALV through vaccination is associated with adverse events. Our inability to demonstrate infectious virus or to find any ALV-EAV sequences in recipients of the U.S.-made MMR vaccine supports the safety of this vaccine product and suggests that these endogenous viruses [contained within the tissues used] are not xenotropic [capable of infecting other species]." The authors conclude their study with a typically rosy assumption. "The proven efficacy of MMR and the absence of evidence of any harm due to MMR vaccination support current immunization policies" (Tsang *et al.*, 1999).

For many years, all live yellow fever vaccines were produced in eggs containing the live avian leukosis. Evidence of exposure to the virus was found in vaccine recipients, but one retrospective study showed no increased risk for cancer in yellow fever vaccine recipients, and therefore chicken leukosis virus in vaccines is considered harmless (Waters *et al.*, 1972).

CHEMICALS IN VACCINES

The chemicals contained in vaccines may be responsible for some vaccine reactions and adverse effects. Many toxic substances are contained within vaccine preparations, including chemicals used in manufacturing processes, toxins of the microorganisms themselves, and various impurities. The interactions of chemical additives contained in the vaccines with the toxins may also produce adverse effects when they are injected into the body. For example, the formalinization of crude toxins polymerizes impurities and other bacterial antigens, and these are not removed by subsequent purification steps (Relyveld, 1980).

Diphtheria and tetanus toxoids are prepared by extraction of toxin from the bacteria and incubation of toxin with formalin (formaldehyde) to produce the toxoid. This toxoid is then adsorbed onto an aluminum salt, and finally a preservative is added to prevent bacterial contaminant overgrowth. Thus, the vaccine contains toxoid, formaldehyde, aluminum, and mercury or another preservative—all with recognized toxicity—that are injected directly into the bloodstream. This chapter summarizes the potential toxic effects of three chemicals commonly injected with vaccine preparations. Other substances added to vaccines include phenol (disinfectant), ethylene glycol (antifreeze), phenoxyethanol (antifreeze), benzethonium chloride (antiseptic), and methylparaben (antifungal, preservative).

Aluminum

Aluminum is added to vaccines as an adjuvant to promote antibody response. The tetanus and diphtheria toxoids and the pertussis bacteria (DTP) are adsorbed onto aluminum salts (aluminum hydroxide, aluminum potassium sulfate, or aluminum phosphate). Adjuvants act by assisting in delivery of antigen to the spleen or lymph nodes, or by activating cells involved in the immune response.

Aluminum adjuvants themselves cause adverse reactions. Concern has arisen that the aluminum content of the DTP vaccine might play a role in the production of hypersensitivity reactions, autoimmune disease, encephalopathy, seizures, and neurologic damage by the vaccine.

One study showed the potentiating effect of aluminum on allergic reactions to pertussis vaccine. In that study, infants initially received either a series of aluminum-adsorbed acellular pertussis vaccine or a series of plain (non-adsorbed) whole-cell pertussis vaccine. When they were two years old, these children received a booster dose of aluminum-adsorbed acellular pertussis vaccine, and their responses were analyzed. The group that had previously received the aluminum-adsorbed vaccine had more severe systemic reactions (fever and fretfulness) and more severe local reactions (swelling and/or redness) in response to the aluminum-containing booster dose compared to children who had previously had the plain vaccine (Blennow & Granström, 1989). The children in the first group (previous aluminum doses) showed production of IgE antibodies to the pertussis toxin, indicating an allergic response, after they received another booster dose containing aluminum. The group that had previously received the plain vaccine did not develop IgE antibodies after receiving a booster dose of either the aluminum-adsorbed vaccine or the plain vaccine (Hedenskog et al., 1989). This suggests that the aluminum precipitated the adverse reactions and the production of IgE antibodies against pertussis toxin.

Other studies have shown that aluminum-adsorbed vaccines cause significantly more adverse reactions than plain vaccines. In a Swedish trial of acellular pertussis vaccines, the systemic adverse reactions to aluminum-adsorbed vaccine were similar to those against placebo containing the aluminum adjuvant alone (Ad hoc group, 1988). Aluminum-containing tetanus and cholera vaccines produced a high incidence of local reactions such as redness, pain, swelling and abscesses at the injection site compared to plain vaccines (Saroso *et al.*, 1978; Collier *et al.*, 1979). This type of lesion in mice was caused by an interaction of aluminum and tetanus toxoid rather than by the aluminum alone (Goto & Akama, 1982). Some reactions to DTP may be due to this interaction between aluminum adjuvant and the bacterial-toxin vaccine components (Gupta & Relyveld, 1991). The toxicity of aluminum adjuvants has led researchers to seek other chemicals as replacements. Calcium phosphate is a normal constituent of the human body, and well-tolerated. Its use as an adjuvant has proved effective, as have the polymerized toxoids without adjuvants (Relyveld, 1980).

Researchers have discovered the ability of injected aluminum to persist in the tissues for weeks or years as subcutaneous nodules (Slater *et al.*, 1982). These tissue deposits from aluminum injections are likely to release the metal for many years (Crapper-McLachlan, 1991).

Aluminum has been implicated as a cause of brain damage and the accompanying symptoms of dementia, Alzheimer's disease, seizures, and comas. The association of aluminum with neurologic symptoms is especially significant, since the aluminum-adsorbed vaccines—diphtheria, tetanus, and pertussis—have all been proven to cause these symptoms as well. The connection of aluminum to encephalopathy— the diverse range of neurologic symptoms caused by inflammation and destruction of brain tissues—has appeared in several contexts.

Aluminum deposition in the brain has been seen in patients with Alzheimer's disease (a form of dementia characterized by memory impairment, disorientation to time and place, and paranoid behavior). Aluminum has been detected in senile plaques in the brain (Candy *et al.*, 1986), in tangles of neurons in brains of patients with Alzheimer's disease (Perl & Brody, 1980), and in sections of different brain regions (cortical and caudate nucleus samples) of persons with Alzheimer's disease (Corrigan *et al.*, 1989). Patients with Alzheimer's disease have significantly higher aluminum levels in their blood compared to people free of the disease (Naylor *et al.*, 1989). Debate still surrounds the question of whether aluminum causes Alzheimer's disease or whether aluminum accumulates in the brains of Alzheimer's patients during the progress of the disease (Eichhorn, 1978). A third proposed possible mechanism is that aluminum can under certain conditions trigger processes that are genetically determined (Eichhorn, 1979).

Exposure to environmental aluminum has been associated with an increased incidence of Alzheimer's disease and dementia. In geographic areas with a high concentration of aluminum in the drinking water, Alzheimer's disease occurs more frequently. This relationship surfaced in counties of the United Kingdom with high levels of aluminum in drinking water. Aluminum sulfate is used as a coagulant in water treatment, to help clear suspended matter. Most aluminum is removed during water clarification, but residual amounts remain. Researchers discovered a 50 percent increase in the risk of Alzheimer's disease in such counties (Martyn et al., 1989). Similar findings have been noted connecting dementia with aluminum content of drinking water in Norway (Vogt, 1986). Another study showed that the relative risk for developing Alzheimer's disease was four times greater for areas with high aluminum content in drinking water (Michel et al., 1990). A further study examined patients in an area of Newfoundland with a cluster of high rates of death from dementia, and discovered a high aluminum concentration in the drinking water (Frecker, 1991). Commentators on these studies have cautioned that other factors in addition to high aluminum consumption might contribute to Alzheimer's disease in these populations (Eichhorn, 1993).

The aluminum exposure from antiperspirants and antacids has also been associated with Alzheimer's disease. In a study that examined the relationship of lifetime exposure to aluminum in antiperspirants and antacids to the incidence of Alzheimer's disease, the risk ratio for Alzheimer's disease in patients who used antiperspirants was 1.6 to 3.2, depending on the frequency of use. For antacids the risk ratio was 3.1 to 11.7, depending on dose (Graves et al., 1990). In another study, patients scheduled for brain surgery were prescribed aluminum-containing antacids for 10 days prior to surgery, and their brain tissue specimens were measured for aluminum content. The patients who took a high-dose antacid had nearly twice the aluminum brain levels as controls (Dollinger et al., 1986).

The neurotoxic properties of aluminum have been confirmed

through several avenues of research. Tests done on primates have shown the ability of aluminum to stimulate convulsions. Aluminum applied directly to nerve tissue caused epileptic symptoms and persisted for years following the initial dose (Kopeloff *et al.*, 1942; Klatzo *et al.*, 1965). Aluminum injected directly into the brains of cats, dogs, or rabbits caused impaired memory and defective learning (Still, 1994). A single injected dose of aluminum causes first a disturbance of learning and memory, and then progressive deterioration of motor control, tremors, and seizures (Crapper-McLachlan *et al.*, 1991).

Aluminum is excreted by the kidneys when the rate of kidney blood filtration is normal (Recker *et al.*, 1977). People whose kidneys no longer function normally must undergo dialysis, in which their blood is filtered by a machine. When patients are exposed to aluminum in dialysis fluids, or when dialysis-dependent patients are treated with aluminum-containing medications to control serum-phosphorus levels, they develop a syndrome labeled dialysis dementia, or dialysis encephalopathy (Mahurkar *et al.*, 1973). Biopsies of brain tissue in fatal cases of dialysis dementia reveal high aluminum deposits in the brain (Alfrey *et al.*, 1976). The symptoms include incoordination of the muscles used in speaking, impaired short-term memory, tremors, spasms, and jerking of muscles, seizures, disorientation, and confusion (Alfrey *et al.*, 1972; Barrett *et al.*, 1975).

The findings regarding aluminum toxicity in dialysis and other types of dementia cases, and in Alzheimer's disease, point to the connection between aluminum and brain damage. The association between aluminum in drugs, in water supplies, and in antiperspirants with Alzheimer's disease suggests toxic exposure as a trigger for brain damage. The similarity between symptoms of dementia and seizure disorders noted in the aluminum toxicity studies and symptoms of reactions to aluminum-adsorbed vaccines suggests that it could be the aluminum in vaccines that triggers these adverse events. Aluminum adjuvants could play a significant role in these reactions. It is possible that the direct assault of aluminum, combined with neurotoxic bacterial products in vaccines, could not only be responsible for the immediate neurologic catastrophes of vaccine reactions but, over a lifetime of repeated injections, could also contribute to a cumulative deposition of aluminum in brain tissue that results in senile dementia and Alzheimer's disease.

Thimerosal (Mercury)

Thimerosal (a mercury sodium salt) is used as a disinfectant. All toxoids, including tetanus and DTP, as well as hepatitis B and Hib vaccines, have contained thimerosal added to prevent bacterial overgrowth. In 1998 the FDA banned the use of mercury in all drugs because of its recognized neurotoxicity and lack of safety. A dramatic and immediate problem with mercury became apparent when calculations determined that an infant who receives all recommended vaccines during the first six months of life would accumulate 187 micrograms of mercury, a cumulative level of exposure higher than that recommended by the Environmental Protection Agency (Committee on Infectious Disease, 1999). In 1999 the US Public Health Service and the American Academy of Pediatrics supported the FDA directive to remove mercury from all vaccines. In May of 2001 Congressman Burton noted that many vaccines still contained mercury, and he demanded that mercury be removed from all vaccines (Burton, 2001). In the wake of these public concerns over mercury toxicity, lawsuits against vaccine manufacturers have been filed by a consortium of ten law firms alleging neurologic damage in children (Waters & Krause, 2001).

Many people have developed allergic sensitivities to thimerosal because of repeated exposure through vaccines. One study of unselected subjects found nearly 9 percent to be allergic to thimerosal on allergen patch testing (Schäfer et al., 1995). A study of patients with eczema showed that 16 percent were allergic to thimerosal (Aberer, 1991). Other studies have shown that up to 37 percent of an allergic population undergoing desensitization treatment with thimerosal-containing allergy shots develop hypersensitivity to the thimerosal (Tosti, 1989). Individuals who are allergic to thimerosal can experience severe reactions to vaccines. Many cases have been reported in the medical literature involving apparent allergic reactions to the thimerosal contained in vaccines (Pierchalla et al., 1987; Tosti et al., 1986). It is probable that some unknown proportion of allergic vaccine reactions are due to thimerosal sensitivity.

- A 29-year-old man with hand eczema was patch-tested for allergens. He was found to be strongly reactive to thimerosal. After receiving a hepatitis B vaccine he developed itching at the injection site, and two days later experienced an eruption of eczema that spread from his arm across his shoulder and back. This eruption persisted for a month and then slowly subsided over the next year.

- A 38-year-old woman developed a widespread itching eruption, beginning at the injection site of a hepatitis B vaccine. Eczema and hives began spreading over her trunk, arms, and legs. Several weeks after the eruption subsided, patch testing revealed a strong reaction to thimerosal (Rietschel & Adams, 1990).

These sensitivities to thimerosal apparently develop as a result of previous vaccinations (Förström et al., 1980). Even the minute amount of thimerosal used in vaccines (.1 to .01 percent) can specifically stimulate the immune system and cause sensitization (Aberer, 1991).

Mercury is a violent poison with many toxic effects. The toxicity of mercury varies depending on the form in which the element appears. Metallic mercury has different effects than inorganic or organic mercury compounds. However, major differences in toxicity are not expected among the different compounds within the inorganic group of mercury salts (Clement, 1992).

The group of inorganic mercury compounds includes thimerosal (an ethyl mercury sodium salt). These compounds are associated with a wide range of health problems, documented in humans and animal studies. The ingestion of inorganic mercury can be fatal to humans and experimental animals (Troen et al., 1951). Lethal doses occur with large amounts of mercury salts (29–50 mg mercury/kg).

The kidney is one of the major target organs of mercury-induced toxicity, apparently involving the immune system. Several investigators have produced autoimmune kidney damage by administering mercuric salts to rats (Druet et al., 1978; Hirszel et al., 1985). Mercury has caused the production of anti-tissue antibodies with a specific anti-kidney activity (Hirsch et al., 1986). Mercuric salts have also caused immune system suppression in mice (Dieter *et al.*, 1983). These effects may have significance for vaccine reactions, since many of the reported adverse effects of vaccines involve autoimmune mechanisms, and immune suppression is a significant concern in relation to vaccines.

The central and peripheral nervous systems are also major target organs for mercury-induced toxicity. Specific neurotoxic symptoms associated with mercury intoxication include tremors, dementia, and memory loss (Chaffin *et al.*, 1973; Davis *et al.*, 1974). These are the same type of neurologic symptoms observed in children following vaccination with the thimerosal-containing vaccines—DTP, pertussis, hepatitis B, and *Haemophilus influenzae*. It is also interesting that the neurologic toxicity symptoms caused by mercury compounds have a delayed onset after exposure (Bakir *et al.*, 1973), which may have significance for the suspected long-term neurologic symptoms of autism, learning disabilities, and behavior disorders associated with vaccines (see page 48). For a complete list of mercury toxicity symptoms, see: *www.autism-mercury/safeminds.htm*.

Formaldehyde

Formaldehyde (formalin) is used to inactivate viruses and detoxify bacterial toxins. It is added to most vaccines and eventually injected into the body. Formaldehyde has carcinogenic potential in humans. Exposure typically occurs through its use in the garment and fabric industries, and contact with wall- and ceiling-insulation materials.

At least 28 studies have found evidence of cancer in people exposed to formaldehyde. One study found an increased incidence of lung, nose, and throat cancer in industrial workers exposed to formaldehyde compared to a control group (Blair *et al.*, 1986). Another study found increased rates of nose and throat cancer in people who had lived ten or more years in a mobile home, especially those mobile homes built in the 1950s to 1970s, when formaldehyde-resins were frequently used in their manufacture (Vaughan *et al.*, 1986). In several studies, risks of nose, sinus, lung, mouth, and throat cancer were found to increase in people exposed to formaldehyde (Acheson *et al.*,

1984; Olsen *et al.*, 1984; Liebling *et al.*, 1984; Blair *et al.*, 1990). The upper respiratory tract is particularly susceptible to the toxic effects of inhaled formaldehyde. Nasal cancers have repeatedly been demonstrated in workers exposed to wood dust (Hayes *et al.*, 1986) and in rats experimentally exposed to formaldehyde (Albert *et al.*, 1982; Kerns *et al.*, 1983). Changes in the structure of nasal cells have even been observed in beginning students of mortuary science exposed to relatively low levels of formaldehyde. Those students were found to have dramatic increases and abnormalities of nasal epithelial cells after performing an average of only seven embalmings (Suruda *et al.*, 1993). Epithelial cell cancers represent the most common carcinogenic effect of formaldehyde (Swenberg *et al.*, 1980; Hayes *et al.*, 1986).

At least 19 studies have revealed an association between leukemia and cancer of the brain and colon with formaldehyde exposure. A significant risk for cancers of the brain and lymphatic tissues has been found in most studies of formaldehyde-exposed professionals (Nelson *et al.*, 1986). In a study of workers in permanent-press garment facilities exposed for at least three months to formaldehyde, leukemia as well as cancer of the mouth were discovered. The incidence of deaths from these cancers increased with the duration of formaldehyde exposure, indicating a dose-related association (Stayner *et al.*, 1988). A study of workers exposed to formaldehyde in a large chemical plant in Massachusetts revealed a significantly elevated incidence of death from colon cancer compared to comparable populations in that county (Liebling *et al.*, 1984).

Formaldehyde exposure following injection, ingestion, or inhalation has also caused liver toxicity and liver damage, as shown in several studies (Beall & Ulsamer, 1984; Stayner *et al.*, 1985).

Animal studies have confirmed the ability of formaldehyde to cause squamous-cell carcinomas (Swenberg *et al.*, 1980; Albert *et al.*, 1982; Kerns *et al.*, 1983). When bacteria, viruses, and mammalian cells have been exposed to formaldehyde, results included gene mutations, chromosomal aberrations, DNA-strand breaks, and inhibition of DNA repair.

CONVENTIONAL VACCINE STUDIES

Before considering each vaccine individually, some general points about vaccine effectiveness should be raised. Critics have charged that adequate studies of vaccine efficacy have not been conducted. The late Dr. Robert Mendelsohn, noted pediatrician, repeatedly questioned the use of any vaccine that has not been tested in a placebo-controlled or longitudinal study of vaccinated vs. unvaccinated groups. Very few studies of this kind have been conducted.

Public health authorities cite the decline in disease occurrence as proof that a vaccine works. In fact, most of the diseases in question have either steadily declined since the advent of general sanitation measures during the twentieth century, or gone through waxing and waning occurrence during epidemic cycles. Critics point out that a coincidental reduction in the number of cases following vaccine introduction in a community does not necessarily prove a relationship to the vaccine.

One set of statistics frequently used to document vaccine efficacy is the increase in pertussis (whooping cough) incidence when vaccine administration is stopped or decreased. This has occurred in Britain, Japan, and Sweden (Cherry *et al.*, 1988). Many critics, however, charge that during times when the number of vaccine recipients decreases, physician sensitivity to the disease increases, and every lingering cough is then reported as pertussis, thereby inflating the actual number of cases (Coulter & Fisher, 1991). During whooping cough outbreaks, any cough that continues for more than 14 days can be labeled "pertussis" without a confirmatory culture (Centers for Disease Control, 1990).

This is because the diagnosis of whooping cough itself presents problems and uncertainties. According to Moskowitz, the statistics of whooping cough incidence should be questioned, especially during supposed outbreaks when the population does not receive the vaccine.

> We should be skeptical about the "outbreaks" that are reported to have occurred. Pertussis, or "whooping cough," is actually rather difficult to diagnose conclusively, as it requires special cultures or antibody tests that many laboratories cannot perform and that many doctors, in the presence of suggestive symptoms, rarely take the trouble to order. Conversely, there are other cases of pertussis with typical signs and symptoms but no detectable antibodies. In other words, whooping cough as a clinical *syndrome* need not be associated with the organism *Bordetella pertussis,* against which the vaccine is prepared, or indeed with any microorganism whatsoever (Moskowitz, 1987).

This possibility of heightened awareness and bias also applies to the polio statistics during the 1950s epidemic. When the vaccine was introduced, dramatic reporting differences occurred, and cases previously reported as polio were now given another diagnosis, such as encephalitis, which appeared to make the vaccine seem more effective (see Polio chapter).

Underreporting of disease incidence creates unreliable statistics. When the widespread use of a vaccine has lulled the medical profession into indifference about a particular disease, a large percentage of actual cases goes unreported. The Centers for Disease Control estimates that only 5–10 percent of pertussis cases are reported each year (Hinman & Koplan, 1984). These errors in reporting create unwarranted faith in a vaccine's effectiveness at preventing disease.

Vaccine proponents assure us that vaccines are safe because adverse effects are rare. This statement arises from the many studies that have investigated vaccine reactions. But the validity of these studies is severely hampered by two limitations. First, most of them have examined the occurrence of symptoms immediately following the vaccine's administration. Often this period has been limited to two days. Some studies have extended this period to a week or two. Any delayed reaction will not be observed in such a study. In fact, delayed reactions and long-term effects are difficult to document. For example, no studies have compared developmental or cognitive functions in vaccinated and unvaccinated children.

The second important limitation of these studies involves the control group. In all of the studies, the adverse effects in a group of children who receive a specific vaccine are compared to these symptoms in a control group, the supposedly "normal" population of children who will provide statistics on the "background" incidence of the adverse effect under consideration. The problem is that the control group is also vaccinated. If the adverse event under consideration is epilepsy or developmental delays, then the control group must be unvaccinated, because any of the vaccines may be capable of inducing these problems. One cannot compare vaccinated children with a population of other vaccinated children and hope to arrive at a valid determination of the risks associated with the vaccine.

Coulter has devised a list of criteria to evaluate studies that attempt to prove that vaccines are safe. In examining the incidence of adverse reactions, the authors of such studies can easily distort statistics through a variety of means. The task of evaluating an epidemiological study may be a daunting exercise in the analysis of research methods, but Coulter warns us against naively accepting the results of such studies.

> Because our medical literature is published in glossy journals, copiously illustrated, and with imposing rows of statistical tables, it may be difficult for the reader to realize that many of the articles are worthless. This is true preeminently of those about vaccination.
>
> For reasons profoundly rooted in the physician's psychology, and not unconnected with his source of income, the childhood vaccination program in the United States has taken on a sacerdotal aura, such that attacks on it are seen as blasphemous. And any statement in their defense, no matter how wildly inaccurate, is accepted at face value. Readers confronted with epidemiologic

surveys purporting to show that childhood vaccines are safe and effective should be intensely suspicious of the author's arguments (Coulter, 1995).

The list below provides examples of Coulter's criteria for examining the methodology of these studies. It is clear from these points that vaccine studies can be skewed through a variety of means.

- How was the sample put together? Is it truly representative of the population being studied, or were the children pre-screened so as to leave out those most likely to suffer vaccine damage? Were any dropped from the study while it was being conducted?

- If children are dropped from the study for having reacted violently, are they included as "vaccine-damaged" in the summary and statistics, or are they just ignored?

- How much "shoe-leather epidemiology" went into the study? Did the authors actually visit the children (rarely, perhaps never), or have they just shuffled Health Department or Blue Cross reports?

- Is the reporting system passive (you wait for the parents to complain) or active (you go out and perform a household survey)? The latter is viewed as a far more effective technique for disclosing vaccine reactions but, being more expensive, is less commonly used.

- How is a vaccine reaction defined? Is it highly restrictive (always) or generous and comprehensive (never)?

Coulter's conclusions are telling:

> My own experience with official American epidemiologic studies leads me to the conclusion that they are filled with half-truths, distortions, and outright lies, partly because of incompetence and partly because of the necessity to reach conclusions palatable to the funding agency. I once called this to the attention of a Public Health Service officer, and he replied, "That's true, but it doesn't make any difference; we already know these vaccines are entirely safe" (Coulter, 1995).

Difficulties Tracking Vaccine Efficacy and Safety

- Decline in disease occurrence prior to vaccine introduction.

- Contradictory findings of vaccine efficacy studies.

- Bias in reporting diseases when vaccines are begun or stopped in a community.

- Deficiencies of studies evaluating vaccine adverse effects: observation period too short, inappropriate control groups, skewed statistics, etc.

ALTERNATIVE MEDICINE: ACHIEVING HEALTH

The Role of Natural Medicine

The growing interest in natural medicine has been accompanied by a shift toward increased self-reliance, an awareness of the principles of self-healing, and the rejection of mechanistic approaches to medicine. Many people have chosen to pursue more life-affirming methods of health care that align with their personal beliefs about wellness, healing, and prevention. They view the methods of allopathic medicine, the pharmaceutical drugs and surgeries, as things to be avoided. They find the concept of drugs used to prevent illness repugnant. If exercise and a healthy diet will prevent bone loss, why take hormones that can cause cancer? Why not rely upon natural methods to treat and prevent illness, when this is possible?

The return to low-tech approaches in health care has gone hand-in-hand with the concepts of recycling, using wind and solar-energy sources, and generally returning to a harmonious coexistence with nature. This is the philosophy that seeks to replace such obsolete notions as nuclear defense, clear-cut logging practices, and heedless toxic-waste pollution with more sensitive and sensible techniques. Similarly, the practices of water fluoridation, routine screening x-rays, and vaccination no longer seem appropriate.

The use of natural medicine implies an inclusive view of health and illness. The principles of homeopathy, Oriental medicine, and naturopathy place disease within a broad perspective. Symptoms and disease processes represent the body's signals that something has become unbalanced and needs to be set in order again. An infection indicates that the body's defenses need reinforcement. Recurrent headaches show that body systems need readjustment to return them to a healthy functioning mode. This may include adjustments of energetic body patterns through diet, acupuncture, physical-body adjustment, or the prescription of a remedy in the form of herbal or homeopathic medicine. The expected result is a stronger, more resilient body, less susceptible to the effects of stress or infections. Such an approach includes emotional as well as physical health.

In relation to infections, the natural healing systems of homeopathy, Oriental medicine, and naturopathy all offer regimens for both preventing and treating diseases. Reliance on one or more of these systems should be the cornerstone of a natural approach to infection. These are the systems accessible to most Americans. Other, more exotic native-healing systems are probably just as effective, but generally inaccessible in our modern culture. Many other natural forms of therapy can assist the body in maintaining health. These include nutritional approaches, Western herbs, Ayurvedic practices, yoga, osteopathic manipulation, chiropractic, and a wide range of energetic and physical forms of massage.

Homeopathy and Oriental medicine each have a long history of successful treatment of infectious disease. Long before the advent of antibiotics, both of these systems successfully managed epidemics and individual cases of complicated infections. The success of both homeopathy and Chinese medicine exists in sharp contrast to the helplessness of allopathic medicine when confronted with viral illnesses, and the ineffectiveness of antibiotics in commonly encountered childhood bacterial conditions such as whooping cough and ear infections.

Practitioners of homeopathic medicine assert that homeopathic treatment itself also affords some protection from disease. Homeopaths suggest that children who receive ongoing homeopathic medical care are less likely to contract serious diseases and will have fewer complications when childhood diseases do occur. Homeopathy claims to support the immune system's functioning, and the plentiful examples of cured cases of allergy and recurrent infection in children in the homeopathic literature support this contention. Since homeopathic medicines appear to work by stimulating the body's defense mechanisms, proponents claim that serious diseases and complications of more common diseases are less likely to occur after homeopathic treatment.

Homeopathy is a system of natural medicine that has become highly developed and accepted in Europe and South America. In the United States, homeopathic medical care is less generally available, though it was quite prevalent and popular during the nineteenth century. Practitioners of homeopathic medicine have effectively treated the common childhood diseases for nearly two centuries. Homeopaths treated measles, mumps, and whooping cough during the 1800s, long before vaccines or antibiotics were available. Clinical studies have not been conducted to document the success of homeopathic treatment in most diseases or in the prevention of disease complications. Nonetheless, practitioners of homeopathy claim success, and express confidence in their treatments based on their 200 years of clinical experience.

Conventional medicine has little to offer when viral diseases occur, and non-homeopathic physicians are anxious to prevent what they cannot treat. The urge to vaccinate children is much stronger when adequate treatment is not readily available. Homeopathic medical providers, however, express confidence in their ability to treat viral diseases and prevent complications of most childhood illnesses. They tend to have less anxiety than conventional physicians about disease complications. If the diseases are less threatening under their care, then the impetus to vaccinate children is less compelling, especially when the potential for serious adverse effects exists in the vaccines. When parents in England who chose not to vaccinate their children were asked why they made that decision, more than 20 percent said they would rather place their confidence in homeopathic treatment of these diseases (Simpson *et al.*, 1995).

Historically, homeopathic treatment has proved effective in a wide range of acute illnesses. During the nineteenth century, homeopathy gained general acceptance because of its ability to cure infectious diseases. During the yellow-fever epidemic of the late nineteenth century in the United States, homeopathy was exceptionally effective compared to the conventional treatment of the time. A report of the Homeopathic Yellow Fever Commission showed that in New Orleans homeopathic treatment resulted in a mortality of 5.6 percent of cases and 7.7 percent of cases in the rest of the South. This compared to an overall death rate of at least 16 percent (American Institute of Homeopathy, 1880). A comparison of mortality rates between homeopathic and conventional medical treatment in the United States and Europe in 1900 showed a two- to eightfold reduction in deaths from life-threatening infectious diseases among the homeopathically treated cases (Bradford, 1900). During the severe influenza epidemic of 1918, homeopathic treatment also resulted in a significant reduction in mortality. These results led to a wide acceptance of homeopathic treatment among the public. Although these studies were conducted in the nineteenth century, prior to the era of double-blind, controlled clinical trials, they serve as a landmark for the recognition of homeopathy as a medical science.

Clinical studies are once again showing the effectiveness of homeopathy—now in carefully controlled trials. Recent publications in major allopathic medical journals have shown the clinical effectiveness of homeopathy in hayfever (Taylor Reilly *et al.*, 1986), asthma (Reilly *et al.*, 1994), acute childhood diarrhea (Jacobs *et al.*, 1994), and ear infections (Jacobs *et al.*, 2001; Frei and Thurneysen, 2001). A review of a large number of homeopathic studies published in the *British Medical Journal* concluded that, based on current research, homeopathy could be established as "a regular treatment for certain indications" (Kleijnen *et al.* 1991).

Homeopathy is a medical system that uses natural (plant, mineral, and animal) substances that stimulate a healing reaction within the body and encourage a curative response to illness. This theoretical framework of cure is in distinction to that of allopathic or conventional medications, which suppress the body's reactions or kill bacteria. Conventional medicines are prescribed with little regard for their detrimental effects on the body. The benefit of the drug is considered worth the risk of side effects. Homeopathic practitioners claim that their medications have no side effects because they are so dilute.

They are assumed to work because of their ability to trigger a reaction within the body; the medicine acts as a catalyst. The healing reaction manifests as a gentle and efficient cure. This has been the claim of homeopathy since its inception. Curative response, according to homeopaths, is not limited to the type of organism responsible for disease. It is assumed to work as well for viral as for bacterial infection. A single dose or a few doses of a homeopathic medicine are usually prescribed to trigger the desired response within the body. The minimal dose possible is employed to effect a cure.

Homeopathic medicine has several practical points that distinguish it from the methods of conventional medicine. A homeopathic medicine is chosen to treat a case of illness when it corresponds to the symptom pattern of the illness in the individual patient. Several different cases of ear infection or measles may require different homeopathic medicines. This is an important practical point: medicines are prescribed for the individual and not for the disease. The symptoms of the individual, in their details and qualities, are compared to the complex of symptoms characteristic of a medicine. When the right match is made and the correct medicine is taken, the curative response begins. In a serious illness, the medicine may need to be changed as symptoms change. The services of a skilled homeopath are required in order to make these decisions.

Homeopathic theory assumes that any drug treatment will either enhance or suppress immune system function. According to homeopaths, a drug will either have a strengthening or weakening effect on the body. Since homeopathic medicines are intended to stimulate the immune system, homeopaths claim that acute illnesses resolve quickly when the body's fight against the disease is strengthened by the correct medicine. The result is a stronger immune system, and resolution of the acute illness without resultant complications. In chronic conditions the body is purportedly encouraged by the appropriate homeopathic medicine to develop a higher level of resistance and less susceptibility to illness.

Homeopaths are generally concerned that antibiotics and vaccinations will suppress the body's fight against disease. Dr. Richard

Moskowitz has proposed that vaccinations may work through a continuous suppressive process. That is, the vaccine stored within the body's cells continually suppresses the ability to respond to a viral or bacterial attack (Moskowitz, 1983).

Several cautions about homeopathic medicines are usually offered by professional practitioners. Although homeopathic medicines are available without prescription, it is advisable to seek medical care from a qualified homeopath whenever a potentially serious acute illness occurs. Various combination homeopathic medicines are also available, labeled with indications for symptoms such as coughs, colds, teething, etc. These are not recommended, since the correct homeopathic medicine for the individual must be chosen carefully. It is unlikely that a medicine that is not appropriately prescribed for the individual case of illness will act curatively.

It is possible for parents to learn to prescribe for simple acute illnesses in their child. Several books are available to help guide parents in the proper use of homeopathic treatment at home. One such book, *Everybody's Guide to Homeopathic Medicines,* provides indications for the correct use of homeopathy in simple illnesses (Cummings & Ullman, 1997). It provides guidelines for safe treatment, and the appropriate times to seek professional medical care. Serious illness always requires consultation with a trained medical practitioner.

There are times when antibiotics or other medications are needed for infectious diseases, and a homeopathic or conventional medical provider can help make these treatment decisions. Tetanus is an example of a disease that requires vigorous, active treatment. It is mandatory that anyone who acquires tetanus receive conventional allopathic care and hospitalization. Similarly, any child who contracts one of the potentially serious diseases of childhood should be evaluated by a qualified medical care provider. He or she will observe your child for complications and the need for intervention.

Oriental medicine refers to those techniques that arose in Asia (China, Tibet, and India). Chinese medicine utilizes a complex theoretical system of understanding energetic influences on the body as its framework for treating acute diseases. The treatment of acute illness usually involves acupuncture and herbs. The purpose of this approach includes the encouragement of natural resistance, the dispelling of pathogenic influences within the body, and the harmonizing of bodily function. This system originated in China over 3,000 years ago.

The use of Traditional Chinese Medicine (TCM) continues in Chinese clinics and hospitals today in conjunction with allopathic techniques. In the United States, colleges of acupuncture and TCM have trained thousands of licensed practitioners to treat children's acute infectious diseases. Studies from around the world have proven the effectiveness of Chinese medical practice, and this record has led to its recognition by the World Health Organization, and to the licensure of practitioners throughout the world. Parents who choose not to vaccinate their children may also choose to utilize Chinese medicine as a means of strengthening resistance to infection and treating acute illness to prevent serious complications.

A problem with TCM techniques involves the acceptability of acupuncture and strong-tasting herbs to children. Although acupuncture techniques have been developed specifically for children (Scott, 1986), and acupuncture has proven effective in treating children's illnesses, homeopathy remains a more palatable form of treatment for the pediatric population.

Naturopathic physicians (N.D.s) have been trained at four-year medical colleges, and have studied both homeopathy and Chinese medicine along with nutrition and Western herbology. They are well qualified to diagnose and treat childhood infections. An individual naturopathic physician often specializes in one area of treatment and utilizes other modalities as the need arises.

- To find a qualified homeopathic practitioner see: *www.homeopathicdirectory.com*

- To find a practitioner of Oriental medicine and acupuncture see: *www.aaom.org* or in California *www.csomaonline.org*.

- To find a naturopathic physician see: *www.naturopathic.org*.

Treatment of Vaccine Reactions

The varied serious reactions to vaccines have no appropriate treatment within allopathic medicine, but homeopaths have treated these successfully for over 100 years. Smallpox vaccine reactions were especially dangerous, and homeopathic medicine developed a reputation for its ability to successfully treat the sometimes lethal effects of the vaccine. A single homeopathic medicine, *Thuja occidentalis,* proved to be efficacious in relieving the symptoms that arose subsequent to adverse smallpox vaccine reactions (vaccinia). During the nineteenth and early twentieth centuries the use of *Thuja* in the treatment of vaccinia as well as wide-ranging symptoms following administration of the vaccine became a commonplace practice (Burnett, 1892). Modern authors have found that the homeopathic preparations of the vaccine or the disease organism itself succeed more often in relieving the symptoms associated with today's vaccine reactions.

The most common clinical finding subsequent to childhood vaccination is weakened immune function with a resulting lowered resistance to infection and increased susceptibility to allergy. These chronic vaccine reactions usually manifest as repeated ear infections in infants and young children, or chronic respiratory congestion and frequent colds. Homeopathic treatment has proven especially effective in treating these conditions. Combining a homeopathic approach with the nutritional guidelines recommended on page 112 should result in a stronger immune system and less frequent infections. The approach of classical homeopathy would usually entail the prescription of a constitutional medicine that corresponds to the total symptom complex of the individual patient. However, some clinicians have also employed homeopathic preparations of the culprit vaccine itself to promote a curative response.

Several case-review articles have been published which describe the successful homeopathic treatment of children whose symptoms began after the receipt of a routine childhood vaccine (Moskowitz, 1983; Moskowitz, 1991; Smits, 1995). Smits recommends using the potentized vaccine in four different strengths (potencies) over four successive days: 30th on day one, 200 on day two, 1M on day three, and 10M on day four (Smits, 1995). Unusually severe vaccine reactions may require a 30th potency, repeated hourly, for one to two days. Other authors have reported success with a single high potency (200, 1M, or 10M) of the vaccine. The dramatic recoveries reported following the administration of the potentized vaccine have led to a high level of confidence in the ability of homeopathy to treat these types of vaccine reactions.

Homeopathy has proven less successful in the treatment of neurologic damage caused by vaccines. Other therapeutic approaches may provide more beneficial effects in cases of autism, brain damage, and epilepsy.

A preventive approach to vaccine reactions has been proposed by several homeopathic authors as well. Smits, for example, recommends that the 200th potency of the vaccine be administered two days before the vaccination and repeated again after the actual vaccine. He further recommends giving the 30, 200, 1M, 10M series on four successive days, one month after a vaccine series has been completed (Smits, 1995). These programs that purport to prevent vaccine reactions have never undergone any type of study to determine their effectiveness. Such a study would require large financial resources, and it is unlikely that any of these programs will be investigated. Parents who proceed with these programs should do so with the knowledge that these regimens are based on clinical experience and have not yet been documented according to the protocols of modern science.

The autoimmune and neurologic reactions to vaccines may require a more comprehensive treatment program to establish significant improvement in symptoms. These clinical conditions include autism, encephalopathies, seizure disorders, attention deficits, and behavior disorders. Treatments include a multifaceted approach that reflects the multiple body system disorders inflicted by vaccines. Adverse vaccine reactions involve the immune system, nervous system, and digestive system. Each requires treatment and support.

Dietary treatment involves a completely gluten- and casein-free diet, accompanied by a supplement program that supports intestinal function and immune system strength. Probiotic supplements are a mainstay of this supplement program (lactobacillus acidophilus and bifidobacteria infantis). Immune system stimulants may include lactoferrin, lactoperoxidase, and concentrated globulin protein. A supplement program may also include dimethylglycine (DMG), an amino acid, as well as vitamin B6 and magnesium. These supplements each have a long history of use and research in autism. For information about these therapeutic interventions see the Autism Research Institute website at *www.autism.com/ari*.

Treatments that require medical supervision are more controversial. They include treatment with the prescription drug Secretin, and intravenous immunoglobulin (IVGG or IGIV). Patients investigating specific immune system treatments will need to obtain laboratory testing to document immune deficiencies and/or elevated antibodies to specific vaccine components. Researcher Teresa Binstock has outlined a list of these types of tests, which can be obtained at *www.jorsm.com/~binstock/tests.htm*. Great Plains Laboratory recommends and performs a range of specific tests for autism patients *(www.greatplainslaboratory.com)*. IVGG therapy is a long and expensive therapeutic process designed for patients with immunodeficiencies. The mechanism of action in IVGG therapy is not known, but treatment is thought to suppress production of antibodies and provide anti-inflammatory effects. Specialists in IVGG treatment can be contacted at the University of California, Irvine, Department of Medicine-Division of Basic and Clinical Immunology, Division Chief, Dr. Sudhir Gupta, at 877 UCI-DOCS or see:

www.ucihealth.com/healthcareservices/medimmu.htm.

For a complete discussion of these treatment methods consult the following resources:

www.healing-arts.org

Seroussi, Karyn. *Unraveling the Mystery of Autism and Pervasive Developmental Disorder*. New York: Broadway Books, 2002.

Shaw, William. *Biological Treatments for Autism and PDD*. Great Plains Laboratory Inc., 2002.

ALTERNATIVE VACCINE METHODS

Conventional vaccines prepared by modern vaccine manufacturers represent only one form of disease-specific prevention. Vaccines and preventive medicines are also available to parents in homeopathic form.

There is a long history within homeopathic medicine of attempting to prevent specific diseases, especially during epidemics. This attempt originated with Samuel Hahnemann, the founder of homeopathic medicine. He used homeopathic dilutions of *Belladonna* to prevent scarlet fever during an especially virulent and deadly epidemic. In 1801 he published a short booklet about the management of scarlet fever, the first presentation of this preventive method to the medical world.

> Three children in a family had succumbed to a very bad attack of scarlet fever; the eldest daughter, who had up to that time been taking Belladonna internally for some other external disease of the finger joints, was the only one who to my surprise refused to sicken with the fever, in spite of the fact that she was always the first to catch any other disease that chanced to be prevalent. After that I did not hesitate to give this providential remedy in very small doses to the remaining children of this numerous family as a preventive . . . and they all remained well and were not attacked in the slightest degree throughout the whole epidemic although among the most poisonous odors from their brothers and sisters, who were still suffering from the fever. . . . I concluded that a remedy which can speedily cure the beginning of an illness must be its best preventive (Hahnemann, 1801).

Since the time of Hahnemann, homeopaths throughout the world have utilized specific remedies for the prevention of disease during an epidemic. These efforts preceded the widespread use of vaccines in the West. Edward Jenner, a contemporary of Hahnemann, had just published his treatise on the smallpox vaccine in 1798. By 1806 the vaccination concept had spread throughout Europe, but enthusiasm subsided as difficulties with production and inoculation made mass vaccine campaigns problematic and dangerous. Not until Louis Pasteur developed more efficient methods of vaccine culture in the late nineteenth century did the concept of vaccination become a significant public issue. Controversy surrounded the early use of vaccines, and protests against vaccination thwarted efforts to conduct large clinical trials.

In the meantime, homeopathic practitioners had success in preventing the spread of epidemics through the use of their medicines. During the nineteenth century, the practice of using a homeopathic medicine that corresponded to the symptoms of a disease epidemic became commonplace. The British homeopaths of the early twentieth century popularized this approach. Dorothy Shepherd and others published books for the lay person outlining the methods involved, and many homeopaths contributed to the literature of epidemic prevention (Shepherd, 1967).

The medicines used in homeopathic form consist of two classes. One class includes those substances obtained from the natural world of plants, minerals, and animal products. The second class, called nosodes, includes substances derived from disease products, tissue samples, mucous, pus from discharges, or pure cultures of microorganisms. Nosodes correspond to the specific diseases associated with the individual bacteria or virus, or the infectious material sample taken from a patient. Both of these classes have been used to prevent disease. Examples of this include *Lathyrus sativa* (a plant) for polio and *Pertussin* (a preparation of the bacteria *Bordetella pertussis*) for whooping cough.

A medicine that has proven effective for a specific epidemic of a disease in the community can be used as the preventive for other cases of that disease, though homeopaths tend to use those medicines that have proven themselves in the past. As a general rule, homeopaths utilize the nosode of the infectious organism to prevent disease. Nosodes are named with the Latin terms for the infection or organism, such as *Morbillinum* for measles, *Diphtherinum* for diphtheria.

This method of homeopathic prophylaxis has been formulated into strategies and rules of two types—short-term prevention during epidemics and long-term prevention.

Prevention During Epidemics

Experience with the use of nosodes during epidemics has led to a level of confidence and optimism about the protective effect of this method. Since the mid-nineteenth century, homeopaths have attempted to prevent or limit the spread of disease during epidemics, with some success. Most of the experience with this approach occurred during the era preceding the availability of vaccines. Homeopaths reported a decrease in the severity and frequency of disease in those patients who received the nosode preventively.

The evidence for effectiveness of this method is primarily anecdotal. A homeopath would experiment with a nosode during an epidemic, and then report that cases had been mild or infrequent. In this way, a level of confidence was established in the method. Clarke referred to the common use of *Morbillinum* and *Parotidinum* to prevent measles and mumps, in the Appendix to his three-volume *Materia Medica* (Clarke, 1925). He described giving the nosode in the 30th potency two to three times a day after exposure. Shepherd popularized the use of nosodes for epidemics that broke out in civilian populations during World War II in Britain.

The reduction or elimination of whooping cough vaccine administration in England and other European countries led to a greater interest in determining the effectiveness of the homeopathic nosode to prevent the disease. A study was conducted giving *Pertussin* 30c every three months during the first year of life, then an eighteen-month dose, and further doses on each birthday until the age of 6. Of the 1,100 children in the initial project, 851 questionnaires were returned, and 694 of these qualified for inclusion in the study. Sixty-seven of these children (9.65 percent) contracted whooping cough during the course of the study. The rate of whooping cough among unvaccinated children in the same community was 27 percent during this same time period. This result suggested a greater than 60 percent reduction in whooping cough incidence in the children who received *Pertussin* compared to the general population. The author concluded that this pilot study provided justification for conducting a more elaborate study (English, 1987a).

The method of homeopathic prophylaxis has never been rigorously tested. Nonetheless, there is some evidence suggesting that homeopathic medicines do act to prevent diseases during epidemics. One study observed the occurrence of meningitis in a group of children who received a homeopathic preventive (*Meningococcinum* 10c in a single dose) during a 1974 epidemic in Brazil. Of the 18,640 children given the homeopathic nosode, 4 developed meningitis (0.02 percent), compared to 32 cases in the 6,340 unvaccinated children (0.5 percent). This represents a significant difference in a controlled study, although the control group was not randomized (Castro & Nogueira, 1975).

Eisfelder reported an uncontrolled study of 50,000 children who received *Lathyrus*, a homeopathic preparation used to treat paralysis, in varying potencies during the polio epidemic of the 1950s. Only one of these children developed (non-paralytic) polio. The general population had a significantly higher rate of polio than 1 in 50,000 (Eisfelder, 1961).

A study of smallpox during an epidemic in Iowa in 1902 also suggests that a homeopathic preparation can prevent the disease. In this study conducted by 15 participating doctors, *Variolinum* 12X and 30X potencies (a homeopathic preparation of a smallpox pustule) was administered to 2,806 participants. Of these, 547 were exposed to smallpox disease, many of them prior to the dosage with *Variolinum*. Only those with definite exposure to smallpox patients were included in this figure; most were members of households or health care workers in direct contact with patients during the disease. Other participants in the study had probable but not verified exposure during this general epidemic. Only 14 people of the 2,806 given *Variolinum* contracted the disease, a truly remarkable number given the virulence and highly contagious nature of the smallpox virus. The author also states that his "experience shows that smallpox occurs after scarification with much greater frequency than it occurs after the use of *Variolinum*" (Eaton, 1907).

These few studies do not prove the effectiveness of homeopathic prophylaxis in epidemics, but many homeopathic practitioners have been convinced by their own experience with this form of disease prevention. The practice of using homeopathic preparations to prevent disease during epidemic exposure may be effective. The medicines cause no adverse effects, and, in the absence of any other form of prevention or a conventional vaccine with significant adverse reactions, they provide a reasonable and promising option.

The dosage of homeopathic preparations for the purpose of prevention during epidemics does not seem to be critical. Some practitioners have routinely prescribed a single dose of a 30X or 30C potency; others have devised more complicated schedules. Grimmer recommended a 30C potency of *Lathyrus* for polio prevention once a month for three months, then two monthly doses of the 200C followed by a 1M two months later (Grimmer, 1952). Shepherd recommended *Pertussin* in a 12C or 30C dose daily for two weeks after contact with a case of whooping cough, and *Pulsatilla* 6C or 30C daily from the third to the 15th day after contact with measles (Shepherd, 1967).

Long-term Prevention

Alternative vaccines in homeopathic form are available for long-term prevention. Several protocols exist for the administration of homeopathic nosodes or the corresponding remedies for the prevention of whooping cough, meningitis, diphtheria, tetanus, polio, and other diseases during childhood. There exists significant controversy within the homeopathic profession about the appropriateness of using these preparations for long-term prevention. This controversy involves the areas of effectiveness, safety, and ethics.

No long-term studies have been conducted to evaluate the efficacy of this form of prevention. There is no reason to assume that these vaccines continue to act preventively years after administration, unless immunity is shown through an objective test or clinical studies. The research that proponents of homeopathic prophylaxis frequently cite to prove an immunizing effect of these remedies involves studies done on diphtheria. An examination of this research is warranted because it represents the only studies used as evidence.

During the early part of the twentieth century, diphtheria research stimulated the investigation of a homeopathic preventive. Following the discovery of the first allopathic vaccine for diphtheria (Smith, 1909), a test was developed to detect immunity (Schick, 1913). The Schick test involves injection into the skin of a minute amount of diphtheria toxin. A positive result consists of redness and swelling around the site within 48 hours and indicates susceptibility to diphtheria. A negative test indicates immunity. It is also necessary to do a simultaneous control test to rule out false positive reactions that occur in response to other proteins in the test material.

The existence of this test for immunity provided homeopathic practitioners with a method to assess the effect of a homeopathic preparation used as a preventive and possibly as a safer substitute for the conventional vaccine. Chavanon published experiments in 1932 with 45 children using homeopathic preparations of the diphtheria toxin and observing its effect on the Schick test reaction. He discovered that *Diphtherotoxinum* 4M and 8M could reverse a positive Schick test result, supposedly conferring immunity (Chavanon, 1932).

In 1941 Paterson and Boyd conducted similar experiments using the Schick test at the Scottish Homœopathic Hospital for Children. Of 33 susceptible children (Schick-positive) who received either the homeopathic diphtheria toxoid 30c (ATP, Alum-Precipitated Toxoid) or the homeopathic nosode *Diphtherinum* 200, 20 children tested negative after the homeopathic preparations. This is a conversion rate of 60.6 percent of children from Schick-positive to -negative following the homeopathic treatment. Proper control tests were also performed on the opposite arm in this study, to rule out false positive reactions. No control group was included in this study, but when these results were compared to similar populations the shift in susceptibility from positive to negative far exceeded that of other groups tested. For example, a study of a similar population of schoolchildren found a conversion rate of 5 percent during the winter, and a conversion rate of 30 percent in a closed community of hospitalized children exposed to diphtheria (Dudley *et al.*, 1934).

These results led Paterson and Boyd to conclude that the homeopathic preparations caused a significant alteration in immunity, based on the conversion of the Schick-test response. They cautioned, however, "that nothing in this research is to be taken as indicating whether potencies of ATP or Diphtheric membrane may or may not have an action which increases the tissue resistance to Diphtheric infection. . . . Our experience of potency action on other lines would make us doubt that a long-lasting immunity could be obtained by any limited doses of a homeopathic potency in the absence of the continual external stimulus of contact with a community morbidity factor" (Paterson & Boyd, 1941). These researchers did not conclude that the homeopathic preparations conferred immunity from diphtheria, yet several authors within the homeopathic profession have cited the studies of Chavanon and Paterson as proof that these preparations do provide immunity. They have continually used these studies as the only documented justification for homeopathic prophylaxis programs.

The question remains whether a conversion of the Schick test from positive to negative in itself indicates immunity or anything at all. The Schick test was used for many years as the primary determination of diphtheria immune status. It has been largely replaced by laboratory measures of circulating antitoxin in the blood because the Schick test proved to be a less accurate measure of immunity (Durbaca and Stoean, 1992).

More relevant is the fact that administration of the Schick test has been known to cause a rise in antitoxin titres (Ferencei *et al.*, 1969). Ferencei and coworkers tested the serum of 22- to 25-year-old subjects for diphtheria antitoxin levels before and after receiving the Schick test. They noted a poor correlation between Schick test results and antitoxin levels measured just prior to the test. More importantly, they found a significant rise in antitoxin levels following the Schick test. The accepted concentration level of diphtheria antitoxin titre that confers immunity is 0.1 IU/ml. (Bannister and Corbel, 1991). In Ferencei's study 21 subjects showed an initial titre less than 0.1 IU/ml. and 12 of them showed an increase of antitoxin levels to 0.1 IU/ml. or higher, five months after the Schick test. This means that the Schick test itself produced immunity that persisted at least five months after the test in 57 percent of subjects. Presumably a repeat Schick test given to these subjects would convert from positive to negative, if the Schick test reaction were accurate, which researchers in the field now recognize it is not. A total of 81 percent of Schick-test recipients in that study showed some increase in antitoxin titre 5 months after the Schick test. No cases of diphtheria were reported in this community during that period, and exposure to disease was eliminated as an explanation for the rise in titre.

Similar findings were noted in another study by Barr and coworkers, who measured antitoxin titres in the cord blood of babies born to tested and untested mothers. They found significantly higher antitoxin titres in the babies of mothers who had been Schick-tested (Barr *et al.,* 1949). All of these studies that question the accuracy and validity of the Schick test were conducted after the homeopathic research of Paterson and Boyd, whose study involved four repetitions of the Schick test. This repetition of the test could easily cause the results that they attributed to the homeopathic medicines. The recent studies would seem to invalidate Paterson's conclusion. If we throw out the Paterson study based on the more recent assessment of the Schick test, then there is no research to support the practice of homeopathic prophylaxis.

Homeopathic preparations have not been shown to raise antibody levels. Smits tested the titre of antibodies to diphtheria, polio, and tetanus in ten children before and one month after giving homeopathic preparations of these three vaccines (DTPol 30K and 200K). He found no rise in antibody levels (Smits, 1995). He speculates that protection afforded by a homeopathic remedy acts on a "deeper" level than that of antibodies. Other homeopaths have stated similar opinions. Golden says, "Unlike conventional vaccines, the Homoeopathic alternative does not rely on antibody formation." He postulates that "Homoeopathic remedies reduce the patient's sensitivity to the dynamic stimulus of the virus or bacteria, thus lessening the patient's predisposition to being overcome by this stimulus" (Golden, 1998).

If homeopathic remedies do not produce an increase in antibody levels, then the only way to measure the effectiveness of homeopathic prophylaxis is through clinical results. This is a formidable undertaking. The cost of long-term studies using homeopathic prophylaxis would be prohibitive, given the present resources available. Ethical problems could also prevent such studies from occurring; it is doubtful that ethics committees would allow children to be deprived of the commonly administered and approved allopathic vaccines. Moskowitz has suggested that the sizable population of unvaccinated children whose parents have refused vaccines could provide a control group to assess the long-term negative effects of vaccines (Moskowitz, 1985). Perhaps this population could also serve as a test group for homeopathic prophylaxis.

Golden has conducted an informal survey of customers who have purchased a kit of homeopathic medicines intended for use in a long-term prophylaxis program beginning in infancy (Golden, 1998). This kit includes the nosodes for whooping cough, diphtheria, measles, mumps, and *Haemophilus,* as well as tetanus toxin and *Lathyrus sativa* (for polio). They are administered in repeated doses, one medicine at a time, during the period from one month of age to five years. For example, *Pertussin* is given at ages 1, 2, 13, and 32 months. Tetanus toxin is given five times at ages 11, 12, 24, 41, and 60 months. The first dose of each remedy is 200 strength, and subsequent doses are 200, 1M, and 10M in succession, every 8 hours in one day. The follow-up survey involves a questionnaire sent yearly from 1988 through 1994, to each of the parents who purchased a kit.

During this five-year span, he received 879 returned questionnaires. Only 2 percent of those children contracted one or more of the diseases covered by the program. Parents were also asked whether a child contracted a disease covered by the program after a known exposure to one of these diseases; they reported that 188 children were exposed to one of these diseases, and 20 contracted the disease. This is an 11 percent failure rate for the homeopathic prophylaxis program with a known exposure to disease. Golden does not specify which diseases the exposure entailed. This very preliminary and limited survey suggests that the 188 supposed exposures may have received some level of protection from the program. Golden notes that symptoms were mild in the majority of cases that did contract the disease. No severe adverse effects were reported in this survey for any of the homeopathic medicines.

The only other evidence cited to support long-term prevention through homeopathy refers to the possible short-term protection it affords during epidemics. It is assumed that repeated doses may provide a protective effect that extends over a span of a few weeks, especially if the child is also challenged during this period with the microorganism that can cause similar symptoms to those produced by the medicine. There is no evidence, however, that any long-term effect accrues from this method.

Dosage schedules for homeopathic prophylaxis vary widely, depending on the practitioner's preference. The schedule, the potencies used, and the number of repetitions are chosen arbitrarily. Golden devised his schedule to approximate the timing of allopathic vaccines, "to reassure parents that their children are being covered by a comprehensive program. . . . " Eizayaga employs 200c potencies of nosodes as homeopathic prophylaxis. His schedule involves giving one nosode twice per day for three days, waiting one week, and then beginning the next nosode in his series. Others advise giving a CM (100,000 dilutions) once, or a 1M (1,000) that will last at least two years (Shepherd, 1967). In the absence of any studies or any way to prove immunity, homeopaths arbitrarily choose dosage schedules.

Disagreement exists among homeopathic practitioners about the safety of introducing a homeopathic medication into the body if there are no clear indications for its use. In general, homeopathic medicines are prescribed on the basis of existing symptoms. These symptoms guide the prescriber to the correct prescription. Classical homeopaths assert that an incorrectly prescribed homeopathic medicine can interfere with the action of other correct prescriptions or disturb the energetic balance of the organism. They generally do not condone the administration of many different nosodes in a single person, as some cases have been rendered apparently incurable by such practices.

Golden has addressed these concerns. He reasons that the damage caused by the administration of the homeopathic nosode is less than the damage caused by conventional vaccines. This is a theoretical assumption that may or may not be true. It is certainly true that homeopathic medicines have never caused the dramatic adverse effects including paralysis, epilepsy, and deaths that are attributed to conventional vaccines. Neither do homeopathic medicines circulate toxic materials in the bloodstream. He further states that the possible adverse consequences of protection using the nosodes are less than the probable adverse consequences of acquiring certain infectious diseases such as polio, diphtheria, and tetanus. Furthermore, even though he finds trust in the protective effect of a constitutional homeopathic medicine attractive in theory, this practice may not prove efficacious, since there are examples of strong and vital individuals and cultures who succumb to infectious disease. His conclusion is that homeopathic vaccines may prove effective, are less toxic than conventional vaccines or the diseases themselves, and are therefore preferable to relying on strictly classical homeopathic prescriptions (Golden, 1989).

Most classical homeopaths would counter that a strong and vital constitution does provide protection from the serious consequences of diseases, unless the disease is different than anything the immune system has ever encountered. Such may be the case with Polynesian islanders exposed to measles, or vital young adults exposed to HIV or the Ebola virus. Parents might also consider this possibility when evaluating needs for protection when children travel to foreign countries with endemic diseases that a child has not previously encountered.

On the other hand, most classical homeopaths will prescribe a preventive medicine or nosode during an epidemic, or following exposure if the effects of the disease could significantly compromise the health of the individual. This practice has some justification, based on the few studies that have been conducted, and on the considerable experience of homeopaths managing epidemics over the past hundred years. In most situations, classical homeopaths tend to rely upon constitutional homeopathic treatment and other immune-enhancing factors in a child's life to develop a strong immune system and prevent serious diseases and their complications, rather than experimenting on patients with unproven preventive medicines that could cause problems. Homeopaths cannot apply a double standard, assuming without any evidence that homeopathic prophylaxis can be used safely and effectively while at the same time criticizing the vaccine industry for exaggerating claims of conventional vaccine effectiveness and minimizing the recognition of adverse effects.

A separate question concerns the advisability of preventing childhood diseases if this will create a greater susceptibility and incidence of the disease in adulthood. Homeopathic prophylaxis results in the same situation as conventional vaccines in this regard. If the homeopathic program is effective, then these nosodes may require repetition throughout the lifespan to protect adults because they have not gained immunity by contracting these infectious diseases during childhood. Since the homeopathic medicines do not apparently act by stimulating measurable antibody responses, there would be no way to determine susceptibility to disease, or the need for repetition of doses. Therefore, the program might require repeated use of these substances on an arbitrary schedule to maintain immunity. Such a maintenance program would be as hopelessly speculative as the dosage schedule is now, since there is no way to document immunity.

The final difficulty with reliance upon long-term homeopathic prophylaxis involves ethical issues. Parents need to understand that there is no evidence to support the use of these homeopathic preparations for long-term prevention. A homeopath who prescribes a prophylactic medicine and assures parents that it will prevent a disease years in the future misrepresents the facts. False reassurance and wishful thinking may dispel parental anxieties about diseases, but they do not represent logical conclusions. There is nothing in the literature that even suggests that homeopathic prophylaxis provides lasting immunity from specific diseases. To claim that they do is an unfounded fabrication.

Some authors have suggested that if parents are given the choice of doing nothing or obtaining the conventional vaccines, then many parents will choose vaccines because they want to do something. Golden forcefully states his argument in this regard. He would "strongly argue that if parents prefer to vaccinate their children rather than provide no specific protection, we as practitioners are professionally obliged to offer them the use of the Homoeopathic alternative. It is then up to the parents concerned to choose between the two options for protection, based on the information available to them" (Golden, 1998). Homeopaths may or may not feel obligated to offer parents a program that has no basis in experience or research. If they do, the information should be accurate and not composed of contrived claims for homeopathic prophylaxis. The decision to use any vaccine rests with the parents. Nonetheless, practitioners cannot advise the use of homeopathic preventives just because they fear that parents will choose conventional vaccines if they offer nothing. This encourages the worst kind of anxieties, and defeats the purpose of a truly informed choice. Fear of disease has bedeviled allopathic medicine for centuries and has led to increasingly toxic methods of suppressing symptoms. Homeopaths would do well to present the facts to parents, and assume that parents have the intelligence and good judgment to come to their own educated opinions. Consumers deserve to have access to all the information available, so that their choice about vaccines, conventional or homeopathic, can be an informed one.

BUILDING A STRONG IMMUNE SYSTEM

Breastfeeding

No discussion of vaccination would be complete without considering the factors that strengthen immune system functions. Several of these influences are under a parent's direct control. For example, breastfeeding protects babies from many infections.

The immunoprotective value of breast milk is unquestionable, but not completely understood. Immunoglobulins in human milk provide passive protection from bacteria. Specifically, secretory IgA found in breast milk blocks the attachment of Streptococci and Haemophilus bacteria to mucous membranes (Hanson *et al.*, 1985). White blood cells in human milk will actively ingest bacteria that invade the infant's body. In addition, lymphocytes carrying specific antibodies pass through breast milk to the baby. Several other chemicals in breast milk (lactoferrin and lysozyme) protect the breastfeeding child from infection by destroying or inhibiting growth of bacteria (Goldman *et al.*, 1982).

Many other resistance factors in breast milk (including interferon) assist the child's developing immune system function (Chandra, 1978). It has been hypothesized that the high levels of prostaglandins found in breast milk may protect infants from infections since prostaglandin E1 decreases inflammatory responses (Backon, 1984). Because of these combined factors, breastfeeding remains one of the best methods of preventing illnesses and their complications in infants.

Several studies have shown that breastfeeding decreases the incidence of acute illness in children. It is well known that in developing countries, infants who are exclusively breastfed have a decreased incidence of diarrheal illness compared to infants who receive supplements of formula, juice, or water (Popkin *et al.*, 1990). However, even in modern nations with excellent sanitation, breastfeeding provides significant protection against acute illnesses in babies. One study of 237 healthy infants followed for three years found a decreased incidence of ear infections in infants who were breastfed for at least six months (Saarinen, 1982). Another study of 1,013 infants followed for the first year of life found a protective effect for single ear infections and recurrent ear infections in those infants breastfed for at least four months (Duncan *et al.*, 1993). A Scottish study of 674 infants similarly found that babies breastfed for at least three months had significantly fewer respiratory and gastrointestinal illnesses over the next year (Howie *et al.*, 1990). Most studies also show that exclusive breastfeeding is more protective than supplemented breastfeeding, and that the protective effect of breastfeeding for the first three to six months persists after children are weaned (Duncan *et al.*, 1993).

Breastfeeding helps to prevent meningitis. Infants who breastfeed for an extended period of time (longer than three months) have a decreased incidence of *Haemophilus influenzae* meningitis compared to infants who breastfeed for a shorter duration. The longer the duration of breastfeeding, the lower the risk of meningitis. The risk decreases for each additional week of breastfeeding (Silfverdal *et al.*, 1997). The protective effect of breastfeeding on meningitis persists for many years. Infants who are breastfed have a decreased incidence of Haemophilus meningitis even five to ten years later (Silfverdal *et al.*, 1999).

Nutrition in Older Children

A person's nutritional status is another prime determinant of his or her general resistance. Malnutrition and undernutrition in underdeveloped countries contribute to low resistance and a higher prevalence of infectious diseases. Similarly, the introduction of refined and processed foods will lower the resistance of a population in a developing country and encourage epidemics.

Good nutrition lays the groundwork for a strong immune system in your child. This includes reliance upon natural foods, and avoidance of chemicals and refined products. Fresh fruits and vegetables provide essential nutrients for the growing child. Processed foods such as canned vegetables and jars of baby food have fewer vitamins, and altered forms of essential nutrients.

Babies should be fed cooked fresh vegetables rather than prepared baby foods whenever possible. The gradual introduction of solids in the form of fresh vegetables, fruits, and grains to supplement breastfeeding (or formula if necessary) during the second six months of life will help develop immune system strength and avoid the weakening effects of food allergies. Each new food should be introduced alone, to observe possible allergic reactions for several days before starting another.

The introduction of potentially allergenic foods too early in an infant's development may predispose him or her to allergic reactions. Avoidance of dairy products, wheat, and egg whites is advisable until a baby has been eating solid foods for at least several months. If a family history of allergies is present, then these foods should be avoided for the first year. Food allergies may predispose children to lowered resistance and frequent infections. The occurrence of chronic congestion or night cough, eczema, frequent colds or ear infections, or behavior problems are possible signs of food allergies. They should be investigated to see if this is the case. Avoidance of the offending foods, a rotation diet, or possibly homeopathic treatment will help the body cope with the physical stresses of viruses and bacteria more efficiently.

Preschoolers and older children may not be the best eaters in the world, but if parents limit refined foods, sweets, and junk-foods, then the result should be a healthy body with a high resistance to infection. Children of all ages develop a sense of values about food. If parents set an example of healthful living and eating, then their children will be more likely to choose healthful foods. This is an important step in the establishment of immune system integrity and a lifelong pattern of wellness.

Most children love sweets, and these should be limited in all situations. Some children are more sensitive to sugar than others. They may develop symptoms of overactivity, distractibility, and poor self-control after eating sugar. Children often crave foods that stimulate allergic reactions in their bodies, and parents should be alert to these cravings as well as food reactions.

Parents should not underestimate their own influence on immune system functioning. The actions that you take can have a direct effect on the immune system. Diet, drugs, medications, and vaccinations all have significant effects. A good diet, avoidance of conventional medications, and the use of natural medicines that stimulate healthy immune system function will provide a good base for high resistance to infection and prevention of complications of illnesses.

A Nutritional Supplement Program

Children who suffer from recurrent infections or allergies can benefit from a nutritional supplement program that strengthens immune function. Any child subjected to the immune assault of vaccines should also take supplements to help prevent immune system deficiencies.

Establishing the proper ratio of fats in a child's diet is one of the most important nutritional adjustments a parent can initiate. Most children have a significant imbalance of fats that contributes to inflammation: too much omega-6 (vegetable oil) and trans fats (hydrogenated oils and fried foods), and not enough omega-3 fats. Since inflammation of mucus membranes is a predominant symptom of allergies and recurrent respiratory infections, any intervention that prevents inflammation will decrease these symptoms. The outer covering of all cells in the body is composed of fats. Maintaining healthy functioning of cells, including the transport of nutrients into cells and the communication between cells through cell membranes, will depend on the quality of the cell's fat composition. Changing the types of fats in a child's diet will help to ensure efficiency of cell function and help prevent inflammation.

Trans fatty acids will cause cell inflammation, and omega-3 fats will prevent inflammation. A balance of omega-6 and omega-3 fats is best, with elimination of as many trans fatty acids as possible. Stop giving trans fatty acids in the diet. Trans fats occur primarily in the form of fried foods, such as French fries, and packaged foods that contain partially hydrogenated fats (chips, crackers, and cookies). Read labels of packaged foods and you will discover that many contain partially hydrogenated oils. You can avoid these fats by shopping at health food stores.

Increase consumption of omega-3 fats. The best sources of omega-3 fats are flax seed oil or ground flax seeds (alpha linolenic acid) and DHA (docosahexaenoic acid) derived from algae. Fish, chickens, and eggs are also sources of omega-3 fats because they eat plants that contain these fatty acids. Therefore, only cage-free chickens that eat green plants or chickens fed algae or fish meal are reliable sources. To be sure that children are getting adequate amounts of omega-3 fats, supplement a child's diet with one teaspoon of flax seed oil or ground flax seeds every day. The best way to do this is to make a smoothie with organic cow's milk or rice milk, fresh or frozen fruit, and flax seed oil. Alternately, grind one teaspoon of organic flax seeds in a small electric coffee grinder and sprinkle on cereal or salads. Do not heat flax seeds or flax oil. Keep oil and seeds refrigerated. Fish, especially salmon, is a good additional source of omega-3 fats, but young children should not take fish oil supplements. A 100 mg capsule of DHA derived from algae will round out the omega-3 supplement program. Children can chew the capsules, or parents can puncture the capsule and mix the contents with food.

Vitamin E will ensure that fatty acids are maintained at optimum efficiency once they are absorbed into cells. In addition, vitamin E has anti-inflammatory effects and increases resistance to infection. Use only natural vitamin E (d-alpha-tocopherol), not the synthetic form (dl-alpha-tocopherol). A mixed tocopherol form of vitamin E is best because children need the gamma as well as the alpha forms.

The only other oils used in the household should be olive oil (monounsaturated fat) and organic canola oil (with a favorable omega-6 to omega-3 ratio of 2:1). Do not use corn oil or other vegetable oils. Olive oil will not cause any health problems, but it does not contain either of the two essential fatty acids, LA or ALA. Canola oil is made from rapeseeds that are often heavily treated with pesticides. Therefore, organic canola oil is the only type that should be used, and it should be cold-processed (expeller-pressed) because heat processing will destroy the omega-3 fats.

The first food a newborn baby receives is colostrum, the clear or yellowish thick fluid secreted from a mother's breasts after childbirth. Colostrum is the greatest immune-enhancing substance known. Colostrum transmits antibodies and other immune-enhancing substances to babies. Older children, and adults, can receive the same beneficial effects by taking cow's colostrum in powdered form as a supplement. Colostrum contains immune defense factors that actively prevent infections and also stimulate the immune system. The most prominent of these factors is an immunoglobulin, IgA, which resides on mucous membranes such as the intestinal lining and protects the body from invading microorganisms. White blood cells, leucocytes, are living cells that respond to infection by ingesting bacteria and releasing IgA. Colostrum and breast milk contain as many white cells as the bloodstream. Lactoferrin, an iron-binding protein found in colostrum, also protects the body from infection by locking onto iron and releasing the iron to red blood cells, thus preventing bacteria from using the iron required for their reproduction. Lysozyme is an agent found in bodily secretions such as saliva that destroys microorganisms on contact. Its presence in colostrum and breast milk has led infant formula manufacturers to add lysozyme to all formulas. Cytokines regulate the intensity and duration of immune responses, boosting T-cell activity and stimulating production of immunoglobulins. Specific sugars including oligo polysaccharides and glycoconjugates bind to bacteria that typically cause ear infections, lung infections, and diarrhea, and block their attachment to mucus membranes. All of these powerful immune factors are available in one simple supplement. Children under the age of six should take at least $^1/_2$ teaspoon of colostrum. Children over six should take 1 teaspoon.

IMMUNE AGENTS CONTAINED IN COLOSTRUM	
IgA:	immunoglobulins protect the body from invading organisms
Leucocytes:	ingest bacteria and release IgA
Lactoferrin:	prevents bacteria from using iron
Lysozyme:	destroys bacteria and viruses on contact
Cytokines:	stimulate immunoglobulins and T-cells
Saccharides:	bind to bacteria and prevent infection

Zinc stimulates immune function, prevents infections, and acts as a cofactor in many enzyme reactions, including the creation of antioxidants. Normal dosage is 10–20 mg. per day. If zinc supplementation is continued over a prolonged period of time, it should be given in conjunction with copper in a ratio of ten to one to prevent copper deficiency.

Children's diets should contain large amounts of natural vitamins A and C derived from fruits (oranges, strawberries, peaches, nectarines, mango) and vegetables (broccoli, carrots, squash, yams, red bell peppers). Vitamin A is also found in fish and eggs. Both vitamins are antioxidants and anti-inflammatories. If children are not eating healthy amounts of these foods, supplements of 5,000 units vitamin A and 200 mg vitamin C can be added to the diet.

Young children can use chewable, liquid, or powdered mineral supplements. Older children can take tablets or capsules.

Immune Supplements for Children—Daily Dosage

	1- TO 6-YEAR-OLDS	6- TO 12-YEAR-OLDS
Flax seed oil or ground flax seeds	1 teaspoon	2 tsp
DHA from algae (Neuromins)	100 mg	100 mg
Colostrum	$1/2$ teaspoon	1 tsp
Zinc	10 mg	20 mg
Copper	1 mg	2 mg
Vitamin E (d-alpha-tocopherol or mixed tocopherols)	100 IU	200 IU

KidShake Recipe

3/4 cup organic rice milk (you can use organic cow's milk if your child is over two years old)

1/2 banana

1/2 cup frozen mango or other fruit (not strawberries unless organic; too many pesticides used on berries)

1 teaspoon flaxseed oil (keep refrigerated)

1 teaspoon colostrum

1 tablespoon liquid calcium/magnesium formula (equivalent to 600 mg calcium, omit if using cow's milk)

1/2 teaspoon honey (optional, use only if your child is over 12 months old)

1/2 teaspoon vitamin C powder (optional, equiv. to 200 mg vitamin C)

Optional: 2 tablespoons whey protein powder (unsweetened, i.e., 0 carbohydrates, equivalent to 10–12 g protein)

SOURCES OF FATTY ACIDS		
OMEGA-6 FAT SOURCES	**OMEGA-3 FAT SOURCES**	**OMEGA-9 FAT SOURCES**
Canola oil	Flax seed	Olives
Safflower oil	Fish	Avocados
Sunflower oil	Algae	
Corn oil	Eggs (cage-free)	

Effect of Living Conditions

Improved sanitation and living conditions have resulted in a steady decline in the incidence of infectious diseases and their complications during the past century. These changes preceded the development of vaccines. Long before the era of antibiotics and specific treatment of infectious diseases, the incidence of complications and deaths from pertussis, measles, smallpox, and scarlet fever had continuously decreased as a direct result of improved hygiene and sanitation practices. These factors are now taken for granted in the United States.

Overcrowding and lower standards of living in a community often accompany a higher incidence of infectious diseases and their complications than in the general population. For example, during the 27,000-case measles epidemic of 1990, over 45 percent of cases occurred in California. Over ten percent of these cases occurred in the San Joaquin Valley east of San Francisco, a low-income, rural farming area. One-third of these cases were in Southeast Asian children, 80 percent of whom were Hmong. It was found that a disproportionate number of these 352 children suffered significant complications (31 percent of these children were hospitalized and suffered a case-fatality ratio of one in every 29 reported cases). A case-control study investigating the reason for this high complication rate revealed that children from families with a lower standard of living had a significantly greater chance of suffering from severe complications or dying during this measles outbreak (California Department of Health Services, 1990).

Similar outbreaks of measles in inner-city populations of New York and Los Angeles accounted for more than 30 percent of the epidemic (Centers for Disease Control, 1991). It is clear that lower-income populations with a lower standard of living remain at greatest risk during epidemics of childhood diseases. This was also proven in a polio outbreak that occurred in Taiwan in 1982. Even though 80 percent of infants were vaccinated against polio, studies of that epidemic of 1,031 cases showed that children were five times more likely to contract paralytic polio if they received water from non-municipal rather than municipal sources (Kim-Farley *et al.*, 1984). This epidemic provides further specific evidence that the level of sanitation rather than the vaccination level in a community fosters the spread of infection and susceptibility to complications.

Finally, mental and emotional health are a key determinant in resistance to infection. Emotional stress is associated with immune system dysfunction, lowered resistance, and more severe forms of infection. The immune system is enhanced in its healthy functions by relaxation, regular rest and sleep, enjoyable activities, and reduction of stress. These factors may be significant for today's children, who have busier schedules and increasing stress from academic demands and parental expectations.

We are now in a position to create environments for children that will foster emotional health and decrease stress. If we promote emotional resilience in children by increasing self-confidence and fulfillment, then a stronger immune system will be the reward. This can be accomplished in many ways. Children thrive when they receive positive reinforcement and praise for their accomplishments and growth. Children want to succeed. Love, attention, and encouragement are the parental tools that stimulate a child's well-being. Learning settings that foster exploration, discovery, and creativity will produce inquisitive minds. Strength of spirit and emotional well-being are associated with healthy physical development. Children who feel confident, strong, and happy are more likely to have an efficient immune system.

LEGAL REQUIREMENTS

Compulsory Vaccination

Vaccines are required by law for children in every state. The specific required vaccines are determined by individual state legislatures in the form of immunization laws that are also periodically amended based on recommendations of national advisory committees. No vaccines are required of adults at the present time, except for those individuals enlisted in military service, and those applying for immigration. However, legal exemptions to vaccines are available for parents, for members of the military, and for immigrants.

Most parents mistakenly believe that their children will not be admitted to schools unless they complete all the state-mandated vaccinations. The school districts, the medical profession, and the media perpetuate this myth. Parents who question the use of vaccines usually receive harsh accusations and bullying tactics from their pediatrician, and relent under this intimidating onslaught. They decide that the issue is not worth the fight and the alienation of their child's doctor. It is usually not laws that force parents to vaccinate, but the professionals, both medical and educational, who care for their child.

The United States government also takes the vaccine campaign very seriously. Parents who make an informed choice about vaccines for their children must contend with compulsory vaccine laws. Conscientious objection to these laws is not handled liberally by the courts. In 1905 the Supreme Court ruled that an individual could not refuse the smallpox vaccine on constitutional grounds of infringement on personal liberty. The court found that an individual's personal liberty must give way to the state's protection of other citizens' health (*Jacobson v. Massachusetts,* 197 US 11, 25; 1905).

Since that time, various state courts have ruled that compulsory immunization statutes cannot be stricken down on constitutional grounds. Every state has a compulsory vaccination law, though the specific requirements for individual vaccines vary from state to state. This means that parents or legal guardians who decide not to give the vaccines will need to seek a legal exemption from vaccines. These come in three varieties: medical, religious, and philosophical. Not all states have philosophical exemptions, so parents in those states must seek either a religious or medical exemption. Usually the issue of a child's unvaccinated status will arise upon registration for school or day-care. Schools require an immunization record, and parents must have proof that their child has been vaccinated, signed by a health care provider. Schools become involved in the vaccination campaign because state and local governments receive federal funding for immunization programs. The federal Public Health Service Act, 42 U.S.C.

§ 262 requires that participating governments must have a "plan to assure that children begin and complete their immunizations on schedule . . ." and "a plan to systematically immunize susceptible children at school entry through vigorous enforcement of school immunization laws" (42 C.F.R. § 5lb.204).

Other situations that may draw attention to an unvaccinated child are visits to an emergency room, clinic, or doctor's office. Parents inform the doctor that the child has not been vaccinated, or they refuse vaccination, and the doctor files a report. When confronted with one of these situations, the parents then seek an exemption. When the exemption is accepted by the school or the health department, the issue is resolved. If a request for exemption is denied, then parents may appeal that decision.

Parents who continue to have difficulty with school and governmental authorities may need to seek legal counsel. One attorney has advised the following legal tactic to avoid litigation if a school continues to refuse admission or if authorities question the parents' legal right to refuse vaccines:

> Some attorneys have prevented litigation by demanding from the school board, the hospital, and the physician administering the vaccine a guarantee that the vaccine will not cause disease, death or injurious side effects. The guarantee usually states that the vaccine will prevent the particular disease for which it is given. It is worded in such a way so as to make the persons signing it not only liable as a representative of the school district or hospital but also individually for damages should any damage in fact occur. To my knowledge no one has ever signed such a document and in each case in which it was used the child has been allowed to return to class without the vaccination (Finn, 1983).

Subsequent to the anthrax terrorist attacks of 2001 and the perceived threat of other biological weapons attacks, a national plan was drafted to manage widespread emergencies of potentially lethal epidemics. The Centers for Disease Control (CDC) presented this plan to state governors, state legislators, and local health officials to guide them in establishing policy. "Emergency health threats, including those caused by bioterrorism, may require the exercise of extraordinary government powers and functions." During such emergencies governors are granted the authority to declare a public health emergency and require vaccinations of all citizens. The plan quotes the 1905 smallpox court decision justifying compulsory vaccination. However, this plan also contains an exemption clause. "To prevent the spread of contagious or possibly contagious disease, the public health authority may isolate or quarantine . . . persons who are unable or unwilling for reasons of health, religion, or conscience to undergo vaccination pursuant to this section" (Center for Law and the Public's Health, 2001).

Exemptions are created within immunization laws because without them the government would be guilty of infringement on personal freedoms, including freedom of religion guaranteed by the First Amendment. This would create potential for lawsuits, and when governments have infringed on these freedoms, citizens have won in court. However, the potential authority to isolate and quarantine those who refuse vaccination represents draconian measures. If such policies were implemented, they would certainly result in lawsuits as well.

Medical Exemptions

All fifty states provide for medical exemption from vaccines. If a physician thinks a child should not have the vaccine, then he or she can provide an exemption. Many doctors are willing to write these, especially if they think the vaccines may have unknown long-term effects that could be detrimental to your child's health. The pediatric literature lists specific medical contraindications for the various vaccines. These conditions are either quite limited in scope (e.g. recent onset of a neurologic disorder or prior serious reaction to the vaccine), or include temporary situations such as an acute illness or a fever.

Physicians may consider themselves at risk if they provide an exemption for any other reason than those on the official lists. One such case was reported by the Centers for Disease Control. A 12-year-old boy acquired tetanus from a splinter and recovered after twelve days of hospitalization. The report was titled, "Tetanus in a Child with Improper Medical Exemption from Immunization—Florida."

> Investigation revealed that the child had received a dose of oral polio vaccine at about 18 months of age but had received no other immunizations. In the school record was a form granting him permanent medical exemption to all vaccines. The form, signed by a health-care provider, gave the reason for exemption as "due to recent medical literature." The provider later stated that the literature referred to "cytotoxic allergies secondary to immunization," but cited no specific references. Review of immunization records in the child's school revealed two other children with similar exemptions granted by this same provider.

They caution that "granting of medical exemptions should not be given indiscriminately." A poor choice of grammar, but such a notice serves as an undisguised warning to the medical profession (Centers for Disease Control, 1985). Medical exemptions have been more carefully scrutinized since the most recent vaccine campaigns of the 1990s.

Wording of the medical exemption is not standardized. A physician can state anything appropriate to the individual child. A simple statement that vaccines are waived indefinitely because of potential adverse effects may suffice. The following alternate wording may help to limit the liability of a health care provider and still release the parents from immunization requirements.

> In the opinion of the parents, vaccines would be inadvisable at this time from a medical perspective. Informed consent was not given for this procedure because of a history of allergic reactions (or low tolerance to medications).

Additionally, the following statement may be added as a verification of the parents' commitment to their decision.

> It is the parents' sincere conviction that vaccine administration would be an invasion of the body's integrity.

Parents who think that their child's medical condition warrants exemption from vaccines should consult an attorney who specializes in this area. Obtaining a medical exemption for a child with a chronic illness may involve complex considerations. An attorney can advise parents concerning case precedent and the best tactics for making the legal argument necessary to obtain a valid medical exemption.

Religious Exemptions

All states except Mississippi and West Virginia allow exemption from vaccination on the basis of parents' religious beliefs. Parents may be members of a religious organization that opposes the use of vaccines, or they can claim an exemption based on their personal religious beliefs that are similar to those of such an organization. Recent legal precedents have established that exemptions should be granted on the basis of parents' personal religious beliefs, and that parents need not be associated with a religious institution opposed to vaccination. These cases have established that the religious exemption must extend to individuals who hold sincere religious convictions against the use of vaccines, and that these convictions may be broad in scope. Religious belief, in other words, need not conform to a specific religion but can encompass spiritual convictions such as a pantheistic view of creative energy in the universe, or beliefs that bear a similarity to those of Eastern religions or Native American traditions.

Several court cases have established that personal religious belief qualifies parents for a religious exemption. School districts and state education departments have lost monetary damage suits for depriving children of their rights to public education when they were denied a religious exemption (*Sherr and Levy v. Northport-East Northport Union Free School District*, 672 F. Supp. 81; E.D.N.Y. 1987). The Massachusetts Supreme Court held that the law granting exemptions to members of a religion that opposed vaccines must also apply to individuals with the same religious beliefs, regardless of their affiliation with a church. The court decided that the law could not grant such preference to certain religious groups (*Dalli v. Board of Education*, 358 Mass. 753, 1971). A similar case in New York found that personal religious beliefs held by the parents constituted grounds for granting an exemption even though the parents did not belong to a church or hold beliefs advocated by any specific religion (*Allanson v. Clinton School District*, No. CV 84-174, slip op. at 5, N.D.N.Y. 1984).

A federal judge has also agreed in a landmark decision that a school district violates a parent's First Amendment rights if a child is prevented from attending school when the parent holds a genuine religious belief that contradicts vaccination (*Curtis v. Hilton Central School District*, United States District Court, Western district of New York, 01-CV-6579T). In the judge's decision of that case, he states that the parent (plaintiff) cited an opposition to vaccines based on "her belief that God has given the body a natural defense system, and that tampering with that system is tantamount to admitting distrust in God's design of, and plan for, the human body." And secondly, "Plaintiff also testified that she opposes immunization on grounds that it subjects healthy children to medical treatment in contravention of Jesus's teaching that 'it is not the healthy who need a doctor, but the sick,' Matthew 9:11." Therefore, "her position that sick children may receive medicine is not inconsistent with her belief that healthy children should not be immunized." And finally, the judge ruled,

> This court may not pass on the wisdom of plaintiff's belief, nor on the manner upon which she came to hold that belief provided that she maintains a sincere and genuine objection to immunization . . . The fact that she may also hold secular beliefs in opposition to immunizations does not preclude her from also holding a sincere and genuine religious belief that immunizations are improper.

Parents seeking a religious exemption need to submit a letter to the school stating their desire for a waiver of vaccines based on their religious belief. The wording of such a letter is important, and should conform to the wording of the statute governing exemptions. It should also state the parents' sincere beliefs, related in such a way that they can be interpreted by the court as religious. The wording of the immunization law can be obtained from the state health department's immunization office.

Parents seeking such an exemption should contact an attorney who specializes in immunization law. They must construct a solid legal case based on their individual situation, their state law, and their own beliefs. Since religious belief can be interpreted broadly, a wide range of personal beliefs and philosophies will qualify parents for a religious exemption. The case that is constructed in the letter must conform to the legal arguments that will be used in litigation if the school and state government authorities reject the parents' petition for exemption. A well-constructed case and an attorney's arguments will usually prevent litigation. The small cost of involving an attorney early in this process will help prevent the major expense of going to court later.

The vaccine campaign and government pressure to vaccinate all children have made schools wary about granting religious exemptions. This is a legal issue of personal choice. If schools deny parents their legal rights, then an attorney will challenge that infringement in a court of law. This is the message that a legal argument will convey to the school district and the state government.

Parents confronted with a denial of their legal rights should not acquiesce because of harassment or intimidation. The law is on your side, and it is not in the school's financial interest to pursue litigation. Letters from an attorney can be very persuasive. All communications should be in writing. Document any phone conversations. Since the common goal of the parents and the school district is to educate the child and abide by the law, a solution to a dispute over vaccine exemption can usually be reached through logic and an appropriate review of the legal requirements. The school must abide by the law.

The medical establishment has repeatedly sought to eliminate the religious exemption on constitutional grounds and through legislation. For example, a federal court case was filed in 1993 on behalf of the California Medical Association (CMA) against the United States Government. The CMA argued that the court should not allow children to be deprived of medical care in the form of vaccinations because their parents withhold consent; that this would be in violation of a child's right to liberty secured by the Fourteenth Amendment to the Constitution, which guarantees that "No State shall make or enforce any law which shall abridge the privileges or immunities of citizens of the United States; nor shall any State deprive any person of life, liberty, or property, without due process of law." The CMA claimed that, "Parents must not be free to expose their children to deleterious health conditions. . . . A child's constitutional right to develop fully must be protected. . . . In fact, the Court has specified that the right to practice religion freely does not include the liberty to expose the community or a child to ill health or death."

They quoted a case precedent to bolster their argument (*Prince*, 321 US at 170). "Elaborating on the issue of parental autonomy, the Court in *Prince* stated: 'Parents may be free to become martyrs themselves. But it does not follow they are free in identical circumstances, to make martyrs of their children before they have reached the age of full and legal discretion when they can make that choice for themselves.'" They requested that the court address "the question of the constitutionality of the religious exemptions provisions currently contained in California child welfare legislation and to hold those provisions constitutionally invalid" (California Medical Association, 1993). Presumably this argument is based on the principle of *"Parens Patriae."* As explained by an attorney who specializes in vaccine law, this doctrine provides for the ability of States to "compel medical treatment necessary to preserve the life or health of a minor citizen notwithstanding vehement parental objection. With its usual deference to the integrity of the family unit and the notion of parental control of minors, the State exercises its power narrowly" (Finn, 1983).

The CMA case was dismissed by the US Court of Appeals in 1994 because of the many case precedents upholding the right of religious exemption, but this challenge to exemptions is not an isolated event. The vaccine industry will continue its attempts to curtail parental rights to make informed health care choices for their children. Similarly, legislation is periodically proposed in various states to eliminate religious and philosophical exemptions from vaccines. These undisguised and unpublicized efforts to limit parents' choices and to undermine parents' fundamental rights continually reveal the motives of the vaccine industry as the guarantee of massive sales and enforced belief in vaccines.

Philosophical Exemptions

A personal or philosophical belief exemption is currently available in 17 states. This means that parents need not justify their preference for avoiding vaccines except to say that they are philosophically opposed to their children receiving them. Parents residing in states that provide a philosophical exemption must sign a form or write a letter that says immunization is contrary to their beliefs. Some states provide a waiver statement on the school district immunization record forms included with registration materials. Other states require a written statement from the parents. Parents need only request the immunization exemption form at their school district office when enrolling their child in school, or present the school district a simple letter. State laws do change, so get a copy of your state's current immunization law from the state health department.

STATES THAT ALLOW A PHILOSOPHICAL EXEMPTION FROM VACCINATION	
Arizona	New Mexico
California	North Dakota
Colorado	Ohio
Idaho	Oklahoma
Louisiana	Rhode Island
Maine	Utah
Michigan	Vermont
Minnesota	Washington
Wisconsin	

Private schools may be bound by state immunization laws. Check the statutes of your individual state (see *http://home.san.rr.com/via/*). Day-care centers, preschools, nursery schools, and private schools can refuse admission to a child for a variety of reasons. Most of these facilities, however, are willing to abide by the recommendations of state health departments concerning immunization requirements, and some states include these day-care and private educational facilities within the statute. A physician's medical exemption should be an adequate waiver in all states, and in states with provisions for religious or philosophical exemptions a parent's signed statement should suffice.

If the director of a private school or day-care center is hesitant about admitting your child, then he or she should be encouraged to contact the medical director of immunizations at the state health department. Refusal to admit a child on the basis of "inadequate" immunization could create a legal liability for a private school in a state where religious or philosophical exemptions exist. That is, parents could take a school to court if the school refuses admission to their child in a state with personal belief exemptions.

Many attorneys and organizations are working to ensure freedom of choice in the area of child vaccination (see Appendix B: Resources). If a parent makes the choice to avoid a required vaccine, then support for that decision is available.

OPTIONS FOR LEGAL EXEMPTION FROM VACCINES

- Use the philosophical belief exemption, if available in your state;

- Find a doctor willing to write a medical exemption; or

- Develop a personal legal case for religious exemption, with the help of an attorney.

Immigration

The Immigration and Nationality Act requires any person seeking an immigrant visa or adjustment of status for permanent residence to show proof of vaccination against certain "vaccine-preventable" diseases. Children must have age-appropriate immunizations as listed in the current Recommended Childhood Immunization Schedule approved by the Advisory Committee on Immunization Practices. Any immigrant over one year of age is required to have varicella vaccine, and adults over 65 must have pneumococcal vaccine and an annual influenza vaccine.

The law includes two exceptions to these requirements. A waiver is available when receipt of vaccine would not be medically appropriate. This waiver can only be given by a civil surgeon, a physician certified by the Immigration and Naturalization Service (INS). An immigrant may also claim that vaccination would be contrary to his or her religious beliefs or moral convictions. In this case the INS reviews the application to determine if the immigrant qualifies for a waiver. The services of an attorney may be necessary to construct the proper wording for a waiver. The text of the relevant section of law follows.

> Illegal Immigration Reform and Immigrant Responsibility
>   Act of 1996
> Pub. L. 104-208
> (b) WAIVER.-Section 212(g) (8 U.S.C. 1182(g))
> (2) subsection (a)(1)(A)(ii) in the case of any alien-

> (A) who receives vaccination against the vaccine-preventable disease or diseases for which the alien has failed to present documentation of previous vaccination,

> (B) for whom a civil surgeon, medical officer, or panel physician (as those terms are defined by section 34.2 of title 42 of the Code of Federal Regulations) certifies, according to such regulations as the Secretary of Health and Human Services may prescribe, that such vaccination would not be medically appropriate, or

> (C) under such circumstances as the Attorney General provides by regulation, with respect to whom the requirement of such a vaccination would be contrary to the alien's religious beliefs or moral convictions

Military Service

All branches of the armed services do have "immunization waivers." Anyone who enlists must state his or her objection to vaccination at that time. The waiver may take the form of religious exemption based on "religious conscience," or a medical exemption, such as allergies or a low tolerance to medication of any kind. Future refusal of vaccination in the absence of this initial objection could result in dire consequences. Anyone who experiences difficulties in obtaining an exemption should follow the same instructions outlined in the section on religious exemptions discussed above in relation to the education system.

Here is the relevant section of the code.

Paragraph 13 of AFJI 48-110

13. Waivers. The respective Surgeons General and CG MPC or Commandant (G-K) grant permanent immunization waivers for military or civilian personnel (employed by the military or training under military sponsorship). Such waivers are granted only in the case of legitimate religious objections to Immunization and are revoked if necessary to ensure the accomplishment of the military mission. Authority to grant temporary waivers is delegated as follows;

13.1. Army only. Medical authority at major commands.

13.2. Air Force only. Major command surgeons.

13.3. Navy and Marine Corps only. The Chief, Bureau of Medicine and Surgery.

13.4. Waivers from private physicians based on personal beliefs or attitudes are not authorized.

13.5. Forward to the appropriate commander or surgeon waivers for religious objections.

13.5.1. Include full name, rank, and SSN; name of recognized religious group and the date of the applicant's affiliation; supporting certification signed by an authorized personal religious counselor. The counselor attests that the applicant is an active member in good standing of the espoused religious group, adheres to tenets consistent with the espoused religious beliefs and the religious group has a tenet or belief opposing immunizations.

13.6. Commanders ensure counseling of the applicant is provided by a medical officer and documented in the health record. The following Information is included in the counseling:

13.6.1. Noncompliance with immunization requirements adversely impact deployability and administrative actions may be taken.

13.6.2. Additional risk to health on exposure to disease against which he/she is not protected.

13.6.3. Possibility he/she may be detained during travel across international borders in accordance with international health regulations.

13.6.4. Possibility that if a waiver is granted the waiver can be revoked if he/she is at imminent risk of exposure to a disease for which an immunization is available. This is in keeping with the tenets concerning involuntary therapeutic care when military mission accomplishment may be compromised.

Part II: The Vaccines

THE DISEASES AND THEIR VACCINES

The following chapters discuss individual diseases and the vaccines currently recommended for children in the United States by the Centers for Disease Control, and vaccines that adults may consider for maintaining immunity and for potential exposure. Each chapter presents a brief summary of each disease, its corresponding vaccine, and the critical factors surrounding its use. Information is included relevant to disease incidence, vaccine efficacy, and adverse reactions to vaccines because these figures are not readily available to the general public. Statistics concerning disease incidence always refer to the United States unless specifically stated otherwise.

Each chapter includes many references to the medical literature because consumers should have facts about vaccines and not just opinions and official recommendations. Our knowledge about vaccines is limited, but the public needs to be involved in the controversy that this incomplete picture generates. Original studies and cases from the medical literature are also included—doctors speaking to other doctors. This is not the picture that parents and patients usually encounter at their doctor's office, where a rosy light is shed upon vaccination.

All vaccines have problems with toxicity and adverse effects, ineffectiveness, and contamination. Full disclosure occurs nowhere— not in the pediatrician's office, not in the pharmaceutical inserts, and not in the medical literature. This data is collected here to provide you with an undisguised view of vaccines. Not all reported cases of adverse reactions to vaccines can actually be attributed to the vaccine. Some symptoms unrelated to vaccines will occur coincidentally following vaccination, and these may be reported in studies along with actual vaccine reactions. The weight of evidence will determine whether a specific effect is caused by the vaccine. I have included the majority of reports for each vaccine so that consumers can see the weight of that evidence for themselves. The major adverse effects of most vaccines are not experienced by a large proportion of vaccine recipients. That is why a vaccine must be used in the field for years before a picture of toxicity develops. Even then the long-term effects will probably never be fully understood.

Throughout the chapters references are made to reports filed with VAERS, the Vaccine Adverse Event Reporting System. VAERS is a passive surveillance system. These are voluntary reports filed by doctors and consumers who suspect that a vaccine may have caused a reaction. They are not confirmed reports. Additionally, it is estimated that VAERS reports represent only a small fraction of actual vaccine reactions, which are significantly underreported. Often no one makes the connection between a symptom's occurrence and a previously administered vaccine. Physicians are reluctant to file vaccine adverse event reports. A 1994 survey of 159 doctors' offices by the National Vaccine Information Center (NVIC) revealed that only 18 percent of doctors said they make a report to the government when a child suffers a serious health problem following vaccination.

There is no question that the incidence of individual diseases has declined, at least in part, because of vaccination. But the cost in adverse effects from vaccines may be too high for us to tolerate given our present level of knowledge about the vaccines and disease occurrence. At the end of each chapter readers will find a suggested personal strategy for each vaccine's use, so that you can begin to develop your own personalized approach to each disease.

The chapters are organized alphabetically by disease name, or by type of disease (for example, meningitis bacteria as a group). For parents' reference, childhood vaccines are usually given in a certain chronological order. You may want to consider each of these as you encounter them at specific ages.

At birth:	Hepatitis
During infancy:	DTaP, Polio, Haemophilus, Pneumococcal
At one year:	MMR, Chickenpox

ANTHRAX

Anthrax is a disease of sheep and cattle. They contract it by eating bacterial spores in the soil. Human infection usually occurs as an occupational disease from contact with diseased animals. The most common form of disease in humans is a skin infection, readily treatable with antibiotics, but a rare form of inhaled anthrax occurs in people who process wool, and this form of the disease is often fatal. A total of only 18 cases of inhalational anthrax occurred in the US in the twentieth century, the last case occurring in 1976 (Brachman, 1980).

A dramatic change in this picture occurred on October 5, 2001, when the first death caused by a terrorist attack with anthrax bacteria occurred in Florida. The threat of anthrax bioterrorism has long been recognized. Research on anthrax as a weapon began over 80 years ago (Christopher, 1997), and the true threat of anthrax became clear to the public when an apparent accident at a Soviet bioweapons facility released anthrax spores into the air in 1979, killing 68 people (Meselson, 1994).

ANTHRAX SYMPTOMS

Human anthrax disease occurs by three routes—through skin contact, by inhalation, and by ingestion of spores. Skin, or cutaneous, anthrax is the most common and the least lethal. Within 2–10 days after exposure, a painless inflamed area develops on the skin, accompanied by fever and tiredness. A round, ulcerated lesion then forms, about the size of a quarter, and forms a blackened base. The name "anthrax" derives from the Greek word for coal, *anthrakis*, because of these black skin lesions. Antibiotic treatment usually results in full recovery. Ingested anthrax occurs after eating undercooked meat from infected animals. Outbreaks have been reported in Africa and Asia (Sirisanthana *et al.*, 1988). The inhaled form of anthrax is the most lethal.

Anthrax bacteria will form spores when the bacteria are deprived of nutrients and exposed to air. These hardy spores can survive for decades (Williams, 1986). They will germinate when they enter a nutrient-rich environment, such as the human lung. The incubation period for recent cases of anthrax disease has been four days. Symptoms begin with a flu-like illness including fever, weakness, chills, profuse and drenching sweats, cough, chest pain, and nausea or vomiting. Then the deadly symptoms hit after a few hours or a few days, characterized by shortness of breath, shock, delirium, and death within another 36 hours. Anthrax meningitis is a frequent complication (Jernigan, 2001). Of those who died as a result of the Soviet accident, 55 percent showed evidence of meningitis on autopsy (Abramova *et al.*, 1979). Laboratory findings include pneumonia, pleural effusion, and a positive blood culture. In recent cases, prompt medical care with multiple antibiotics has resulted in a fatality rate of 64 percent (Jernigan, 2001). Historically, fatality rates have been 85 percent (Brachman, 1980).

BIOLOGICAL WEAPON

Japan developed anthrax biological weapons in the 1930s and reportedly used them against the Chinese in World War II (Williams & Wallace, 1989). The United States and Great Britain developed anthrax for biowarfare in the 1940s (Bernstein, 1987). During the 1980s the Soviets built bioweapons facilities capable of producing two tons of anthrax per day (Alibek, 1999). US intelligence sources estimate that Iraq concealed at least 2,650 gallons of liquid anthrax, and maintains the ability to produce more anthrax for biological weapons attacks in at least six production facilities.

Anthrax would probably work well if dispersed through the air over unprotected troops during a war, but it is not an ideal terrorist weapon. First, it is not contagious, so it only kills those exposed to the spores. Second, the spores are difficult to get into the air for people to breathe. They must be dried, powdered, and dispersed in some manner, but they are difficult to aerosolize because they tend to block spray nozzles. And third, terrorists handling and spraying anthrax spores would need excellent protection to prevent them from succumbing to their own terrorist weapon before they could dispense it. Anthrax would be extremely effective as a weapon of war because a jet could easily dump a large quantity over enemy troops. This would result in mass deaths unless the troops were protected by dust masks and able to decontaminate their clothing. A similar attack could occur against a civilian population. These wartime scenarios require sophisticated laboratory and transport facilities only available to nations with technological capabilities.

Terrorist acts using anthrax are clandestine and silent. Since anthrax spores will persist virtually forever, they require no bioreactors or culture techniques to keep them alive as do viruses. Powdered anthrax spores will disperse into the air when handled, and this capability has allowed terrorists to kill civilians by dusting letters with spores and sending them through the mail. During the period October 5, 2001, through November 21, 2001, a total of 11 people contracted inhalational anthrax as a result of handling mail intentionally contaminated with anthrax spores. Seven of the victims died (64 percent) (Jernigan *et al.*, 2001; CDC, 2001c).

ANTHRAX VACCINE

Animal vaccines for anthrax were first developed in 1880. Human vaccine was licensed in 1970 as a six-dose primary series with annual booster doses, but no controlled studies have ever been conducted on vaccine efficacy (Nass, 1999). In 1997 the Department of Defense announced mandatory anthrax vaccination for all military personnel. More than 511,000 service members have been vaccinated with more than 2 million doses of the vaccine since March 1998. Because of concerns about adverse vaccine reactions, the Pentagon changed the vaccine strategy in June 2002. The current plan includes vaccinating all military personnel stationed in the Persian Gulf, Korea, and other areas of the world with a significant risk of biological attack. Stockpiles of anthrax vaccine will also be kept in reserve for use by rescue squads, police, and civilians who live or work in areas exposed to anthrax as a result of terrorist attacks.

Military experts, however, agree that current vaccines are unlikely to prevent disease caused by weapons-grade anthrax, since Iraq and other potential aggressor nations have the ability to engineer strains of the virus resistant to current vaccines and antibiotics (Kadlec *et al.*, 1997). Even naturally occurring strains of anthrax routinely overwhelm the currently used vaccine when tested in laboratory animals.

Vaccine Reactions

Many concerns have arisen concerning the vaccine's safety as a result of the experience with its use in the military during the Persian Gulf War. Reactions following the anthrax vaccine given to military personnel include illness that persists for three weeks or longer. Symptoms include nausea, severe headache, lassitude, and vomiting of blood. In one case reported by the Navy, a 24-year-old serviceman developed Guillain-Barré syndrome following his third anthrax vaccination. This autoimmune reaction has been reported following many other vaccines and consists of destruction of the sheath surrounding nerves by the body's own immune mechanisms, causing paralysis (Newcomb, 1998). As of April 2000, 428 reports were received by the passive surveillance Vaccine Adverse Event Reporting System (VAERS). Of these, 311 (73 percent) concerned systemic reactions (CDC, 2001c). The CDC admits that adverse events are probably underreported because of concerns among service members that a report will render them unable to complete the vaccination series, thereby limiting career advancement options (CDC, 2001c).

According to one survey at an Air Force base, "many who are experiencing problems are afraid to report their symptoms. . . . The military and civilian career implications of losing flight status are so great that for many individuals, living with the problems seems to be a better alternative than reporting them." Of 252 surveys sent out to service personnel at the base, 81 respondents (32 percent) fell into the category of having a probable systemic reaction. Typical comments include statements such as "since initiating the anthrax series, I have been 'weaker' and more ill than any other period in my life." And "My immune system just cannot seem to keep up anymore since I started the series." "I used to get one cold per year. Since I had the shots I've had 8–10 bad colds. One cold got so bad they thought I had spinal meningitis." The survey responses are peppered with symptoms such as persistent tiredness and decreased endurance, severe headaches, and numbness. Less than 20 percent of those with systemic reactions completed a VAERS report, and less than 45 percent sought medical attention (Captain Jean Tanner, Dover Air Force Base Survey, *www.anthraxvaccine.org*).

Between 130,000 and 150,000 US military personnel received the anthrax vaccine during the 1991 Persian Gulf War (Desert Storm). At least 15,000 Gulf War veterans have reported a long-term disease, subsequently named Gulf War Syndrome (GWS), characterized by fatigue, muscle and joint pains, neurological abnormalities, autoimmune thyroid disease, headaches, memory loss, skin rash, diarrhea, and sleep disturbances (Fukuda *et al.*, 1998).

Three studies of GWS in veterans have found an association between the disease and exposure to bioweapons vaccines, as well as other toxic exposures during the war. The United Kingdom deployed over 53,000 military personnel to the Persian Gulf War. The rates of symptoms associated with GWS occurring in more than 4,000 British Gulf War veterans were compared to the rates in the same numbers of service personnel participating in the Bosnia conflict, and a similar number of personnel serving at the same time but not deployed. The UK veterans of the Gulf War were about three times more likely to experience the symptoms of GWS and chronic fatigue than the control groups. Additionally, "servicemen who received vaccinations against biological warfare agents were more likely to report long-term symptoms" (Unwin *et al.*, 1999).

A survey of over 1,500 Gulf War veterans from the state of Kansas studied the relationship of vaccines to GWS symptoms. That study also found an increased incidence of GWS in veterans who received vaccines for biological weapons compared to non-exposed veterans.

GWS occurred in 34 percent of Gulf War veterans, 12 percent of veterans who received vaccines but were not deployed to the Gulf, and only four percent of veterans who did not receive vaccines (Steele, 2000). A study of Canadian Gulf War veterans found a significant association between receiving vaccines for anthrax and plague and several symptom-defined outcomes including chronic fatigue (Goss Gilroy, 1998).

French troops participating in the Gulf War conflict did not receive anthrax vaccine or other protective vaccines and drugs for biological warfare. According to a report delivered to the British subcommittee on national security, only 140 of the 25,000 French veterans of the Gulf War reported illnesses related to their service in the Gulf, compared to approximately 10 percent of US and British troops who received vaccines (*Guardian*, 2002).

A clue to the possible mechanism involved in the production of GWS symptoms appeared in studies conducted on Gulf War veterans. Antibodies to a dangerous vaccine additive were found in those veterans with the disease. Squalene is a synthetic polymer added to vaccines to improve absorption and immune response. It is not approved for use in human vaccines, but it has been used in animal trials of the anthrax vaccine and several human vaccine experiments (GAO Report, 1999). However, one study has found evidence of antibodies to squalene in affected Gulf War veterans. Of those veterans in the study suffering from GWS who were deployed to the Gulf, 95 percent had serum antibodies to squalene. One hundred percent of those with GWS who were not deployed but received vaccine exhibited squalene antibodies. None (0 percent) of the Gulf War veterans without disease showed antibodies to squalene. And neither civilian patients with autoimmune disease nor healthy controls had antibodies. Positive controls consisted of individuals who had participated in experimental tests of squalene-containing vaccines (Asa *et al.*, 1999).

The Department of Defense (DOD) has denied the use of squalene in human anthrax vaccine, although the DOD has conducted five clinical trials with vaccines containing squalene. Two of these trials occurred prior to the Gulf War. The Government Accounting Office

(GAO) has stated, "We cannot say definitively whether or not Gulf War-era veterans were given vaccines with adjuvant formulations containing squalene. . . . Although DOD officials told us they did not administer such vaccine, they stated they did not have documentation on the process and results of decision-making related to the administration of vaccines at the time of the Gulf War" (GAO Report, 1999).

Gulf War Syndrome has been attributed to abnormal immune responses similar to the response in those patients suffering from silicone exposure. Women with breast implants develop multisystem symptoms similar to GWS, including joint pain, muscle pain, and neurological disorders. Several studies have found that injected squalene triggers arthritis and other immune system afflictions in animals (Lorentzen, 1999). Squalene can induce increased levels of interleukin and interferon associated with autoimmune disease (Valensi et al., 1994). When squalene was used in influenza vaccine and HIV vaccine it caused severe systemic reactions including fever, chills, nausea, and swelling of lymph nodes (Keutek et al., 1993; Keefer et al., 1996).

Other manufacturing problems have continually plagued the anthrax vaccine. Only one manufacturing facility exists for the production of anthrax vaccine. In 1998 a company known as Bioport took over the production facilities previously operated by the state of Michigan in Lansing. The anthrax vaccine was approved for use in 1970, two years before efficacy data were required for FDA approval of vaccines. The vaccines produced at the state-operated facility were never approved for human use. No safety and efficacy studies were conducted, and a 1997 FDA report found the facility had significant lapses in quality and safety standards. The Bioport facility also failed FDA safety inspections in both 1999 and 2000, and was unable to produce more vaccine despite the government's investment of $126 million in this facility over a ten-year period beginning in 1991. The 1999 FDA report listed 30 areas of manufacturing problems and deficiencies at the Bioport plant (www.anthraxvaccine.org/bpeval.htm). To make matters worse, conflict of interest issues have surfaced. Bioport was founded by former Joint Chief of Staff member Admiral William Crowe, who holds 19 percent of Bioport's stock. The military is Bioport's only customer. Despite the unanswered questions about squalene and other production problems, the government decided to continue the use of stockpiled vaccine for military personnel until new supplies became available.

Amid reports of an association between GWS and anthrax vaccine and the government criticisms of the vaccine's production facilities, about 400 service people have refused to take the vaccine and have been disciplined or expelled because of that stance. Hundreds of pilots in the National Guard and reserve units have resigned rather than take the shots. A congressional committee convened to investigate the anthrax vaccine program concluded in its report that:

> Safety of the vaccine is not being monitored adequately. The program is predisposed to ignore or understate potential safety problems due to reliance on a passive adverse event surveillance system and DOD institutional resistance to associating health effects with the vaccine.
>
> Efficacy of the vaccine against biological warfare is uncertain. The vaccine was approved for protection against cutaneous (under the skin) infection in an occupational setting, not for use as mass protection against weaponized, aerosolized anthrax. (Subcommittee, 2000)

ANTHRAX FACTS

- Disease is acquired by contact with bacterial spores. It is not contagious.

- Skin anthrax is readily treatable with antibiotics. Inhaled anthrax is often fatal.

- Unlike smallpox, the vaccine may not be effective for different strains of anthrax.

- Anthrax vaccine has been associated with significant immediate adverse effects such as Guillain-Barré syndrome and long-term systemic disease such as Gulf War Syndrome.

A Personal Strategy

There is no proof that the anthrax vaccine has the ability to prevent anthrax disease in humans, particularly for strains engineered as biological weapons.

People in high-risk jobs such as mail handlers can use a HEPA dust mask (3M Corp mask for TB prevention), which will filter 95–99 percent of particles in the anthrax size range. In addition, disposable latex gloves will help to prevent skin exposure.

Inhalational anthrax is unlikely to occur more than 60 days following exposure (based on data from animal experiments). Therefore, those people with known exposure can take a 60-day course of preventive antibiotics. Traces of live spores have been found in the lungs of exposed animals up to 100 days following exposure, though no animals developed disease later than 60 days post-exposure. Theoretically, these live spores could result in anthrax disease, and an additional 40 days of antibiotics might provide further protection.

Homeopathic preparations also exist for the prevention of anthrax. Their effectiveness has not been documented. However, for those individuals who decline antibiotic treatment, homeopathic prophylaxis is an option. There is no known interaction between homeopathic preventives and antibiotics, so both forms of prevention can be used simultaneously. For information about homeopathic prevention in epidemics see page 97.

Further Reading

See *www.anthraxvaccine.org* for research and information about the adverse effects of vaccine.

CHICKENPOX (VARICELLA)

Chickenpox is universally recognized by parents as a mild and benign disease of childhood. Anyone infected develops permanent immunity. The disease is caused by the varicella-zoster virus, a member of the herpesvirus family.

The symptoms of chickenpox usually include a fever and runny nose, followed by the appearance of the typical eruptions. These are small, flat, pink areas that soon fill with a clear fluid, and then open and crust over within 2–3 days. They appear in crops, and persist as active lesions for a week. During this time children are usually uncomfortable and itching, especially if they have many eruptions or if these occur on mucous membranes. The disease usually ends uneventfully after a week, except in adults. For them, chickenpox is more troublesome. Symptoms and lesions tend to persist for a month in adults.

Treatment is directed at making children comfortable. Homeopathic treatment may be helpful for the itching and other bothersome symptoms. Allopathic treatment consists of acyclovir, an antiviral drug. One study found a moderate improvement of symptoms in children treated with acyclovir. They had fewer skin lesions (average 294 versus 347 in the placebo group) and had fever for a day or two less than the placebo group (Dunkle *et al.*, 1991). Another study found a similar reduction in skin lesions, but no reduction in complication rates or transmission rates to other children (Balfour *et al.*, 1990). These are modest gains for an expensive drug that has its own set of associated adverse effects. It is estimated that treating 4 million children with chickenpox per year in the United States with acyclovir would cost $128 million each year (Preblud, 1986).

DISEASE COMPLICATIONS

Complications of chickenpox include secondary infections of the skin and neurologic disease. Encephalitis occurs infrequently in children— once in every 4,000–10,000 chickenpox cases. Many of these cases are mild, and hospitalization is required once in every 10,000 to 15,000 cases (Guess *et al.*, 1986). The incidence of encephalitis and associated deaths has been decreasing. An average of 58 cases of encephalitis per year was reported between 1972 and 1979. This was reduced to an average of only 28 cases reported between 1980 and 1983 (Preblud, 1986). Reye syndrome, a dangerous encephalopathy characterized by convulsions and coma, is another rare complication of chickenpox, and its incidence has also declined dramatically in recent years. The avoidance of aspirin during chickenpox illnesses may be responsible for the reduction in Reye syndrome.

Deaths from chickenpox complications occur in less than 50 children per year. The risk of death from chickenpox in healthy children is 0.0014 percent (Preblud, 1986). Children with a disease that compromises the immune system are more likely to develop complications from chickenpox. These children include cancer and leukemia patients undergoing chemotherapy, and those with inborn immune deficiencies, but the vaccine is contraindicated in these children (Committee, 1995).

With the advent of a vaccine for chickenpox, vaccine experts have attempted to maximize the emphasis on disease complications in order to convince doctors that mass vaccination is worthwhile. A particularly heinous tactic of vaccine-industry rhetoric is the omission of incidence rates of complications, which tends to distort the medical view of a disease and overemphasize its seriousness. For example, contemplate the eye-opening title of one review of chickenpox in the *New England Journal of Medicine*: "Varicella and herpes zoster: changing concepts of the natural history, control, and importance of a not-so-benign virus" (Weller, 1983). In another review published in the *Journal of Infectious Diseases* researchers note, "Varicella is not necessarily benign even in healthy children. . . . The records of 96 children hospitalized for varicella [found] that 81 were immunologically normal"

(Gershon *et al.*, 1992). They neglect to inform readers in that article that only one in every 10,000–15,000 cases of chickenpox requires hospitalization.

Adults who contract chickenpox generally have a more prolonged and serious illness. The complication rate is also higher in adults than in children. A severe form of encephalitis occurs more commonly in adults. This diffuse encephalitis is associated with a high mortality rate (5 to 35 percent). Women who contract chickenpox during the first 16 weeks of pregnancy may have children with congenital malformations. The estimated risk in one study of 150 women infected during pregnancy was less than 1 percent (Siegel *et al.*, 1966). Babies who are born within five days of their mother contracting chickenpox have a high risk of death. Severe illness often occurs in these babies during the first five to ten days after birth. The risk of death is estimated at 31 percent (Meyers, 1974).

VARICELLA VACCINE

The foisting of the chickenpox vaccine on the American public qualifies as one of the great public relations marketing scams of all times. The idea of preventing chickenpox in healthy children is ludicrous. The selling of this vaccine to the American public could only be due to an unequivocal belief that any vaccine is worthwhile, or the outright avarice of the pharmaceutical industry. After all, as reported in *The Wall Street Journal,* Merck invested over $5 million in chickenpox vaccine development. Their sentiments are aptly expressed by Samuel Katz, Duke University's pediatrics chairman and head of a vaccine panel at the National Academy of Sciences: "Merck isn't going to make back its investment in that vaccine by just distributing it to kids with cancer. They're going to be interested in pushing for use in the normal population" (Wessel, 1985).

The most frequently stated purpose of the chickenpox vaccine is not to protect children from this benign childhood illness, but to keep parents at their jobs rather than missing a few days of work to care for their sick child at home. According to a leading varicella vaccine researcher, "It is clear that we can reduce the cost of chickenpox by routinely immunizing normal children, primarily by reducing the loss of parental income" (Brunell, 1991). Prior to vaccine licensure it was estimated that vaccination of the entire population would save an estimated $380 million dollars in lost income and wages (Preblud, 1986). Parents lose 0.5 to 1.8 days of work outside the home while caring for their child with chickenpox (Sullivan-Bolyai *et al.*, 1987). The population is being subjected to this mass experiment, risking the potential long-term adverse effects of the vaccine, so that parents can avoid missing an average of 1 day of work. Economic interests have spurred the adoption of a chickenpox vaccine. This travesty is being perpetrated in the name of public health.

Much more alarming to parents are media reports about chickenpox-associated deaths. According to the CDC an average of 43 children died each year from chickenpox in the years 1990–1994, just prior to the vaccine's licensure in 1995. In 1997 the CDC reported six chickenpox-related deaths, three in children and three in adults. One of the children and one of the adults had been taking inhaled or oral steroid medication for the treatment of asthma, a medication that suppresses the body's ability to fight infections (CDC, 1997; CDC, 1998). During 1998 six fatal cases of chickenpox in Florida were reported to the CDC. Four of these people had been taking immune-suppressive drugs, including steroids, at the time (CDC, 1999).

Parents would be well advised to seek alternative medical care rather than relying on steroid medications to treat symptoms of asthma and allergies.

The varicella vaccine was developed in the 1970s, and licensed for children 12 months or older in 1995. Studies have evaluated the use of the vaccine in combination with the measles, mumps, and rubella shot (Brunell *et al.*, 1988), and it is now recommended that the four vaccines be given simultaneously (Committee, 1995).

Vaccine Efficacy

The vaccine seems to be at least 90 percent effective in producing antibodies to the varicella-zoster virus (Arbeter, 1986). These antibodies persist at protective levels for several years. The persistence of immunity over longer periods has not been determined because the vaccine has not been tested in large enough trials for long enough periods of time. During eight years of study the rate of varicella after vaccination averaged from 1 to 3 percent per year, compared to an annual varicella rate of 7 to 8 percent in unvaccinated children (Watson *et al.*, 1993). Although researchers assert that when chickenpox occurs in children previously vaccinated their cases are usually mild (Gershon, 1992), unusually severe cases of chickenpox do occur in those previously vaccinated. For example, a 3.5-year-old boy who had previously developed protective levels of antibodies in response to varicella vaccine contracted chickenpox and aseptic meningitis 21 months later (Naruse *et al.*, 1993). This was the first reported case of such a dramatic vaccine failure.

We can predict the results of mass chickenpox vaccine usage from our experience with measles and mumps vaccines. Just as those diseases have become increasingly more prevalent in adults compared to children, with more likelihood of serious disease and resulting complications, so we are likely to see chickenpox become more common in adults. Persistence of vaccine effectiveness declines over time. Unusual cases of varicella-zoster illness may also occur, as they do after measles and mumps vaccine. These possible effects are unknown, but they do concern vaccine researchers. Dr. Philip Brunell, in his introduction to a state-of-the-art report on varicella vaccine, describes the reluctance to use the vaccine in normal children because "chickenpox, which is relatively mild in childhood, might increase in frequency during adult life when it is much more severe" (Brunell, 1986). He later stated, "Our present performance in immunizing adults is not good. If we were to find that the protection conferred by varicella vaccine was not durable, re-immunization to prevent chickenpox in adults would be an unreliable solution" (Brunell, 1991). The experience with measles and mumps would seem to justify this cautionary note. Another vaccine researcher stated this concern in even stronger terms:

> One would not, however, want to vaccinate against varicella routinely in childhood if immunity wanes and thereby creates a population of varicella-susceptible adults. . . . Practically, however, the only means to determine whether waning immunity will

be a problem is to vaccinate a large number of healthy children and follow them for many years. Therefore, only post-licensure surveillance of vaccinated children can be utilized to determine if this will be a significant problem (Gershon, 1987).

The vaccine industry is now conducting this colossal experiment.

VACCINE REACTIONS

Like most newly licensed vaccines, prelicensing studies of varicella vaccine showed only mild adverse reactions. The more severe reactions began to appear during the postmarketing safety surveillance phase of the mass vaccination campaign. Reports of adverse reactions trickle in slowly, especially with the present voluntary reporting system.

More than 9,500 reports of adverse reactions to varicella vaccine were submitted to the Vaccine Adverse Event Reporting System (VAERS) in the period March 1995 through January 2000 (Wise *et al.*, 2000). Since varicella vaccine is often administered at the same visit as the MMR vaccine, some reports are difficult to attribute to one particular component. On the other hand, the simultaneous administration of several vaccines could potentiate more severe adverse reactions (Jaber *et al.*, 1988; Hirsch *et al.*, 1981; Nicholson *et al.*, 1992). However, the number of reports following the varicella vaccine given alone makes it clear that this vaccine has some serious consequences.

Several **deaths** have been reported following varicella vaccine.

A 12-month-old boy received varicella vaccine (VV) at a well-baby visit. He had no significant previous medical history. Three days after vaccination he developed a fever and irritability, and a rash appeared one week after vaccination. Five days later his mother heard a shrill cry and found the boy convulsing. By the time he reached the emergency room, he was dead.

A 15-year-old boy with cerebral palsy and mental retardation developed severe varicella pneumonia and sepsis one month after varicella vaccination, and died ten days later (Wise *et al.*, 2000).

Many **neurologic reactions** have occurred following VV administration. Reports for 193 such reactions were registered with VAERS during the first five years after licensure. Bell's palsy, a partial facial paralysis, occurred in 15 patients. Another 15 patients developed demyelinating syndromes including Guillain-Barré syndrome, transverse myelitis, and encephalomyelitis. Convulsions were recorded in 163 reports. "In 25 reports, patients with no prior seizure history received only varicella vaccine and had no evident pathology to account for convulsions" (Wise *et al.*, 2000).

> A 16-year-old boy had an absence seizure three days after receiving a varicella vaccine. He had no previous history of seizures. One month later he received his second dose of VV and experienced two generalized tonic-clonic seizures.

This case seems to confirm the causal relationship between the vaccine and subsequent convulsions.

Autoimmune reactions following the vaccine included joint pain (45 patients), thrombocytopenia (a decrease in blood platelets with resultant bleeding) (31 patients), and erythema multiforme (a severe and potentially fatal skin lesion consisting of varied eruptions) (46 patients). Two patients developed aplastic anemia two months after VV, which required bone marrow transplantation.

Varicella-zoster virus can be stored in nerve cells after natural chickenpox infection, and cause a recurrence of infection sometime later in the person's life. This subsequent infection is known as *herpes zoster* or *shingles*. It consists of a very painful skin eruption (the Danish term is "Hell's fire"), which may persist for several weeks. Reports of 251 cases of herpes zoster were filed with VAERS subsequent to vaccination.

The most common reaction has been a generalized rash that resembles naturally acquired chickenpox. This eruption occurs in at least 5 to 10 percent of vaccinees (Arbeter, 1986). Such eruptions have spread to susceptible contacts of vaccinees. In studies of vaccinated children with leukemia, 2 to 10 percent of siblings developed varicella vaccine virus eruptions (Gershon, 1984; Gershon, 1986).

No one knows the possible effects of latent vaccine virus stored within the nervous system. Varicella-zoster virus may be a cause of **cancer**. This association has never been proven, though varicella-zoster-infected human cells have transformed mouse cells to cancerous cells in a laboratory setting (Yamanishi *et al.*, 1981) and varicella-zoster virus-infected cells produced cancers when inoculated into hamsters, which also developed viral antibodies (Gelb *et al.*, 1980). Such findings have led reviewers to comment, "Although no clinical association between the virus and cancer in human beings has even been suggested, the remote possibility of such a relation should be considered in planning long-term surveillance of trials of live-virus vaccines" (Weller, 1983). The possible long-term effects of this herpesvirus vaccine remain unknown.

Mass vaccination of children will be a monumental experiment. Once again, we are injecting children with a live virus that can cause encephalitis and has the ability to remain latent for an entire lifetime. This experiment is being conducted on your children, and the proposed goal is saving money from lost parental wages.

CHICKENPOX FACTS

- Chickenpox is a mild disease of childhood; complications of the disease are rare in healthy children.

- Adults almost always have more severe infection than children, and disease complications are more common.

- Long-term efficacy of the vaccine is unknown. Widespread vaccine usage may shift the age distribution of chickenpox from children to adults.

- Adverse reactions are common, and long-term effects of the vaccine are unknown.

A Personal Strategy

Varicella vaccine has questionable usefulness, and introduces a persisting live virus into the body, which has unknown long-term adverse effects. A more sensible strategy is to purposefully expose your children to others who have active chickenpox so that they contract the disease and develop lifelong immunity. By contrast, those children who receive the vaccine may become susceptible to the disease as adults when symptoms are much more severe. Tampering with the immune system in order to save parents' and the corporate world's time and money is patently ridiculous. This is a clear instance of the vaccine industry's desire to sell a product that we do not need.

DIPHTHERIA

Diphtheria is an acute infectious disease caused by a bacterium. The disease is characterized by a sore throat and the development of a membrane that may cover the throat. It can become a dangerous disease if this membrane makes it difficult or impossible to breathe. Complications of diphtheria include (1) myocarditis (infection within the heart), which can lead to heart failure, and (2) transitory paralysis of the limbs, muscles of respiration (sometimes causing death), or muscles of the throat or eye. The incubation period is two to four days.

INCIDENCE

Diphtheria is now an extremely rare disease in the United States. The number of cases has steadily declined during the past century. Between 1900 and 1920 the mortality rate from diphtheria declined by 50 percent, before the widespread use of diphtheria vaccine (Mortimer, 1978). The toxoid vaccine was invented in 1923 and came into widespread use over the next 15 years. Prior to that time, a toxin-antitoxin preparation had been used in more limited settings after its discovery in 1914. During the 1940s, reported diphtheria cases numbered 15,000 to 30,000 per year in the United States. By the 1960s the number of cases declined to 200 to 1,000 per year. And in the 1990s there were 0 to 4 cases per year. Despite the absence of diphtheria from the population during the past twenty years, the vaccine is still given to infants beginning at two months of age, and to adults whenever they receive a "tetanus booster."

VACCINE EFFICACY

There is some question about the effectiveness of diphtheria vaccine. A classic situation occurred in Germany during World War II. When diphtheria vaccination was made mandatory, there was a 17 percent increase in the number of cases and a 600 percent rise in the number of deaths from diphtheria. When the vaccine was stopped at the end of the war, the incidence of diphtheria dramatically declined, despite the poor living conditions and malnutrition. During an epidemic of diphtheria in Chicago during 1969, 25 percent of the cases had been fully vaccinated, and an additional 12 percent showed serologic evidence of full immunity, though they had received less than the full series of shots (Mendelsohn, 1978).

Vaccine Reactions

Diphtheria toxoid is given only in combination with tetanus toxoid, and reactions are therefore impossible to attribute to one or the other vaccine. Reactions that do occur are usually attributed to tetanus because tetanus toxoid, when given alone, causes these reactions also. Early studies of diphtheria toxoid showed that vaccination caused severe local and systemic reactions (fever, muscle aches, fatigue, headaches, and chills). These problems were alleviated by improved manufacturing methods and reduction of the dose of vaccine (Edsall *et al.*, 1954; Myers *et al.*, 1982).

Diphtheria Facts

- Diphtheria is a potentially serious disease, but extremely rare in the United States, with an incidence of less than 4 cases per year.
- The vaccine has questionable effectiveness.
- Long-term effects of the vaccine are unknown.

A Personal Strategy

At the present time this vaccine seems unnecessary due to the low incidence of disease and questionable vaccine efficacy. However, consumers often have difficulty locating a medical facility that stocks tetanus toxoid alone. Persistence may be necessary to find tetanus vaccine without diphtheria, or patients can ask doctors to order a series of tetanus vaccine for their individual use.

FLU

Everyone knows about the flu and the flu vaccine. What people do not know is that flu vaccines are nearly useless in preventing flu, they will cause the flu, and they often result in nervous system damage that can take years for the body to repair. Other nations chuckle at Americans' infatuation with the flu vaccine. The joke would indeed be funny, if it weren't for the damaging effects caused by the vaccine.

The history of the flu vaccine reads like one stumbling fiasco after another. Take an example. Ever wonder how the particular viruses are chosen for next year's vaccine? The answer could be drawn from a 1930s film noir of Shanghai villainy. Scientists kill migrating ducks in Asia, culture the viruses, and put those in next year's vaccine, because they have seen an association between bird and pig viruses and the following year's human flu epidemics. Perhaps this desperate guesswork is responsible for so many years when the flu vaccine's viruses had nothing in common with circulating viruses. According to a CDC report of the 1994–1995 flu season, 87 percent of type A influenza virus samples were not similar to the year's vaccine, and 76 percent of type B virus were not similar to the virus in that year's vaccine. During the 1992–1993 season, 84 percent of samples for the predominant type A virus were not similar to the virus in the vaccine.

Here is a list of the most common side effects of the flu vaccine as stated by the CDC—fever, fatigue, muscle aches, and headache. Sound familiar?

The primary targeted population for flu vaccine is the elderly, yet the vaccine is notoriously ineffective in preventing disease in that population. According to the CDC, the effectiveness of flu vaccine in preventing illness among elderly persons residing in nursing homes is

30–40 percent (CDC, 2001b). Other studies have shown an even lower efficacy of 0–36 percent (averaging 21 percent). The CDC proudly notes that for those elderly persons living outside of nursing homes, flu vaccine is 30–70 percent effective in preventing hospitalization for pneumonia and influenza. Yet the Department of Human and Health Services found that, with or without a flu shot, pneumonia and influenza hospitalization rates for the elderly are less than one percent during the influenza season. Regardless of vaccination status, 99 percent of the elderly recover from the flu without being hospitalized. The ineffectiveness of flu shots in the elderly led the CDC in 2000 to begin recommending the shots for all persons age 50 years and older. The rationale being that one third of Americans have a risk factor or chronic disease that puts them at risk of increased morbidity from the flu.

Annual flu vaccination is recommended for those individuals with asthma and other chronic respiratory and cardiovascular disorders. However, those people with impaired immune systems are the most likely to suffer adverse autoimmune reactions.

Children are the next frontier for the lucrative flu vaccine campaign. Vaccination is currently recommended for children over six months of age with high-risk medical conditions, but is not recommended for healthy children. Experts in the field suggest that parents of children age six months to two years "be informed that their children are at risk for serious complications of influenza, and allowed to make individual informed decisions regarding influenza immunization for their children" (Neuzil *et al.*, 2001). This statement was made by Marie Griffin (and others), the same author who was implicated in the flawed study that supposedly exonerated the pertussis vaccine of nervous system damage. She is also a paid consultant to one of the world's largest vaccine manufacturers, Burroughs Wellcome. The children's market is the next big hope for vaccine campaigners. A 1998 working group began investigations to not only support, but also to "recommend" flu vaccine for young children.

The next big change in flu vaccines will be the introduction of a live intranasal flu vaccine, a dose that is actually sprayed into the nose. This vaccine has already been tested on young children. Live intranasal vaccine was found 93 percent effective in preventing influenza in children age one to six years old (Belshe *et al.*, 1998). Unanswered questions about the live vaccine include the possibility of transmitting other, more dangerous viruses through the vaccine, the possibility of enhanced replication of the attenuated virus in individuals with compromised immune systems, and the possibility of bacterial superinfection if the replicating live virus disrupts nasal membranes (Subbarao, 2000). This vaccine waits in the wings for its chance as the next big gun in the vaccine arsenal aimed at our children.

GUILLAIN-BARRÉ SYNDROME

In 1976 the flu vaccine was dealt a near fatal blow when reports appeared that the vaccine caused Guillain-Barré syndrome (GBS), an autoimmune nervous system reaction characterized by unstable gait, loss of sensation, and loss of muscle control. A mass vaccination program was mounted that year by the US Government, and 45 million Americans received the swine flu vaccine. Statistical studies have confirmed a causal relationship between the vaccine and GBS. During that year the rate of GBS in Ohio was 13.3 per 1,000,000 in vaccine recipients compared to 2.6 per 1,000,000 in nonrecipients (Marks & Halpin, 1980). A follow-up study also showed a significantly increased incidence of GBS during the first 6 weeks following receipt of the vaccine in patients residing in two other states. The rate of GBS was 8.6 per million vaccinees in Michigan and 9.7 per million vaccinees in Minnesota (Safranek *et al.*, 1991). This episode, which became known as the swine flu catastrophe, left doctors extremely reluctant to administer flu vaccine, and shattered the public trust in the flu vaccine campaign.

The association between GBS and flu shots was not unique to the swine flu. Earlier reports had also summarized cases of nervous system disorders occurring soon after the flu vaccine (Flewett & Hoult, 1958; Horner, 1958). More recently, an increased risk for GBS occurring in patients during the six weeks following the flu vaccine was revealed in the 1992–1993 and the 1993–1994 flu seasons (Lasky *et al.*, 1998).

PREGNANCY

One of the most bizarre twists on the flu vaccine saga is the CDC recommendation of 2001 that all pregnant women receive the vaccine in their second or third trimester. This recommendation even has doctors confused, since the vaccine remains a category C drug (unknown risk for pregnancy). No adequate studies have been conducted to monitor safety of the vaccine for mother and fetus. The only studies of adverse effects in pregnancy were conducted in the 1970s (Heinonen *et al.*, 1973; Sumaya & Gibbs, 1979). Some flu vaccines still contain mercury as a preservative, despite a 1998 FDA instruction to remove mercury from all drugs. According to the CDC, two groups are most vulnerable to methylmercury—the fetus and children ages 14 and younger. An article published in the *American Journal of Epidemiology* in 1999 stated, "the greatest susceptibility to methylmercury neurotoxicity occurs during late gestation" (Grandjean *et al.*, 1999). How did CDC committee members determine that flu vaccines were safe for pregnant women? They did not. The committee, despite its own recommendation, states, "additional data are needed to confirm the safety of vaccination during pregnancy" (CDC, 2001b).

FLU FACTS

- Flu vaccine manufacturers are notoriously inaccurate at predicting the appropriate viruses to use in an individual year's vaccine, rendering the vaccine ineffective.

- Flu vaccine is relatively ineffective in those patients most at risk of flu complications.

- The vaccine has caused GBS in recipients during several different flu seasons.

- Those most at risk of flu complications probably share a higher risk of adverse reactions to the flu vaccine as well.

A PERSONAL STRATEGY

Avoid the flu vaccine. Risks are not worth the slim chance of vaccine effectiveness.

HEPATITIS A

Hepatitis A is caused by a virus spread by the fecal-oral route in person-to-person contact or through ingestion of contaminated food or water. In adults the infection has an abrupt onset of symptoms that include fever, tiredness, loss of appetite, abdominal pain, dark urine, and jaundice. Signs and symptoms usually last less than two months, though 10–15 percent of symptomatic cases have prolonged or relapsing disease lasting up to six months (Glikson *et al.*, 1992). Between 11 and 22 percent of symptomatic cases are hospitalized (CDC, 1996), and adults who become ill lose an average of 27 days of work (CDC, 1999b). Virus is shed through the stool, and usually the period of infectivity ends with the onset of jaundice.

Up to 70 percent of children less than six years of age have no symptoms, and often hepatitis A in children goes undetected because infection is not usually accompanied by jaundice. Infants and children, however, are able to shed the virus for up to several months after the onset of illness (Rosenblum *et al.*, 1991). Day-care centers, where diapers are changed, are a frequent source of hepatitis A spread.

Infection with hepatitis A confers lifelong immunity.

INCIDENCE

The Centers for Disease Control reported an average of 25,000 cases of hepatitis A disease each year during the period 1990–2000, although these figures probably reflect substantial under-reporting because of asymptomatic cases (CDC, 2001). One third of cases occur among children less than 15 years of age. Rates of hepatitis A are substantially higher in the western United States (California, Arizona, New Mexico, Oregon, and Washington), and among populations that have frequent contact with persons from countries where hepatitis A is endemic (e.g. Mexico and Central America). The overall incidence of hepatitis A has declined over a period of several decades as a result of improved sanitation and living conditions. Disease rates are highest among ethnic groups with poor living conditions and crowding.

Approximately 50 percent of people with hepatitis A infection do not have a source identified for their infection. In studies where testing of adults' household contacts was performed, 25–40 percent of contacts less than six years of age had evidence of acute hepatitis A infection. Household or sexual contact accounts for 12–26 percent of new hepatitis A infections. International travel is responsible for 4–6 percent of cases, and 11–16 percent of cases occur among children or employees in day-care centers. About a third of the US population has serologic evidence of prior hepatitis A infection (CDC, 1999b).

The prevalence of hepatitis A among children has led to a vaccine campaign targeting children to control outbreaks and to prevent spread among the population.

VACCINE STRATEGY

Hepatitis A vaccine (HAV) was first licensed for use in 1995. This is an inactivated vaccine similar to that used for polio, administered in a two-dose schedule. The vaccine is licensed only for individuals over two years of age. Since children are a major source of disease transmission, they have been targeted for routine vaccination. This would prevent infection in the age group with the highest incidence, eliminate the spread between children and between children and adults, and eventually protect adults since immunity is assumed to be long-lasting. However, this strategy does not target children under two years of age, a large proportion of those in day-care settings.

In 1996 CDC recommendations included vaccinating children living in communities with the highest rates of infection. Recommendations of 1999 stepped up the campaign to include the routine vaccination of children in states, counties, and communities with hepatitis A rates that are twice the 1987–1997 national average or greater (i.e., greater than or equal to 20 cases per 100,000 population), and consideration of routine vaccination in areas with 10–20 cases per

100,000. Others in high-risk situations are also recommended to receive vaccination, including travelers to endemic areas of the world, illegal-drug users, and men who have sex with men (CDC, 1999b).

If HAV is revealed to be as devastating to the immune system of children as HBV, then the current strategy will result in the following trade-off. Thousands of children will experience lifelong immune system damage in order to prevent a disease that usually causes no symptoms in those children who contract hepatitis A. Vaccination of children in an entire state, such as California, will result in untold numbers of adverse reactions in children who would never be exposed to hepatitis A. Previous vaccination strategies have involved going into communities with a high incidence of disease, and vaccinating children (e.g. Alaskan or Asian villages).

A more prudent and far less risky public health strategy for disease prevention would be to identify specific communities with a high incidence of hepatitis A, and target specific improvements in their living conditions.

Vaccine Efficacy

Hepatitis A vaccine was found to be 94 percent effective in protecting against clinical disease in a study conducted in Thailand among approximately 40,000 children 1–16 years of age living in villages that had high rates of hepatitis A (Innis et al., 1994). A study of approximately 1,000 children 2–16 years old in a New York community with a high rate of hepatitis A showed a protective effect against clinical hepatitis A of 100 percent (Werzberger et al., 1992). Both of these studies were double-blind, placebo-controlled, randomized clinical trials.

Long-term effectiveness has not been evaluated for such a recently licensed vaccine. Antibody levels have only been observed over a six-year period (CDC, 1999b). As with other diseases, maintaining adequate levels of immunity may require booster doses of vaccine.

Vaccine Reactions

Reports of adverse reactions are comprised of pre- and post-licensing periods. In prelicensure clinical studies, no serious adverse effects could be attributed to HAV. Prior to the 1995 HAV licensure in the US, an estimated 1.3 million people in Europe and Asia were vaccinated. Reports of serious adverse events included anaphylaxis, Guillain-Barré syndrome, brachial plexus neuropathy, transverse myelitis, multiple sclerosis, encephalopathy, and erythema multiforme (CDC, 1999b). These are the same types of autoimmune reactions common to the vaccine's more familiar cousin, the hepatitis B vaccine (see page 174).

During the period beginning with HAV licensure in 1995 through June 1997, the Vaccine Adverse Event Reporting System (VAERS) received 428 reports of adverse events occurring within 30 days of HAV administration. These reports included neurologic, hematologic, and autoimmune syndromes. Serious events were noted in 93 reports, and 19 of these occurred in people who received only HAV (Niu, 1998).

Like most newly licensed vaccines, adverse event reports trickle into the medical literature and VAERS slowly. As more children receive the vaccine, a more complete picture of vaccine reactions will emerge.

HEPATITIS A FACTS

- Hepatitis A is spread by the fecal-oral route in person-to-person contact or through contaminated food or water.

- Children often spread hepatitis A through communities because they usually have no symptoms of disease, and diaper changing is a common route of transmission to adults.

- International travel and sexual contact are also common sources of exposure to hepatitis A and disease transmission.

- Routine vaccination of children will result in untold numbers of dangerous adverse immune system reactions in individuals who have little likelihood of exposure to a disease caused by poor living conditions.

A Personal Strategy

If you reside in a community with a high incidence of hepatitis A, consider having yourself and your children tested for antibodies to hepatitis A. Those who have adequate antibody levels from previous exposure do not need to receive the vaccine. If you do not have antibodies, then consider getting the vaccine and giving it to your children. Others in high-exposure situations, such as men who have sex with men, may also consider being tested for antibodies. No studies of HAV for prevention of the disease due to sexual contact have been conducted (Koff, 2001).

Always wash hands after changing diapers and using the bathroom to prevent spread of hepatitis A and other diseases contracted by the fecal-oral route. International travelers may consider either the hepatitis A vaccine or IG (Immune Globulin) injection (see Travel, page 265).

HEPATITIS B

Hepatitis B is a viral infection usually acquired during adolescence or adulthood as a result of sexual contact, injection drug use, or occupational or household exposure. The virus is spread through bodily fluids including blood, semen, vaginal secretions, and saliva.

Hepatitis B infection usually goes unnoticed. Acute infection may have no symptoms, or it may be characterized by flu-like symptoms—weakness, loss of appetite, diarrhea, and right upper abdomen pain. Jaundice may accompany these symptoms, with dark urine, light-colored stools, and yellowing of the eyes and skin. Most cases recover fully. In 5 to 10 percent of cases, infection can persist for many years in a chronic form and cause liver damage or liver cancer. In rare cases of acute infections, liver failure may occur with possible coma and death. Approximately 1 to 3 percent of identified hepatitis B cases progress to liver failure.

Infants born to hepatitis-B-infected mothers are at high risk of contracting hepatitis. The risk of an infant acquiring hepatitis depends on the mother's hepatitis B antigen status. Infants who become infected at birth have a 90 percent risk of chronic infection, and up to 25 percent will die of chronic liver disease as adults (Beasley & Hwang, 1984). Children do not commonly contract hepatitis except through family exposure.

Screening pregnant women for HBsAg (hepatitis B surface antigen) will identify those infants at risk of acquiring hepatitis. If a mother is HBsAg negative, then it is extremely unlikely that a child will contract hepatitis B.

INCIDENCE

The Centers for Disease Control reported an average of 11,000 cases of hepatitis B disease each year during the period 1990–2000 (CDC, 2001). Less than 1 percent of hepatitis B cases occur in children younger than 15 years (Alter *et al.*, 1990).

VACCINE STRATEGY

Hepatitis B vaccine (HBV) is given as a three-dose series, beginning as early as the first day of life. However, a two-dose series administered at an interval of six months results in antibody levels similar to the three-dose schedule (Gellin *et al.*, 1997). Prior to the 1991 CDC recommendation for universal vaccination of children beginning at birth, medical providers used the vaccine primarily for the following high-risk groups: people with multiple sex partners, health care workers, populations with a high incidence of hepatitis, users of illicit injectable drugs, etc. This strategy did not lower the incidence of hepatitis B. The failure of the hepatitis vaccine strategy was attributed to the low compliance in high-risk populations (Centers for Disease Control, 1991c).

Not everyone agreed with the idea of preventing hepatitis in teenagers and adults by vaccinating all infants at birth. Parents often saw no reason to vaccinate their child if they knew the mother was not infected with hepatitis. Why not just give the vaccine to infants whose mothers showed a positive blood test for hepatitis antigen? Since hepatitis is not a childhood disease, the expense and the addition of yet another series of shots to the schedule of vaccines made little sense. Many physicians agreed. Following the CDC recommendation in 1991 that all infants receive hepatitis vaccine, only 32 percent of pediatricians in North Carolina responding to a survey questionnaire thought the vaccine was warranted for all newborns (Freed *et al.*, 1993). A study to determine whether family practitioners agreed with the new recommendation found similar results (Freed *et al.*, 1993a).

The new policy came under fire for a variety of reasons. The expense of such a project seemed less than cost-effective. Family physicians argued, "Given that 4 million infants are born in this country each year, a universal vaccination program costing only $50 per infant will cost $200 million each year. Since the majority of the program's effect will not be seen for 15–20 years, the nation will spend $3 to $4 billion before a significant effect on hepatitis B is seen" (Ganiats *et al.,* 1993). Targeting high-risk infants and teenagers, it is argued, would provide more immediate and cost-effective protection.

Several authors have pointed out the absurdity of vaccinating infants to protect them from a disease of adulthood, since the protective effect of the vaccine decreases significantly over time. When addressing the question of persistent immunity after hepatitis B vaccination, the American Academy of Pediatrics Committee on Infectious Disease members casually remarked that "immunologic memory . . . persists for at least 10 years in normal adults and infants" (Hall & Halsey, 1992). Yet several studies report consistent declines in hepatitis B antibody. One study found that only 52 percent of vaccinees maintained antibody levels above the recommended level after 4 years (Pasko & Beam, 1990). Another study produced similar findings showing that over 60 percent of vaccine recipients had sub-protective levels 4.5 years after vaccination (Street *et al.,* 1990). The CDC recommendations statement admits that "follow-up studies of children vaccinated at birth to prevent perinatal HBV infection have shown that a continued high level of protection from chronic HBV infections persists at least 5 years" (Centers for Disease Control, 1991c).

If protection from the vaccine only lasts 5 years, and hepatitis is a disease of adults, what is the point of vaccinating children? The point is selling more vaccine. Vaccinated infants obviously will need a booster at adolescence. How much more vaccine will be sold if everyone were vaccinated twice? The CDC statement affirms that booster doses of vaccine are not recommended, but then admits, "the possible need for booster doses will be assessed as additional information becomes available." Many critics ask, "Why not just vaccinate the adolescents?"

Vaccine policy officials had given up on vaccinating adolescents. The American Academy of Pediatrics Committee on Infectious Disease decided to vaccinate infants because "achieving adequate coverage and compliance [in adolescents] was thought to be problematic"

(Hall & Halsey, 1992). The logic in this argument has been questioned by other physicians: "What about the CDC's argument that teenagers are too hard to vaccinate? Would you really implement a childhood vaccination program that may not work when needed just because the program is convenient?" (Ganiats *et al.,* 1993). If you can't get adolescents to take the primary series, what makes anyone think they will accept a booster?

Nonetheless, the program to vaccinate all children beginning at birth continues. The vaccine campaign of infants began in 1991. Each child now receives three doses of vaccine. In 2020 these children will be adults. Then we may have some follow-up to see if the strategy worked. In the meantime, the cost of giving these vaccines remains enormous in terms of financial commitment and adverse effects.

VACCINE EFFICACY

How effective is the hepatitis B vaccine? Two different types of vaccines have been developed. A plasma-derived vaccine was licensed by the FDA in 1981 and subsequently abandoned because of fears that vaccine obtained from human serum could transmit unrecognized viruses, particularly HIV (Institute of Medicine, 1994). The first synthetic recombinant vaccines were licensed in 1986. Adequate antibody levels are achieved in 95 percent of vaccine recipients, and the vaccine is assumed to be close to 95 percent effective in preventing HBV infection and clinical hepatitis (Koff, 2001).

Different individuals mount different levels of antibody response to the vaccine, and then these antibody levels steadily decline. It is generally assumed, based on study results, that immunity persists for 5 to 9 years following the three-dose series of vaccine (Stevens *et al.,* 1992). Some of these studies may be methodologically flawed because of inadequate follow-up, but it is clear that the vaccine does protect individuals at risk, including children born to hepatitis antigen-positive mothers (Lo *et al.,* 1988) and men who have sex with men (Hadler *et al.,* 1986), at least on a short-term basis.

It is not surprising to find reports of vaccine failure sprinkled throughout the medical literature. For example, a 26-year-old man suffered acute hepatitis B infection 2 years after full HBV vaccination

(Ballinger & Clark, 1994). A 60-year-old woman on hemodialysis received a kidney transplant 18 months after vaccination with HBV. Six months later she developed hepatitis B. Similarly, a 37-year-old woman contracted hepatitis B five months after receiving a kidney transplant, despite vaccination with HBV one year prior (Goffin *et al.*, 1995).

Hepatitis vaccine has only been available for a relatively short period of time. It is probable that declining levels of antibody in vaccine recipients and continued reports of vaccine failure will result in future recommendations for repeated booster doses with unknown effectiveness, even though experts now decline to recommend booster vaccinations (Hall, 1993).

VACCINE REACTIONS

The viral vaccines seem to be the most dangerous and reactive. Hepatitis B vaccine has built a dramatic reputation for devastating adverse reactions. Studies and case reports have consistently identified Guillain-Barré syndrome, arthritis, demyelinating nervous system disease, and anaphylaxis as reactions to hepatitis B vaccines. In recent years, associations have also been made between HBV and diabetes, as well multiple sclerosis.

During the period July 1990 through October 1998 nearly 25,000 HBV adverse events were reported to VAERS. Over 17,000 of these reports were in individuals who received only HBV without other vaccines. Nearly 6,000 were reports of serious events, including 146 deaths. More than 2,000 adverse events, including 1,200 serious events, were reported for children under age 14 after receiving HBV.

Death in newborns following HBV occurred in 18 reports to VAERS during the period 1991–1998. The mean age of these babies was 12 days. The median time from vaccination to onset of symptoms was two days. The median time from onset of symptoms to death was 0 days. Twelve of these 18 cases revealed no obvious cause of death upon autopsy, and were therefore recorded as death from SIDS (Niu *et al.*, 1999).

A peculiar reaction to the hepatitis B vaccine is massive hair loss. In a review of 60 case reports of sudden unexpected hair loss associated with vaccines between the years 1983 and 1995, 46 had received the hepatitis B vaccine. Hair loss occurred after revaccination in 16 of these cases, confirming the cause as the hepatitis B vaccine. Severe hair loss including more than half of the head, the eyebrows, and eyelashes occurred in 16 of 37 cases that could be evaluated through follow-up phone interviews. Most cases recovered, but four reported persistent baldness (Wise *et al.*, 1997).

A disturbing number of reported **autoimmune reactions** have occurred following vaccination with HBV. A 39-year-old woman developed jaundice, loss of appetite, tiredness, and vomiting four weeks after receiving her first dose of recombinant HBV. Antibodies to DNA were detected on blood testing. She recovered within four months (Lilic & Ghosh, 1994). A 43-year-old woman developed swelling of both legs two weeks after a first dose of HBV. Laboratory tests were consistent with systemic lupus erythematosus (Tudela *et al.*, 1992). Two cases of **thrombocytopenic purpura**, another suspected autoimmune phenomenon that causes bleeding into the skin, mucous membranes, and other organs due to decreased blood platelets required for clotting, were reported in the same issue of *Lancet*. A 15-year-old girl developed isolated purpura four weeks after receiving the third dose of HBV. A 21-year-old woman developed purpura and an enlarged spleen three weeks after receiving the second dose of HBV (Poullin & Gabriel, 1994). A 33-year-old man developed acute abdominal pain, multiple inflamed joints in his hands and feet, chills, and fever two days after HBV vaccination. Blood tests showed decreased platelets and anemia caused by an autoimmune mechanism (Martinez & Domingo, 1992). This combination of hemolytic anemia and thrombocytopenia in the same patient is extremely unusual. In Canada, 30 self-reported cases of chronic fatigue syndrome (CFS) were alleged to be associated with HBV. No cause-effect relationship was determined (Report, 1993).

Cases of **Guillain-Barré syndrome (GBS)**, another autoimmune phenomenon, following HBV were identified in a large surveillance study of 850,000 vaccine recipients during the three-year period 1982 to 1985. This study identified nine cases of GBS that occurred within seven weeks of a hepatitis B vaccine dose (Shaw *et al.*, 1988). The rate of GBS incidence in the vaccine group proved to be significantly higher than the background incidence in the general population. Several isolated cases of GBS following hepatitis B vaccine have been reported in the medical literature (Ribera & Dutka, 1983; Morris & Butler, 1992). Fourteen cases of GBS were reported to the Vaccine Adverse Event Reporting System (VAERS) during 1990 to 1992 (Institute of Medicine, 1994). Despite these studies and reported cases, the Vaccine Safety Committee declined to recognize a causal relationship between hepatitis B vaccine and GBS (Institute of Medicine, 1994).

Many cases of other **central nervous system demyelinating diseases** following HBV have been reported as well. A 28-year-old woman developed muscular weakness and partial paralysis six weeks after receiving HBV. A diagnostic MRI revealed hyperintense lesions in the white matter of the left cerebral hemisphere, indicating multiple sclerosis. A follow-up MRI revealed extension of this lesion, and an additional area of demyelination. At three months she remained partially paralyzed (Herroelen *et al.*, 1992). A 26-year-old woman with a previous history of relapsing multiple sclerosis and complete recovery after these episodes received the HBV vaccine. Six weeks later she had a recurrence of multiple sclerosis symptoms, but this time the symptoms did not improve. Four years later she continued to suffer from partial paralysis (Herroelen *et al.*, 1992). An 11-year-old girl developed headache, back pain, leg weakness, and urine retention three weeks after a hepatitis vaccine injection. Her muscle weakness of the legs improved, but she was left with apparently permanent inability to normally empty her bladder (Trevisani *et al.*, 1993). Two cases of multiple sclerosis were reported to the Institute of Medicine in 32-year-old and 37-year-old women who developed symptoms three and two weeks following HBV (Waisbren, 1992). Fourteen additional cases of demyelinating disease were reported in VAERS prior to 1994 (Institute of Medicine, 1994). Needless to say, the Vaccine Safety Committee refused to recognize a causal relationship between HBV and any demyelinating disease.

A study published in 1999 followed eight patients over a period of 18 months who demonstrated central nervous system inflammation occurring less than 10 weeks after HBV. These authors determined that persistent inflammatory activity evident on MRI studies was comparable with that usually observed in multiple sclerosis (Tourbah *et al.*, 1999). In October 1998, France became the first country to stop hepatitis B vaccination requirements for schoolchildren after reports of chronic arthritis, symptoms resembling multiple sclerosis, and other serious health problems following hepatitis B vaccination became so numerous that the Health Minister of France suspended the school requirement. A French court ruled that there was sufficient evidence to conclude there was a connection between a vaccine produced by British drug maker SmithKline Beecham and multiple sclerosis symptoms. The French government consequently compensated three recipients of hepatitis B vaccine for their development of MS.

An association has been made between the rising incidence of **diabetes** in children and the hepatitis B vaccine. Christchurch, New Zealand, has the only existing diabetes registry in the country. A massive hepatitis B vaccination program began in 1988, and over 70 percent of children in Christchurch were vaccinated (Classen, 1996). The annual incidence of type–1 diabetes in persons 0–19 years of age rose from 11 cases/100,000 in 1982–1987 (preceding the vaccine) to 18 cases in 1989–1991, a 60 percent increase (Classen, 1996; Classen, 1997). Dr. Bart Classen has postulated that the most likely mechanism for the onset of diabetes after vaccination is the release of interferons, since vaccines can cause the release of interferons that produce autoimmune reactions including diabetes (Huang *et al.*, 1995; Stewart *et al.*, 1993).

Since the publication of these findings, a follow-up study failed to show any association between vaccination and diabetes (DeStefano *et al.*, 2001); however, the fact that the onset of diabetes may occur several years after vaccination could explain the lack of a clear correlation. Long-term reactions and delayed reactions are difficult to study for this very reason. Classen has suggested that it may take up to four years to develop diabetes following the insult of vaccination. A vaccine assault will destroy some percentage of pancreatic islet cells, and it may take several such assaults by vaccines or other agents to deplete the ability of the pancreas to produce insulin (Classen, 1996a).

Italian researchers presented findings at the American Diabetes Association annual meeting in 2000 that suggest HBV does have an association with type 1 diabetes in children. To assess the risk of developing type 1 diabetes in children after HBV vaccination, 400,000 children vaccinated at age 12 were compared to an unvaccinated group. Children vaccinated with HBV had a diabetes rate of 17.8 per 100,000 compared to 6.9 per 100,000 in the unvaccinated. For 150,000 children vaccinated at age three months, the rate of diabetes was 46 per 100,000 in the vaccinated group compared to 34 per 100,000 in the unvaccinated (Moyer, 2000).

Arthritis following hepatitis vaccine is another well-recognized phenomenon. The 1994 IOM report noted that the Vaccine Adverse Event Reporting System (VAERS) had received 57 well-documented reports of arthritis developing within two months after receipt of HBV between 1990 and 1992 (Institute of Medicine, 1994). Other reports have appeared in the literature as well. A 15-year-old girl developed severe pain, swelling, and redness in her left knee, which spread to the right knee, ankles, and jaw. Six months later, at the time of the report, arthritis still persisted in her knee (Gross *et al.,* 1994). A 20-year-old woman experienced pain and swelling of her right wrist and fingers four days after a hepatitis vaccination. The pain and swelling resolved, but returned again six months later with more severe swelling and pain following a second hepatitis vaccination. Nine years later, X-ray of the hands showed erosive destruction throughout her wrist joints (Gross *et al.,* 1994). A 19-year-old man developed sudden left-ankle arthritis two weeks after receiving HBV. Symptoms resolved until he received a second HBV dose and developed swelling of his right knee and left ankle. On blood tests, HLA-B27 antigen was found, which confirmed his diagnosis of reactive arthritis (Hachulla *et al.,* 1990). A 49-year-old woman developed arthritis of her hands within 24 hours of her first HBV vaccination. Her symptoms progressed, with pain and stiffness of wrists, hands, and ankles. Blood tests revealed an elevated RF (rheumatic factor) titre, confirming her diagnosis of rheumatoid arthritis (Vautier & Carty, 1994). A 41-year-old nurse developed migratory arthritis two weeks after receiving a single dose of HBV vaccine. Symptoms persisted for seven months (Hassan & Oldham, 1994). Despite the large number of cases submitted to the Vaccine Safety Committee, they have refused to acknowledge that HBV vaccination causes arthritis.

Eighteen cases of **anaphylaxis** were reported in VAERS between 1990 and 1992. Five of these were well-documented reactions that met the Vaccine Safety Committee's strict definitions of anaphylaxis. Others included "anaphylactic-type reactions (cardiovascular collapse associated with wheezing)," that either did not occur within 4 hours of vaccination or had no recording of low blood pressure accompanying the report.

HEPATITIS B FACTS

- Hepatitis B is primarily a sexually transmitted disease. Other common sources of transmission include exposure to infected blood, injected-drug use, and occupational or household contacts.

- Infants can contract hepatitis B from their infected mothers.

- Women can be tested during pregnancy to determine if they are infected, and infants born to infected mothers can receive hepatitis B vaccine and hepatitis immune globulin at birth.

- Only those children exposed to infected mothers are at risk. Antibody levels produced by vaccination will probably decline to non-protective levels before children reach the age when they are sexually active or exposed to other risk factors.

- Hepatitis B vaccine has been associated with severe, debilitating, and life-threatening adverse reactions.

A Personal Strategy

If a child's mother is hepatitis antigen-positive, then parents may choose to give hepatitis vaccine soon after birth, accompanied by hepatitis immune globulin. Other infants do not need protection. There is no reason for parents to consider hepatitis B vaccine until children are sexually active. Adolescents should be counseled concerning risk factors for hepatitis B, including sexual activity, exposure to blood products, and intravenous-drug use. Adolescents, their parents, and adults can choose whether the risk of acquiring hepatitis B seems greater than the risk of reactions to the vaccine, some of which are known and others possibly yet to be discovered. Safe sex practices (including condoms) will prevent most sexually transmitted diseases, including hepatitis A, B, and C. For individuals at high risk, including those with multiple sex partners, or exposure to blood in health care settings, vaccination with hepatitis B may be prudent.

LYME DISEASE

Lyme disease is contracted from the bite of an infected tick. Only one species of tick, the Ixodes, carries the spirochete *Borrelia burgdorferi* that can infect humans. These ticks are most prevalent in the northeastern United States, but occur in other areas of the country as well. Between 15 and 30 percent of Ixodes ticks in the most problematic areas are infected. Human infection is unlikely to occur before 36 hours of tick attachment, so daily checks for ticks and prompt removal will help prevent infections. Other measures of prevention include tucking pants into socks or boots, and applying insect repellents to clothing.

Lyme disease derives its name from the town in Connecticut where it was first identified. Symptoms usually begin with a characteristic solitary rash and generalized feelings of malaise, headache, muscle aches, and joint pain, though some infected individuals have no specific symptoms. The incubation period is typically 7–14 days from onset of infection to appearance of the rash. Some days to weeks after appearance of the rash the disease can spread and affect the nervous system, musculoskeletal system, or rarely the heart. The symptoms of this stage include meningitis, nerve palsies, and joint or muscle pain. The final stage, which can occur weeks to months after infection, includes swelling and pain in the large, weight-bearing joints (e.g. the knee).

Diagnosis is accomplished by observation of symptoms and a blood test. Standard treatment includes a regimen of antibiotics. Approximately 12,000 cases of Lyme disease are reported each year to the CDC.

Lyme Vaccine

A vaccine was licensed for prevention of Lyme disease in December 1998 in individuals 15 to 70 years of age. The vaccine has not been evaluated in children under 15, or in pregnant women. The vaccine's effectiveness decreases in elderly people. Three doses of vaccine are required for protection (at 0, 1, and 12 months), which does not reach optimal levels until 12 months following the first dose. According to the CDC recommendations, the vaccine "should be considered" for people who engage in activities that result in frequent or prolonged exposure to tick-infested habitat, and "may be considered" for people whose exposure is neither frequent nor prolonged. Exposure generally means hiking through the woods or performing property maintenance in tick-infested areas. Since antibody levels decline rapidly, booster doses may be needed every 1–2 years, but the safety of booster doses is unknown (Rahn, 2001). In 2002, however, production of the vaccine was stopped by the manufacturer as reports of severe vaccine reactions accumulated.

Vaccine Reactions

More than 1,000 reports of adverse events in people who received the vaccine were reported to VAERS from December 1998 through October 2000. Of these, 133 reported arthritis, 13 cases reported facial paralysis, and 37 were possible allergic reactions.

The vaccine's safety has been questioned in a class action lawsuit against the vaccine's manufacturer, SmithKline Beecham (Cassidy v. SmithKline Beecham, No. 99-10423, *www.sheller.com/complaint.htm*). More than 350 people claiming harm from the vaccine are represented in the suit. At least four lawsuits were also filed by people who had participated in the vaccine trials. One case was settled for an undisclosed amount. The class action suit alleges that the vaccine stimulates an autoimmune reaction that results in treatment-resistant arthritis. The problem stems from similarity between a bacterial protein and a protein found on human blood cells. The main bacterial protein used in the vaccine stimulates antibodies that fight off future invasion by the Lyme bacteria; however, those same antibodies can also attack the body's own cells. This human protein is present in 30 percent of the population. The lawsuit alleges that SmithKline knew about the similar protein, yet did not warn vaccine recipients to get a blood test that can identify who will be at risk from the vaccine. The lead researcher for the SmithKline vaccine, Dr. Allan Steere, had published a paper in *Science* six months before the vaccine was approved, which showed that the body's immune system might mistakenly attack its own cells in those people with the similar protein (Gross *et al.*, 1998). In a study of hamsters, 100 percent of those that received the vaccine developed "severe destructive Lyme arthritis" when infected with Lyme bacteria. By comparison, none of the unvaccinated hamsters developed higher than normal levels of arthritis typical of hamsters with Lyme disease. Those authors concluded that the human vaccine should be modified to eliminate the protein responsible for the autoimmune reaction (Croke *et al.*, 2000).

Here are the words of one participant from the Lyme vaccine trials conducted in 1994.

> I became ill three days after the second injection, and contacted the study people as they had required participants to do. I was dismissed as having the flu. . . . This was in December 1994, and I have never had a "well" day since. By the summer of 1995, I required knee surgery and . . . the doctor who performed the surgery informed me he found Lyme spirochetes in my synovial fluid. . . . At my surgeon's urging, I found a doctor willing to treat me for Lyme and a lawyer willing to take on the drug company. . . . I was on IV antibiotics for two years during which time I had surgery on my other knee and stopped working because I was required to use a wheelchair. . . . I still get letters almost weekly from new vaccine sufferers asking me to give them some encouragement. I have none. My last bone scan showed both ankles, knees, shoulders, and wrists are completely destroyed by inflammatory disease. An MRI of my back indicated I have the spine of an 80-year-old (I am 47).
>
> A.E.S., July 8, 2001

In the face of multiple lawsuits and plummeting sales of the vaccine, GlaxoSmithKline stopped production of Lyme disease vaccine in February 2002. The pharmaceutical giant also withdrew an application with regulators to market a pediatric version, and the company has halted all research into Lyme disease.

Lyme Disease Facts

- Lyme disease is transmitted to humans from ticks that carry the bacteria, although ticks attached to the skin for less than 36 hours are less likely to infect those bitten.
- Lyme disease is usually treatable with antibiotics.
- The vaccine may be capable of causing persistent arthritis that is treatment-resistant in recipients who possess a protein similar to the protein of the vaccine.
- In response to lawsuits and minimal demand for the vaccine, the manufacturer, GlaxoSmithKline, ceased production of the vaccine.

A Personal Strategy

Those individuals who decide to receive a Lyme disease vaccine series should first obtain a blood test to determine if they are positive for HLA-DR4 (approximately $400). This is the cell-surface protein that is similar to the bacterial protein in the vaccine that could be responsible for autoimmune reactions and persistent arthritis.

As an alternative to vaccination, those who hike or work in wooded areas should take precautions against tick bites. Tuck pants into socks or boot tops. Apply DEET or a permethrin insecticide to clothing. Wear long-sleeved shirts. Check the skin for ticks on a daily basis, and remove ticks promptly by grasping the tick's body with a tweezers and slowly pulling straight out of the skin without twisting.

MENINGITIS VACCINES

Three types of vaccines are licensed for the prevention of bacterial meningitis and other forms of invasive disease caused by these bacteria: *Haemophilus influenzae* type B (Hib), a meningococcal vaccine, and a pneumococcal vaccine. Only the Hib and pneumococcal vaccine are recommended for routine use in children. Invasive disease refers to the invasion of usually sterile sites in the body by pathogens, specifically the blood and the nervous system.

Haemophilus Influenzae Type B (Hib) Meningitis

Haemophilus influenzae bacterial infections occur frequently in childhood, accounting for a large percentage of common sinus, throat, and ear infections. They usually resolve on their own without treatment. However, one strain of Haemophilus, the type b encapsulated strain, is capable of causing invasion of infections to deeper levels in the body, particularly the spinal fluid, lungs, heart, and blood. Vaccines have been developed because Haemophilus can cause meningitis, pneumonia, epiglottitis, and other complications. The bacteria has no relationship to influenza. It was named *influenzae* because early researchers found the bacteria in people with flu, but did not recognize until later that Haemophilus is a normal resident of mucous membranes.

Meningitis in children often begins with flu-like symptoms including fever, headache, nausea and vomiting, tiredness, and irritability. This may be followed by a change in alertness, stiff neck, and seizures. Between 20 and 30 percent of children with bacterial meningitis have seizures. Arthritis, pericarditis, and pneumonia are common complications (Kaplan & Fishman, 1988). Disease of sudden onset with rapid progression is usually associated with a different bacteria, *Neisseria meningitidis,* which has a much higher risk of death. A sudden change in level of alertness or severe headache in children is cause for concern.

Mortality from Hib meningitis is 3 to 8 percent (Sell, 1987). Sensorineural (permanent) hearing loss occurs in approximately 10 percent of meningitis cases (Dodge *et al.,* 1984), though this is most common with pneumococcal meningitis. Appropriate treatment of Hib meningitis includes the use of a cephalosporin (or other) antibiotic, administered intravenously.

Several studies have observed long-term cognitive effects of previous *Haemophilus influenzae* meningitis on children. Most recent studies have found no differences in IQ scores or academic success of children with a history of meningitis compared to their sibling controls (Tejani *et al.,* 1982; Feldman & Michaels, 1988; R.D. Feigin & P.R. Dodge, unpublished data). But several previously conducted studies did find that learning disabilities, reading problems, and lower IQ scores occurred more frequently in postmeningitic children compared to randomly selected peer-group controls (Sell *et al.,* 1972; Pate, 1972). This may indicate that Hib meningitis is associated with learning problems, but the validity of this association is still in question.

INCIDENCE

The estimated incidence of Hib meningitis was about 12,000 cases per year prior to the licensing of Hib vaccines, plus an additional 7,500 cases of invasive disease (lungs, heart, etc.). Prior to the Hib vaccine, approximately 1 in 350 children younger than 5 years of age developed Hib meningitis (Sell, 1987). In 1995, five years after the vaccine became available for infants, the total reported incidence of invasive disease was 1,300 cases (Bisgard *et al.,* 1998). This 98 percent reduction in Hib invasive disease has been attributed to the vaccine campaign.

Native American and Eskimo children are particularly susceptible to Hib meningitis. Incidence had increased over the three decades preceding vaccine availability. Some observers associated this increase with the administration of other vaccines and their apparent ability to impair immune system resistance. Sporadic outbreaks of invasive Hib disease have continued to occur in Eskimo children despite nearly universal vaccination. In 1996–1997, ten cases of invasive Hib disease occurred in Alaska Native children, compared to only nine total cases in the preceding five-year period (Galil *et al.*, 1999).

Children under 6 months are protected by maternal antibodies, and breastfeeding reduces incidence rates (Istre *et al.*, 1985; Cochi *et al.*, 1986). The peak incidence of meningitis occurs in children 6 to 7 months of age. The attack rate decreases rapidly with increasing age. Fifty percent of cases occur in infants under 1 year of age. Only 25 to 30 percent of cases occur in children over 18 months old (Broome, 1987).

The congregation of infants in day-care settings creates a significantly higher risk of infection (Istre *et al.*, 1985; Cochi *et al.*, 1986; Fleming *et al.*, 1985). In one study, 50 percent of all invasive disease caused by *H. influenzae* type b was attributable to day-care settings (Cochi *et al.*, 1986). In these studies more of the children with Hib had attended day-care than children without the disease. Later studies attempting to show the transmission of Hib in day-care settings did not reveal a pattern of disease spread between children. Two studies failed to find cases of *H. influenzae* invasive disease in contacts of children with primary infections in day-care settings (Osterholm *et al.*, 1987; Murphy *et al.*, 1987).

Perhaps the increased incidence among infants attending day-care has more to do with those infants who do not breastfeed. The protective effect of breastfeeding on Hib meningitis in infants is well known (Cochi *et al.*, 1986). Infants who breastfeed for an extended period of time (longer than three months) have a decreased incidence of *Haemophilus influenzae* meningitis compared to infants who breastfeed for a shorter duration. The longer the duration of breastfeeding, the lower the risk of meningitis. The risk decreases for each additional week of breastfeeding (Silfverdal *et al.*, 1997). The protective effect of breastfeeding on meningitis persists for many years. Infants who are breastfed have a decreased incidence of Haemophilus meningitis even five to ten years later (Silfverdal *et al.*, 1999).

Several different *Haemophilus influenzae* type b (Hib) vaccines are manufactured. The quality of efficacy studies varies, and the findings can only be applied to the specific form of the vaccine being evaluated.

In 1985 the first Hib vaccine, a purified form of the polysaccharide capsule (called PRP, from the chemical name of the capsular substance), was licensed. The PRP vaccine was not effective in children under 24 months old, and these children represented 80 percent of Hib meningitis cases (Ward, 1987). The development of the vaccine was enthusiastically heralded as a great step in prevention of Hib invasive disease, but hopes for its success were soon dashed.

The effectiveness of the PRP vaccine was called into question by a case-control study published in the *Journal of the American Medical Association*. This study found that 41 percent of Hib cases occurred in vaccinated children. The vaccine's protective efficacy was minus 58 percent. In other words, children were much more likely to get the disease if they had received the vaccine (Osterholm *et al.*, 1988). Apparently the vaccine had lowered their resistance and created an environment that encouraged the spread of the disease to the nervous system. This is precisely what one would predict if the vaccines do suppress immune system function.

In other studies, vaccine efficacy ranged from 41 to 88 percent. An active surveillance study which included a population of 2.5 million children under five years of age identified 1,444 cases of invasive Hib disease. Vaccine efficacy in this group was found to be 62 percent compared to controls—again a much lower figure than expected by researchers (Harrison *et al.*, 1989). As improved forms of vaccine were developed, the PRP vaccine was abandoned.

Vaccine researchers found that when the PRP form of the vaccine was joined to a protein carrier, then the vaccine was more effective, and developed antibody responses in younger children. These "conjugated" forms are now used beginning in infancy. In 1990, the first conjugate vaccines were licensed for use beginning at two months of age.

Evaluating the efficacy of the conjugate vaccines has been complicated by the different versions of protein carriers studied in varied populations with several different types of study methods. The technology of conjugate vaccines has developed rapidly over a short period of time. Several conjugate vaccines have been rushed through licensure, some with only one or two efficacy trials. The field trials evaluating the PRP-T conjugate vaccine in 5,200 infants were terminated early because another Hib vaccine was licensed during the study period, and all controls subsequently received the new Hib vaccine (Vadheim *et al.*, 1993). PRP-T was licensed nonetheless, despite the findings in this study that PRP-T vaccine caused a higher incidence of seizures, crying, and high fevers than the control vaccines in these children (Vadheim *et al.*, 1993).

The dismal failure of the previous unconjugated PRP vaccine spurred the adoption of the newer conjugate versions, sometimes with only one or two efficacy trials. The effectiveness of the various conjugate vaccines as measured in these studies has varied. For example, the PRP-D conjugate vaccine showed an efficacy of 74 to 96 percent in various studies (Centers for Disease Control, 1993), but in a study of Alaskan Natives the efficacy was only 35 percent, indicating that it did not confer immunity. The vaccine proved entirely ineffective in either stimulating protective antibody levels or preventing Hib disease in these infants (Ward *et al.*, 1990). The authors eliminated the possibility that genetic factors played a role in this vaccine failure because they detected no differences in genetic markers that could distinguish susceptibility to Hib disease in Alaskan Natives compared to controls (Petersen *et al.*, 1987). They concluded, "The findings of this study indicate that three doses of PRP-D vaccine induce marginal immune responses in young infants, and in infants at high risk three doses fail to provide significant protection. The most likely reason for these results is an intrinsic limitation in the immunogenicity of the PRP-D vaccine, at least in young infants" (Ward *et al.*, 1990).

In another study, 90 percent of children vaccinated with the PRP-D conjugate vaccine responded with antibody levels considered to be protective, but only 60 percent produced levels of antibody indicating long-term protection (Berkowitz *et al.*, 1987). Nonetheless, millions of children are vaccinated with PRP-D. Other conjugate vaccines (PRP-OMP and HbOC) have shown high levels of efficacy in the few trials conducted. One study of the PRP-OMP conjugate vaccine showed a 93 percent efficacy (Santosham *et al.*, 1991). The HbOC vaccine was evaluated in two studies that showed a 100 percent (Black *et al.*, 1990) and 97 percent (Eskola *et al.*, 1990) level of efficacy. It must be remembered, however, that these studies were each conducted over a one- or two-year period. The continuing protective effect of Hib vaccines is unknown.

Regardless of the reported efficacy rates of conjugate vaccines, they were quickly credited with a drop in reported cases of Hib-invasive disease, a 98 percent decline since the pre-vaccine era. One report claimed that "Hib disease has been nearly eradicated in a fully immunized population" (children enrolled in a particular HMO health plan). These authors report that the incidence of Hib disease for infants decreased in Los Angeles the year *prior* to the licensure of vaccine for this age group, yet they audaciously attribute this declining incidence of Hib during that year (1990) to the vaccine. They speculated that this decline could be due to less transmission of Hib from older children who *were* vaccinated (Vadheim *et al.*, 1994). The argument that declining disease incidence is caused by the introduction of vaccine in a community may or may not be true. Many epidemiological factors could contribute to the decline of a highly infectious disease.

Similar spectacular results of the Hib vaccine campaign have been claimed in Finland, where over 90 percent of infants are vaccinated. During the 1950s, the incidence of Hib meningitis in greater Helsinki averaged 8 cases per year. This increased to an average of 22 cases per year during the period 1976–1985. After the introduction of Hib vaccine in 1985, the incidence declined to the previous levels of 3–9 cases per year (Peltola *et al.*, 1992). Comparable declines in Hib disease were reported in Minnesota (85 percent decline) and Dallas, Texas (92 percent decline); however, the decline in Dallas Hib cases began prior to the introduction of vaccination, and efficacy studies in Minnesota showed Hib vaccines to be ineffective (Murphy *et al.*, 1993). These figures may merely indicate a peak of Hib meningitis cases in the 1980s that began to decline prior to and coincident with the introduction of Hib vaccination. The celebration of Hib vaccine effectiveness may need to wait for more definitive and long-term studies.

VACCINE REACTIONS

Evaluating reactions to the Hib conjugate vaccines presents problems because Hib vaccines are given together with the DTP vaccines, sometimes in the same shot. Reactions, therefore, could be attributable to any of these four vaccines. The most reliable indications that Hib vaccines cause significant reactions come from field trials where the vaccine is given alone. The withdrawn PRP vaccine caused significant adverse effects including seizures, anaphylactoid allergic reactions, serum sickness-like reactions (joint pain, rashes, and edema), and one death within 4 hours of vaccination. These effects were reviewed in a study of 152 spontaneous reports of vaccine reactions submitted to the FDA during the first year of vaccine availability, 1985–1986 (Milstien *et al.*, 1987). Only reactions to the newer conjugate vaccine are reviewed here.

The most common and potentially significant Hib vaccine reaction has been the **increased incidence of Hib disease** following vaccination. The older PRP vaccine caused Hib disease within the first 7 days following vaccination in children over 18 months of age. This was confirmed in 4 case-control studies conducted in 1988 that all found a 2- to 6-times increased chance of contracting Hib disease in the first week after vaccination compared to controls (Black *et al.*, 1988; Harrison *et al.*, 1988; Osterholm *et al.*, 1988; Shapiro *et al.*, 1988).

The new conjugate vaccines also cause a decline in antibody levels immediately following vaccination (Daum *et al.*, 1989). Ten cases of early Hib disease following vaccination with conjugate vaccines were reported through VAERS between 1990 and 1992. All cases occurred within 5 days of vaccination. Investigators have postulated that increased susceptibility to infection in the immediate post-vaccination period might be related either to a transient decrease in pre-existing antibody or to transient suppression of antibody synthesis (Marchant *et al.*, 1989; Sood & Daum, 1990).

The conjugate vaccines have been associated with the onset of **Guillain-Barré syndrome (GBS)**. Many cases have been reported in the medical literature and through VAERS. Some of these children received other vaccines concurrently, but several cases occurred when the Hib vaccine was given alone. A 4-year-old girl developed progressive weakness of the legs, pain in the legs and feet, and gradual inability to walk 10 days after Hib vaccination. On the fifth day she had swallowing difficulties, facial weakness, and a monotonous voice. Her symptoms gradually improved, and within three weeks she could walk with help (Gervaix *et al.*, 1993). Two cases were reported after PRP-D alone (D'Cruz, 1989), and three cases following the HbOC conjugate vaccine were reported through VAERS prior to 1992 (Institute of Medicine, 1994).

Cases of **transverse myelitis,** a paralyzing disease of the spinal cord, following Hib vaccine have been reported through VAERS. One child developed a 105° temperature, extreme floppiness, and toxic appearance within 24 hours of the HbOC conjugate vaccine given alone. Two other children received HbOC accompanied by DTP and OPV vaccination. One of these children developed persistent paralysis and spinal cord lesions. The other baby was unable to crawl following vaccination. Further details were not presented (Institute of Medicine, 1994).

In a study examining the safety of Hib conjugate vaccine (PRP-T) compared to hepatitis B vaccine, in which all infants were also given DTP, five infants developed **seizures** within 48 hours of vaccination in the PRP-T group, compared to none in the control group (Vadheim *et al.*, 1993). Three additional infants had seizures between 3 and 14 days after Hib vaccination, compared to two infants who received hepatitis B. Two children in the PRP-T group died from possible vaccine reactions. One child developed symptoms of muscle weakness one week after vaccination, which progressed to muscle wasting over the next five months and eventually resulted in death at seven months of age. A second child died at 14 months from central nervous system demyelination, a frequently encountered reaction to vaccines. Since these children all received DTP and OPV concurrently with the Hib vaccine, it is difficult to attribute their reactions to Hib vaccination alone. However, the significant differences in the two groups suggests that the Hib vaccine could have caused these reactions, or potentiated the adverse reaction to DTP.

Thrombocytopenia, a decrease in blood platelets responsible for clotting and consequent spontaneous bleeding, has been reported following Hib conjugate vaccination. Five cases of thrombocytopenia were reported in VAERS between 1990 and 1992 in children who also received DTP or MMR in addition to Hib vaccines (Institute of Medicine, 1994). In an early research study of 15 subjects who received the PRP-D conjugate vaccine, extensive blood testing of vaccine recipients revealed an asymptomatic fall in blood platelet count in one study subject (Granoff *et al.*, 1984). A postmarketing survey of the earlier PRP vaccine revealed three cases of low platelet counts or bleeding into the skin following Hib vaccination (Milstien *et al.*, 1987).

Diabetes has been associated with Hib vaccine in several broad-based population studies. Finland has the highest rate of type-1 (juvenile onset, insulin dependent) diabetes in the world. The incidence of diabetes in children aged 0–4 rose 62 percent between the years 1980–82 and 1990–92 following a widespread Haemophilus influenza vaccine campaign begun in 1986 (Tuomilehto *et al.*, 1995; Classen and Classen, 1997). A later study in Finland compared the effect of four doses of Haemophilus vaccine to 0 doses and noted a relative risk of 1.26 for the onset of diabetes in the vaccinated group compared to those not vaccinated (Classen, 1999; Karvonen *et al.*, 1999). A similar phenomenon occurred in the US. In Allegheny County, Pennsylvania, the Haemophilus vaccine was introduced in 1985. This county has the oldest type-1 diabetes registry in the US. An epidemic of diabetes occurred in the 0–4 age group during the years 1985–1993, following introduction of the vaccine. The annual incidence of diabetes in these children rose 60 percent during the postvaccine years (1985–1989), compared to the prevaccine years (1980–1984) (Dokheel, 1993). This temporal association does not prove a causal relationship, but it is certainly suspicious, especially when considering an identical rise in diabetes following the hepatitis vaccine.

Haemophilus influenzae B (HIB) MENINGITIS FACTS

- Hib meningitis is a potentially life-threatening disease, and long-term sequelae of infections (hearing loss, learning disabilities) occur.

- Long-term effectiveness of the vaccines has not been determined, and reports of short-term effectiveness vary considerably; however the incidence of disease has dramatically declined since the introduction of the vaccines.

- Serious vaccine-associated reactions have been reported.

- Disease is more common in children who attend day-care and less common in infants who breastfeed.

A PERSONAL STRATEGY

This new vaccine, relatively untested and questionably effective, presents a difficult decision for parents. Meningitis is not a mild childhood disease. Haemophilus meningitis was not uncommon prior to widespread use of the vaccine. Parents must make a choice about the Hib vaccine based on a few facts and vague uncertainties about the vaccine.

One issue remains clear: if a child stays home with a parent in the first 12 to 18 months of life, when Hib disease occurs most often, then the likelihood of exposure decreases dramatically compared to a child who attends a large day-care center. Breastfeeding significantly reduces the risk of invasive Hib disease.

Parents should weigh the likelihood of exposure against their feelings about the known adverse effects of Hib vaccine, including the ability of the vaccine to suppress immune system function and cause an increased susceptibility to Hib disease. A parent's philosophy about immune system competence, unknown effects of vaccines, and the politics of vaccine campaign promotion will always enter into the decision process when a new vaccine is marketed for a serious disease.

Meningococcal Vaccine

Neisseria meningitides (Meningococcus) bacteria are responsible for about 2,000 cases of meningitis per year in the US. There are 13 meningococcal serogroups, but serogroups A, B, and C cause 90 percent of disease worldwide, with serogroups B and C responsible for most disease in Europe and the Americas. Approximately 20 percent of all cases occur among children under one year old. The case fatality rate is 10 percent, and another 10–20 percent of cases suffer permanent neurologic symptoms. Those factors that increase the risk of meningococcal disease include patients taking corticosteroids and household crowding. Race and income level were not associated with increased risk (CDC, 2000). Explosive and deadly outbreaks have earned meningococcal meningitis a fearful reputation.

Vaccine Strategy

Vaccine licensed for use in the US contains four serogroups (A, C, Y, and W-135) and is used primarily to control epidemics. No vaccine exists for the B serogroup, which is responsible for more than half the cases in infants less than one year of age. The vaccine is relatively ineffective in children under two years of age. Current recommendations suggest that when three cases of serogroup C meningococcal disease occur in three months or less in a community, mass vaccination of persons two years of age and older should be considered (CDC, 2000). In addition, because of one study published in 1999 that found college freshmen living in dormitories to be at higher risk than other undergraduate students (Bruce *et al.*, 1999), the CDC recommends that parents and college students be informed about possible benefits from the vaccine.

Long-term protection from existing vaccines is unlikely. Among children under four years of age, a single dose of serogroup A vaccine provided clinical protection for less than three years (Reingold *et al.*, 1985). And studies have shown that multiple doses of vaccine result in a decrease in antibody response (Granoff *et al.*, 1998).

Vaccine Reactions

In November 1999 a meningococcal C vaccine was introduced into the routine infant vaccination schedule in the United Kingdom, and immediately ran into a firestorm of controversy. By June 2000, six months after the program's initiation, nearly 5,000 adverse events were reported, including seizures, recurrent blackouts, and severe headaches, amounting to one adverse reaction in every 3,000 recipients. By August 2000, 16,000 adverse reactions had been reported, including 11 deaths. The British paper, *The Observer*, on August 27 accused the British government of a cover-up to hide the safety issues associated with the vaccine. One week later *The Observer* reported the government's admission that four public health officials and medical advisers were paid consultants of the vaccine's manufacturers. *The Times* quickly attempted to reassure the public that none of the reported deaths could be directly attributed to the vaccine, though several were categorized as unexplainable SIDS. Upon the heels of those stories, parents began phoning *The Observer* with reports of their children's severe reactions and collapse following the meningitis vaccine. They also complained of efforts by government officials to keep them from telling their stories.

Vaccine Facts

- Meningococcal serogroups B and C are responsible for most cases of meningitis, but no safe vaccine exists for serogroup B.

- Approximately 10 percent of the 3,000 meningococcal meningitis cases per year are fatal.

- Vaccine probably provides only short-term protection during outbreaks, and cannot be used in anyone under two years of age.

- Routine vaccination is not recommended by the CDC at this time.

A Personal Strategy

The history of dramatic and numerous adverse reactions in the United Kingdom should give anyone pause before allowing vaccination with the highly experimental and expensive meningococcal vaccines.

Pneumococcal Vaccine

Streptococcus pneumonia (Pneumococcus) is a bacterium associated with many cases of meningitis, bacteremia (systemic infection in the bloodstream), pneumonia, and ear infections. At least 10 to 25 percent of all pneumonias culture *S pneumonia* (Williams *et al.*, 1988) and approximately one-quarter of all ear infections in children are associated with *S pneumonia* growth (Bluestone and Klein, 1988). It is estimated that the Pneumococcus causes approximately 17,000 cases of invasive disease each year among children under the age of five years (Poland, 2001). The overall case fatality rate for bacteremia is 15–20 percent. Up to 40 percent of the 6,000 children with pneumococcal meningitis suffer death or disability each year (Baraff *et al.*, 1993).

The rate of invasive disease is highest among children under two and adults over 65 years of age. Black adults have a threefold to fivefold higher overall incidence of pneumococcal bacteremia than whites, and the risk rises at an earlier age (CDC, 1997). Cigarette smoking is the single most important risk factor for the development of invasive disease (Nuorti *et al.*, 2000).

At least 90 serotypes of pneumococcal bacterium are known, and up to one third of all US types demonstrate moderate to high-level resistance to antibiotics (Breiman *et al.*, 1994). Several pneumococcal vaccines exist, incorporating various combinations of serotypes. In 1977, a pneumococcal vaccine was licensed that contained 14 types of *S pneumonia*. This was replaced by a vaccine of 23 types in 1980. These early polysaccharide vaccines met with limited success. A conjugate vaccine that contains the seven serotypes responsible for 80 percent of invasive disease in children was licensed in 2000 for use in infants and children, and is now recommended for use in all infants (CDC, 2000b).

Those recommended for vaccination by the CDC include people over 65 years old and people with chronic illness (such as diabetes, heart disease, emphysema, alcoholism, HIV, chronic liver disease, and immune deficiency diseases). All children under two years of age and children aged two through five years old with an increased risk of pneumococcal infection are also advised to receive a series of pneumococcal vaccine (CDC, 2000b).

Vaccine Efficacy

The pneumococcal vaccine is notoriously ineffective. Many studies have demonstrated a lack of effectiveness in adults (Austrian, 1981; Simberkoff *et al.*, 1986), including studies that failed to demonstrate efficacy in preventing pneumonia in the targeted elderly population (Forrester *et al.*, 1987, Ortqvisdt *et al.*, 1998). Other studies show an effectiveness ranging from 40 to 100 percent. A review of randomized trials revealed that the vaccine has a modest effect in preventing pneumonia among low-risk subjects, and no effect in high-risk subjects (Fine *et al.*, 1994).

A large study of conjugate pneumococcal vaccine involving 38,000 children was conducted at a California HMO. The vaccine, which consists of only seven serotypes, was approximately 95 percent effective in preventing invasive disease, and 33 percent effective in preventing pneumonia (Rennels *et al.*, 1998). However, the vaccine reduced the incidence of ear infections by only six percent. Another study of 1,700 children showed that ear infections caused by one of the pneumococcal serotypes present in the vaccine were reduced by 57 percent, but the vaccine group had 33 percent *more* ear infections caused by non-vaccine serotypes compared to the control group (Kilpi, 2000). Previous studies with the polysaccharide vaccine also showed fewer episodes of ear infections associated with the types of *S pneumonia* present in the vaccine, but children in the vaccine and control groups had the same total number of ear infections (Karma *et al.*, 1980; Makela *et al.*, 1980, 1981; Sloyer *et al.*, 1981; Teele *et al.*, 1981). The use of this pneumococcal vaccine has merely caused a shift in the bacterial types associated with childhood ear infections, as well as a shift in bacterial serotypes that colonize the nose. Researchers have concluded that "since non-vaccine serotypes are already present in the community as the etiology of acute purulent OM [ear infection], it is predictable that these non-vaccine serotypes will become more common especially in children less than two years of age" (Pelton, 2000).

Vaccine Reactions

Early studies of the polysaccharide pneumococcal vaccine reported a higher than expected frequency and severity of both systemic and local adverse reactions in those receiving a second dose (Borgono *et al.*, 1978; Lawrence *et al.*, 1983). One study noted that adverse reactions were more prevalent in those recipients with higher prevaccination antibody levels (Sankilampi *et al.*, 1997). During the HMO trial of the children's conjugate vaccine, the vaccinated group had twice as many seizures within three days of the vaccine compared to the control group. The vaccinated group also had significantly more asthma and gastritis than the control group (Black, 2000).

Pneumococcal Vaccine Facts

- *Streptococcus pneumonia* is associated with a large percentage of ear infections, meningitis, pneumonia, and bacteremia in children, and invasive disease in elderly adults.

- The vaccine is relatively ineffective in adults (it does not prevent pneumonia), but is effective in preventing pneumonia and other invasive disease in children.

- The vaccine does not prevent ear infections.

A Personal Strategy

Like all newly licensed vaccines, the conjugate pneumococcal vaccine for children will only reveal its safety record and adverse reactions once large numbers of children become part of the vaccination campaign. In the meantime, parents cannot be well informed about the risks associated with the vaccine. The widespread use of vaccine may cause shifts in disease pathogens to serotypes not contained in the currently licensed vaccine, thus leaving the overall incidence of problems caused by the bacterial group relatively unchanged.

Elderly patients are not served well by this vaccine because of its ineffectiveness in that age group.

MMR (MEASLES, MUMPS, AND RUBELLA)

Vaccination for these diseases is usually given as a single shot of combined live viruses (the MMR vaccine) at 12 months of age or older. Mass vaccination of children for mumps, measles, and rubella has resulted in a shift in the pattern of these diseases. The age distribution has changed significantly since the vaccines were introduced in the 1960s. Now these are increasingly becoming diseases of adolescents and young adults. This is a problem, since the diseases themselves cause more complications in this older population.

The vaccines seem to have caused atypical forms of the diseases to appear. It should also be remembered that the natural occurrence of each of these viral diseases generally confers permanent immunity against subsequent attacks.

Measles

Measles was a common disease of childhood prior to the widespread use of measles vaccine. The disease is transmitted by a virus that is highly contagious. The symptoms of measles are cold symptoms, cough, irritated eyes, and high fever, with the appearance of a rash on the fourth day of illness. The symptoms, including the rash, reach a climax on about the sixth day and then subside in a few days.

Measles occasionally sets the stage for other diseases. These complications include ear infections, pneumonia, infection of lymph nodes, and encephalitis, but they are not common. In the past, deaths from measles were not uncommon during epidemics. Now the disease has become milder and deaths are rare. Measles is usually a self-limited disease. Encephalitis is reported to occur in one out of 1,000 cases, though this figure is probably exaggerated. Of these encephalitis cases, 25 to 30 percent show manifestations of brain damage.

Orthodox medicine has no specific treatment for measles or measles-associated encephalitis. Homeopaths feel confident about their ability to prevent complications, though no efficacy studies have been conducted.

INCIDENCE

Measles was contracted by most children prior to vaccine licensure. Following the licensing of measles vaccine in 1963, the incidence of measles declined to an average of 3,000 cases per year in the 1980s (Centers for Disease Control, 1994). However, in 1989, a resurgence of measles occurred in the United States, constituting an epidemic that brought levels back up to the 1970s rate of 27,000 reported cases per year. The epidemic continued in 1990, primarily in preschool-age children. In fact, nearly 20 percent of measles cases in 1990 and 1991 occurred in children less than 1 year of age. What did researchers blame for this resurgence of cases in babies? The vaccine. "The cause of the increase in measles cases among children <15 months of age is . . . earlier susceptibility to measles due to transplacental transfer of lesser amounts of measles antibody from young mothers whose measles immunity is from vaccine rather than wild measles virus" (Centers for Disease Control, 1992b). Mothers, in other words, who grew up in the measles vaccine era do not pass antibodies to their babies because immunity from the vaccine disappears over time. Now the shift has occurred from measles as a childhood disease to measles as a disease of adults—and infants born to these adults. Both groups tend to have more complications.

During the late 1990s the incidence of measles again mysteriously decreased. Approximately 100 cases per year occurred between 1997 and 2000 (CDC, 2001).

VACCINE EFFICACY

The vaccine has apparently resulted in a dramatic decline in measles cases. In the light of these promising statistics, a national goal was set to eliminate measles by 1982. Notwithstanding these hopes, reports of epidemics in fully vaccinated populations have appeared periodically and consistently since the vaccine's introduction (Shasby *et al.*, 1977; Weiner *et al.*, 1977; Hull *et al.*, 1985).

A typical example was reported by Dr. Tracy Gustafson and colleagues in the *New England Journal of Medicine*. During the spring of 1985, a measles outbreak occurred in two fully vaccinated secondary-school populations (greater than 99 percent of students vaccinated). On serologic testing, 95 percent of students showed immunity to measles. The epidemic occurred in the remaining 5 percent, all of whom had been "adequately" vaccinated (Gustafson *et al.*, 1987).

Some authors have postulated that a waning immunity over time is responsible for these outbreaks among older children (Shasby *et al.*, 1977). Others blame primary vaccine failure. In any case, the public health goal of eradicating measles in the United States by 1982 was not met, despite rigorous vaccine programs.

Gustafson concluded in 1987 that such a goal is impossible to meet. She was right. In an attempt to counteract the resurgence of measles, CDC announced a two-dose measles schedule (Centers for Disease Control, 1989i), but a new epidemic again foiled the goals for measles eradication. Nonetheless, a new date was set for elimination of measles in 1996 (Centers for Disease Control, 1994c). In frustration, other researchers also admitted that eradication of measles may not be possible since transmission continues to occur in adolescents and adults who have been fully vaccinated. Their understated and plaintive response was, "Measles elimination has proved more difficult than previously predicted" (Hersh *et al.*, 1991).

Measles cases now consistently occur in the vaccinated. A review of measles outbreaks in the United States during 1985–1986 revealed that a median of 60 percent of cases in school-age children occurred in vaccinated individuals (Markowitz *et al.*, 1989). Similarly, a review of 1,600 cases of measles in Quebec, Canada, between January and May 1989 showed that 58 percent of school-age cases had been previously vaccinated (Centers for Disease Control, 1989a). In states with comprehensive (kindergarten through 12th-grade) immunization requirements, between 61 and 90 percent of measles cases occur in persons who were "appropriately" vaccinated (Markowitz *et al.*, 1989).

The official response to measles vaccine failure and epidemics has varied. Within the first ten years after widespread vaccination, the vaccine failures prompted public health authorities to repeatedly raise the recommended age for vaccination. In 1969, the age for vaccine administration was raised to 12 months or older (Albrecht *et al.,* 1977). Because of continued vaccine failure, the age for administration was subsequently raised to 15 months (Centers for Disease Control, 1989b). During 1988, an epidemic in Los Angeles prompted a reconsideration of vaccine recommendations when statistics showed that 38 percent of cases were less than 16 months old (Centers for Disease Control, 1989c). The age for vaccine administration was then lowered again to 9 months in areas with recurrent measles transmission (Centers for Disease Control, 1989d). These children would then require revaccination at 15 months.

The fact that a large percentage of measles cases occurs in school-age children and adolescents resulted in the recommendation of mass revaccination. The American College Health Association recommended that all colleges and universities require documentation of both measles and rubella immunity as a prerequisite to matriculation (ACHA, 1983). And finally, the Centers for Disease Control and American Academy of Pediatrics announced that the measles vaccine failures necessitated a second dose of vaccine (Centers for Disease Control, 1989i).

VACCINE REACTIONS

The list of adverse reactions associated with the measles vaccine is shamefully long. The measles vaccine has proven to be a failed and tragic experiment. Vaccine apologists assure us through statistics that natural measles would cause the same effects as vaccination, but in greater numbers. This is small compensation to parents of children who have been injured by the measles vaccine.

The problems caused by the measles vaccine read like a neurologic textbook. Encephalitis, meningitis, autism, subacute sclerosing panencephalitis, seizure disorder, sensorineural deafness, optic neuritis, transverse myelitis, Guillain-Barré syndrome. The human tragedy described in the thousands of reports is staggering. This vaccine is dangerous. Yet the final twist on this extravagant failure is that the Vaccine Safety Committee ignores their own findings and would have us believe that inadequate evidence exists to prove an association between vaccination and these devastating diseases. The only conditions attributed to the MMR vaccine are thrombocytopenia and anaphylaxis (Institute of Medicine, 1994). Such denial amounts to a travesty of adverse event reporting. Why report these events at all, if the vaccine industry chooses to ignore them?

The adverse reactions described below sometimes occurred following measles vaccination alone. When measles vaccine is administered in the combination MMR vaccination, attributing reactions to one vaccine is difficult unless specific antibody studies confirm the specific cause. Reactions to MMR vaccine are included in this chapter.

Acute encephalopathy resulting in brain injury or death has been clearly associated with the measles vaccine. Researchers reviewed medical records of claims from the National Vaccine Injury Compensation Program for children who developed encephalopathy within 15 days of a measles or MMR vaccine. A total of 48 children developed seizures, motor and sensory deficits, and retardation on days eight or nine following the measles vaccine. Eight of these children died. The evaluators determined that a causal relationship between measles vaccine and encephalopathy may exist (Weibel *et al.*, 1998).

Reports of central nervous system disorders following measles vaccination abound throughout the worldwide medical literature. A review of cases reported to the Centers for Disease Control from 1963 to 1971 revealed 59 patients with extensive neurologic disorders (Landrigan & Witte, 1973). In the United Kingdom, 47 cases of encephalitis were reported between 1968 and 1974, and 122 febrile convulsions occurred following measles vaccinations (Beale, 1974). Another report from England identified 26 cases of convulsions between 1975 and 1981 after vaccination (Pollock & Morris, 1983). A report of adverse events associated with measles vaccine in Japan from 1978 to 1983 described 12 cases of encephalitis (Hirayama, 1983). Cases reported through VAERS included 17 suggestive of encephalopathy or encephalitis (Institute of Medicine, 1994).

One of the most dangerous reactions caused by measles vaccine is an inflammatory response in the brain known as subacute sclerosing panencephalitis (SSPE). This disease causes demyelination of nerve sheaths and a slow, progressive, deteriorating condition, resulting in death, often within one to two years. Its association with natural measles infection is well established.

The first reported case of SSPE following measles vaccine occurred in 1968, in a child with onset of symptoms within three weeks of vaccination. The child died 18 months later (Schneck, 1968). Within five years of that report, 22 additional cases of measles vaccine-associated SSPE were reported in the medical literature (Jabbour *et al.*, 1972). In 1969, a registry was established to document cases of SSPE and its association to measles vaccine. The registry now includes data on more than 575 patients (Institute of Medicine, 1994). Although the annual incidence of SSPE has declined since the 1970s, accompanying the decline in natural measles, the proportion of cases with an antecedent history of measles vaccination has increased (Dyken *et al.*, 1989).

Other neurologic problems have been seen following measles vaccination. **Guillain-Barré syndrome (GBS)**, an autoimmune disease characterized by paralysis and demyelination of nerve sheaths, occurred in a 19-month-old girl after measles vaccine. Within one week following vaccination she was unable to stand. A second girl, aged 10 months, developed GBS within four days of measles, DTP, and OPV vaccination (Grose & Spigland, 1976). A 12-year-old girl was diagnosed with GBS following MMR vaccination (Norrby, 1984) and a total of 17 cases developed GBS following measles or MMR vaccination in the MSAEFI and VAERS reporting systems between 1979 and 1992 (Institute of Medicine, 1994). Cases continue to be reported. In 1994 a report appeared describing a 16-month-old girl who became "clumsy," with a tendency to fall over, 10 days after MMR vaccination. Over the next two weeks she became progressively more weak, and was unable to stand without support. Her cough and cry became weak with inability to swallow. She required nasogastric feeding for 4 weeks (Morris & Rylance, 1994).

In recent years the onset of **autism** in children has been associated with the measles vaccine. A study by Wakefield and 13 other researchers showed that 12 children who simultaneously developed intestinal disease and autism had elevated levels of IgG measles antibodies compared to controls, and measles-specific antigens in cells of the colon (Wakefield, 1998). A follow-up study conducted by Wakefield, O'Leary, and others also showed the presence of persistent measles virus and inflammatory bowel disease in children with developmental disorder. A total of 91 children with developmental disorder and bowel disease were compared to 70 developmentally normal controls, some of whom also had inflammatory bowel disease, Crohn's disease, or ulcerative colitis. Among the children with developmental disorder 75 of 91 (82 percent) had persistent measles virus, presumably from the MMR vaccine, compared to 5 of 70 (7 percent) developmentally normal children (Uhlmann *et al.*, 2002).

Dr. Vijendra Singh has identified specific antibodies that produce an autoimmune attack on brain tissue in response to measles vaccine (Singh, 1996; Singh, 1998). Brain injury from the measles vaccine has long been suspected, and a recent report has verified the causal relationship between permanent brain injury and the vaccine (Weibel *et al.*, 1998).

A questionnaire administered to mothers of autistic children revealed another alarming connection to vaccines. This time the effects were apparently passed from mother to infant. Of the 240 mothers surveyed, 25 had received a rubella vaccine or MMR vaccine during the postpartum period, and 20 of these women (80 percent) had children with autism. Nine of these children were born just prior to the vaccination, and it is presumed that transmission occurred through the mother's breast milk (Yazbak, 1999). Seven women in this survey received a rubella, measles, hepatitis B, or MMR during pregnancy. "Six out of the seven children (85%) who resulted from these pregnancies were diagnosed with autism, and the seventh, whose mother received a measles vaccine, exhibits symptoms which suggest autistic spectrum. This child's twin brother was stillborn" (Yazbak, 1999a).

In the fall of 2000, the National Institutes of Health (NIH) established a committee to investigate the relation between MMR vaccine and autism. Despite the findings of clinical studies showing the association, the committee's report concluded that "the evidence favors rejection of a causal relationship at the population level between MMR vaccine and autistic spectrum disorders (ASD)" (Institute of Medicine, 2001).

Deafness caused by nerve damage following MMR vaccine has been reported by many authors. A 7-year-old girl developed total deafness in the left ear 11 days after MMR vaccine. She did not recover (Nabe-Nielsen & Walter, 1988). A 3-year-old girl was diagnosed with moderate to severe bilateral deafness, accompanied by muscle inco-ordination, attributed to an illness 10 days following MMR vaccination (Brodsky & Stanievich, 1985). A 27-year-old woman developed joint pain, fever, headache, and gait unsteadiness beginning 3 days after measles and rubella vaccination. Progressive hearing loss began 22 days following vaccination. Profound and permanent bilateral hearing loss resulted (Hulbert *et al.*, 1991). A recent review reported six additional cases of profound hearing loss attributed to MMR vaccine in 1- to 6-year-old children (Stewart & Prabhu, 1993).

Optic neuritis accompanied by blindness or partial vision loss has also occurred following MMR vaccination. A 6-year-old boy developed optic neuritis 18 days after MMR injection. He recovered fully after several weeks (Kazarian & Gager, 1978). Marshall and colleagues reported the following case.

> A 16-month-old baby girl . . . had been previously healthy and developmentally normal. . . . In September, 1983, 14 days after measles, mumps, and rubella vaccination, she had subjective fever, cough, conjunctival injection, and a generalized macular erythematous rash. Two days later, the majority of these symptoms abated, but the conjunctival injection worsened, her pupils became dilated, and she began walking into objects. . . . On admission to the hospital, examination revealed a vigorous toddler who would not reach for objects and had only minimal light perception. Ophthalmologic examination showed a diffuse chorioretinitis with perivascular retinal edema, mild papilledema, and a stellate macular configuration. . . . Repeat fundoscopic [eye] examination several days later demonstrated evolution into a

"salt and pepper" pigmentary pattern distributed radially along the retinal veins. These changes were most consistent with measles retinopathy. . . . On follow-up examination 7 months later, her visual acuity had improved; she was able to ambulate freely but still sat close to the television set and held objects close to her face. Fundoscopic examination revealed macular scarring (Marshall et al., 1985).

Thrombocytopenia, a decrease in blood platelets responsible for blood clotting with accompanying spontaneous bleeding, has been acknowledged by the Vaccine Safety Committee as an adverse reaction to measles vaccine, based on overwhelming evidence (Institute of Medicine, 1994). During early research on the measles vaccine, it was discovered that vaccination resulted in a dramatic decrease of platelet counts in 86 percent of vaccinated subjects (Oski & Naiman, 1966).

Many clinical case reports have confirmed the incidence of thrombocytopenia following measles vaccination. Swedish health authorities received reports of 16 cases of thrombocytopenia following MMR vaccination in a three-year observation period between 1982 and 1984 (Bottiger *et al.*, 1987). Eleven cases of thrombocytopenia occurred following measles vaccination between 1976 and 1989 in Germany (Fescharek *et al.*, 1990). In Canada, a passive surveillance system received reports of 5 thrombocytopenia cases following MMR vaccination during 1987 (Koch *et al.*, 1989). Finland reported 23 cases of thrombocytopenic purpura occurring within a mean of 19 days of vaccination during a campaign that involved 700,000 children (Nieminen *et al.*, 1993). The VAERS reporting system received 7 case reports of thrombocytopenia following measles or MMR given alone during the period 1990–1992 (Institute of Medicine, 1994).

Anaphylaxis, a severe, acute, systemic, and potentially fatal allergic reaction, has occurred following measles and MMR vaccines. Many reports have documented these reactions. Egg proteins contained in the measles and mumps vaccines may play a role in severe hypersensitivity reactions, since some individuals are exquisitely sensitive to eggs. However, other components of live attenuated virus vaccines, especially the antibiotics contained in these preparations, have been implicated in triggering severe allergic reactions.

In a report from England, nine reactions categorized as anaphylaxis with collapse occurred following measles vaccine during a seven-year period (Pollock & Morris, 1983). The Drug Reactions Advisory Committee of Australia received 15 reports of reactions occurring within 30 minutes of measles vaccination during the period 1980–1982 (McEwen, 1983). A measles vaccine grown in monkey kidney cells rather than chicken embryo cells caused six severe hypersensitivity reactions in a Norwegian report (Aukrust *et al.*, 1980). The Canadian passive surveillance system reported 30 allergic reactions to MMR during 1987 (Koch *et al.*, 1989). And nine cases of possible anaphylactic reactions were reported through VAERS during 1990–1992 (Institute of Medicine, 1994).

A disturbing syndrome of **atypical measles** has occurred in children previously vaccinated. This consists of an illness with exaggerated rash, muscle weakness, peripheral edema, and severe abdominal pain with persistent vomiting (Cherry *et al.*, 1972). These reactions, though rare, have also occurred following vaccination (St. Geme, 1976).

Recent research has shown an association between measles vaccine and **inflammatory bowel disease**. In one study individuals who had received measles vaccine in the 1960s were more likely to suffer from chronic intestinal disease including Crohn's disease (characterized by deep ulcers, holes, and thickening of the intestinal lining) and ulcerative colitis thirty years later compared to controls (Thompson *et al.*, 1995). This is not surprising since persistent measles virus infection has been located in intestinal tissue affected by chronic inflammation, particularly in Crohn's-disease-affected bowel (Wakefield *et al.*, 1995). These researchers found an incidence rate of 1 case of inflammatory bowel disease for every 140 persons vaccinated for measles, compared to an incidence of 1 in 400 controls (Thompson *et al.*, 1995).

Measles vaccine has also been associated with **immune system suppression**. This mechanism could explain the severe neurologic symptoms and pathology following measles vaccination. For example, after measles vaccine, the number of lymphocytes, a type of white blood cell that fights disease, decreases (Nicholson *et al.*, 1992), and certain lymphocyte functions essential to their role in fighting pathogenic organisms are depressed (Hirsch *et al.*, 1981).

MEASLES FACTS

- Measles has historically been a common childhood disease with rare complications.

- Mass vaccination has resulted in a dramatic decline in measles incidence, but outbreaks now occur in older populations and in infants born to women whose immunity from vaccination has deteriorated. Periodic epidemics continue to occur.

- The vaccine is associated with serious adverse reactions including permanent nervous system damage and autism. Long-term effects are unknown.

A PERSONAL STRATEGY

Parents must decide whether they are willing to risk the many known and the unknown adverse effects from the measles vaccine in order to prevent the rare complications of natural measles. Parents might choose to rely on alternative healing systems to treat measles infections in children if the disease should occur. Then their children would also obtain lifelong immunity following the natural infection.

Mumps

Mumps was a common and very mild disease of childhood that went unnoticed in an estimated 30 percent of cases prior to widespread vaccine use. The illness begins with fever, headache, and fatigue, and within 24 hours the child complains of earache near the lobe of the ear. The next day the salivary gland in front of the ear becomes swollen. Within one to six days, the illness runs its course.

Infection of the testicles, ovaries, and other organs is not unusual but occurs much more commonly in adults. Infection of the testicle occurs in 20 to 30 percent of mumps cases in adolescent or adult males (Philip *et al.*, 1959). Sterility following such an illness is extremely rare. Encephalitis and meningitis complications during epidemic out-breaks occur at a rate of 2 to 4 cases for every 1,000 reported cases of mumps (Centers for Disease Control, 1972). However, only an estimated 70 percent of mumps cases are reported. Deaths from mumps are rare, but about half of mumps-associated deaths have been in persons over 20 years old (Centers for Disease Control, 1989g).

INCIDENCE AND VACCINE EFFICACY

A live mumps virus vaccine was licensed in 1967, and recommended for routine use in 1977. It apparently resulted in a decline in the incidence of mumps cases. Subsequent outbreaks of mumps, however, have caused a re-evaluation of the previous optimistic vaccine success reports. The number of mumps cases had decreased during the early 1980s to 3,000 to 5,000 cases per year, a dramatic decline from the 100,000 cases per year of the early 1970s. However, during 1986, 7,800 cases occurred, and during 1987 there were nearly 13,000 reported mumps cases. During the early 1990s the number of reported cases continued to decline to a low of 300–400 cases per year in 1999 and 2000 (CDC, 2001).

The most disturbing factor in these statistics is the shift in mumps cases to older age groups who are much more susceptible to the complications of testicular and ovarian infection. During the period 1967–1971, the annual average of cases in persons 15 years of age or older was 8.3 percent; this age group accounted for 38.3 percent of cases in 1987. This represents a greater than eightfold increase (Centers for Disease Control, 1989e). The proportion of mumps in adolescents and adults remained at that level (34 percent in 1993). Although we are assured that the risk to adolescents is still less than in the pre-vaccine era, this trend is disconcerting. It is thought that the rise in cases among adolescents is due to a lack of vaccination in children born between 1967 and 1977, and not to waning immunity in persons vaccinated previously (Cochi, 1988). Nonetheless, this shift to older populations is worrisome. Mumps in young children is a mild, benign disease. In adolescents and adults, it is a disease associated with more complications. The response of public health authorities is to revaccinate those who are susceptible during adolescent years.

The efficacy of mumps vaccine has ranged from 75 to 95 percent in various studies.

VACCINE REACTIONS

The mumps vaccine is associated with adverse effects similar to the measles vaccine. Since mumps vaccine is usually administered in combination with measles vaccine, reactions are difficult to accurately attribute to one or the other. Two conditions are associated with the mumps virus and not with measles. These are meningitis and diabetes. It has been associated with fevers, seizures, encephalitis, and severe, atypical mumps disease.

Meningitis is clearly associated with mumps disease. Cases of aseptic meningitis (not caused by bacteria) reported after administration of mumps vaccine have led researchers around the world to investigate mumps vaccine as a possible cause of meningitis as well. In Canada, the sale of mumps vaccine was suspended in 1990 after the mumps-vaccine virus strain was isolated from eight children who developed meningitis following MMR vaccination (Colville & Pugh, 1992). The rate of virologically-confirmed mumps vaccine-associated meningitis was one case per 3,800 doses, significantly higher than the incidence of meningitis in children not recently vaccinated. In Yugoslavia, a review of childhood aseptic meningitis cases occurring between 1979 and 1986 revealed that 115 children developed meningitis within 30 days of mumps vaccination. This was an attack rate of one case per 1,000 immunized children (Cizman *et al.*, 1989).

In Japan a surveillance program was instituted during 1989 after a public outcry over mumps vaccine-associated meningitis. This study revealed 311 suspected cases of vaccine-associated meningitis. One-third of these suspected cases were later confirmed by laboratory analysis of spinal fluid; however, the authors stated that "Most of the unconfirmed cases were likely to have been vaccine-related, because the two groups (i.e., confirmed and unconfirmed cases) were closely matched in the time of occurrence, the time interval between vaccination and the onset of illness, the age distribution and the clinical manifestation of the illness." Those researchers calculated the incidence rate as one in 2,000 people who received MMR (Sugiura

& Yamada, 1991). The Vaccine Safety Committee has recognized mumps vaccine as a cause of aseptic meningitis because the vaccine-virus strain can be isolated and positively identified from patients with meningitis following vaccination (Institute of Medicine, 1994).

Diabetes, specifically insulin-dependent diabetes mellitus (IDDM), is characterized by an insufficiency of insulin secretion by the pancreas. Diabetes is thought to arise in response to both genetic and environmental factors. Viruses represent one of the most important environmental triggers of diabetes (Maclaren & Atkinson, 1992). Many studies have proven that natural mumps infection causes pancreatitis (infection of the pancreas) and stimulates the onset of diabetes. This has been shown in the reports of clusters of diabetes following epidemics of mumps disease (Dacou-Voutetakis *et al.,* 1974) and in large epidemiologic studies that demonstrate parallel curves between outbreaks of mumps disease and new cases of diabetes (Sultz *et al.,* 1975).

Mumps vaccination has similarly stimulated the onset of diabetes. The postulated mechanisms of diabetes onset that include autoimmune processes or persistent infection suggest that there may be a prolonged interval between vaccination and the onset of diabetic symptoms (Institute of Medicine, 1994). Nonetheless, many cases of diabetes have been reported following recent mumps vaccination.

One study revealed 20 cases of diabetes occurring after mumps vaccine given during the period 1976 through 1989 in Germany. Twelve cases began within 30 days of vaccination (Fescharek *et al.,* 1990). Another report included 7 children who developed diabetes in the second to fourth week following mumps vaccination (Helmke *et al.,* 1986). A third report cited 3 cases of diabetes beginning 10 days to 3 weeks after mumps vaccination (Otten *et al.,* 1984). Five cases of diabetes following receipt of MMR or mumps vaccine were reported through VAERS during the period 1990–1992 (Institute of Medicine, 1994). During interviews with 112 parents of diabetic children in Erie County, New York, the onset of diabetes was noted by parents to follow mumps disease in almost 50 percent of the children and by mumps vaccination in 11 percent (Sultz *et al.,* 1975).

Several individual cases of diabetes after mumps vaccination have been reported, and one case of pancreatitis occurred in a 19-year-old woman 11 days after MMR vaccination accompanied by abdominal pain and vomiting, and confirmed by abnormal pancreatic enzyme levels on blood tests (Adler *et al.*, 1991). The Vaccine Safety Committee declined to accept diabetes as a consequence of mumps vaccine despite these reports (Institute of Medicine, 1994).

Mumps Facts

- Mumps is generally a benign disease of children. Complications of mumps do occur, but an estimated 30 percent of cases go unnoticed.

- Mumps has increasingly become a disease of adolescents and adults since the widespread use of the vaccine.

- Complications of mumps occur much more frequently in adults.

- The vaccine has caused significant adverse reactions, including vaccine-associated meningitis, in as many as one per 1,000 doses.

A Personal Strategy

Use of the mumps vaccine, which has been associated with serious adverse effects, seems unjustifiable. Administering the vaccine during adolescence may simply prolong the problem of waning immunity, and shift the disease and its complications to an even older population.

Rubella (German Measles)

Rubella is a mild childhood illness that consists of fever, rash, and tiredness lasting for a few days. It has no serious complications except in very rare instances.

The purpose of vaccination is to prevent pregnant women from contracting rubella, since abortion, stillbirths, and deformities can result from illness during the first three months of pregnancy. Between 20 and 50 percent of babies born to women who contract rubella during the first three months of pregnancy will have birth defects (eye defects, deafness, mental retardation). This vaccine is unique in that children are vaccinated to interrupt circulation of the virus and reduce the risk of exposure to susceptible pregnant women.

Prevention of rubella using the live-virus vaccine can be accomplished in one of two ways: vaccinate susceptible women of child-bearing age, or vaccinate preschool and school-age children to prevent disease transmission. The question has persistently arisen whether the rubella vaccine should be given to children or to susceptible adolescent and adult women, with many experts on both sides of this controversy.

Drs. Otto Sieber and Vincent Fulginiti, recognized vaccine experts, argued against routine vaccination of children (Fulginiti, 1976; Sieber & Fulginiti, 1977). When reports appeared that antibody titers decreased after childhood rubella vaccination, they stated, "one might argue that immunization of adolescents or adults might be a more appropriate strategy than our current emphasis upon vaccination of infants. . . ." If the protective effect of the vaccine decreases over time, then a girl who is vaccinated during childhood may become susceptible once again as an adult. If the vaccine has significant adverse effects, then vaccinated children could be needlessly exposed to this risk. Both of these factors argue against the use of rubella vaccine in children.

Another reason for vaccination of susceptible adult women rather than children was put forward by Dr. Stephen Schoenbaum and colleagues in 1975, in the *Journal of the American Medical Association*. They discovered that children may not be the major source of rubella spread to pregnant women. They tested a hypothesis:

If children were an important source of contagion for pregnant women, it should be reflected by one of the following: First, the percentage of women with detectable antibody titers, signifying previous experience with rubella, should rise with increasing parity [number of children born to a woman] more than one would expect on the basis of age alone. Second, the incidence of rubella among susceptible pregnant women should increase with increasing parity and should be reflected by an increasing frequency of babies with rubella syndrome among children born of later pregnancies.

In other words, mothers should show evidence of more exposure to rubella than other women. Their study found the opposite to be true.

To summarize the serologic data, there was no evidence of a decrease in susceptibility with increasing parity. These data, therefore, offer no support for the presumption that the number of susceptible adult women materially decreases after the first pregnancy. . . . This finding is consistent with the concept that most persons who contract rubella as adults do so through contact with other adults (Schoenbaum *et al.,* 1975).

If children are not the primary source of infection for pregnant women, then children should not be targeted for prevention. They come to the logical conclusion that "We . . . would prefer the alternative policy of selectively and efficiently vaccinating adolescent girls."

INCIDENCE

The incidence of rubella and congenital rubella syndrome (infants with defects due to maternal infections) has declined dramatically since the vaccine was licensed in 1969. Previous levels of 20,000 to 60,000 reported cases of rubella per year declined to several hundred per year in the 1980s and an average of 200 cases per year in the period 1990–2000 (CDC, 2001).

VACCINE EFFICACY

The protective effect of rubella vaccine has been estimated as 77 percent in one study (Hough *et al.,* 1979). A continuing concern is the gradual reduction in an individual's antibody titer following rubella vaccination. The effectiveness of the vaccine may decrease, so that women who were not susceptible as children become susceptible again as adults. In fact, the disease has shifted to older age groups. During the three-year period before vaccine licensure (1966–1968), 23 percent of rubella cases occurred among persons 15 years of age or older. In 1987, 48 percent of cases occurred in persons 15 or more years old (Centers for Disease Control, 1989f). Serologic surveys of postpubertal populations have found that rates of rubella susceptibility are comparable to the prevaccine years (10 to 20 percent lack evidence of immunity) (Crowder *et al.*, 1987; Bart *et al.*, 1985). The proposed solution to this problem of shifting age-occurrence has again been to revaccinate susceptible women of childbearing age.

VACCINE REACTIONS

Adverse effects of the rubella vaccine include encephalitis-type symptoms, meningitis, and Guillain-Barré syndrome (muscle paralysis and sensory nerve deficits). In addition, at least 12 to 20 percent of women develop arthritis symptoms after receiving the vaccine. These may begin several weeks after the administration of vaccine (Fulginiti, 1976). They may persist for weeks, months, or years. In some cases, women develop rheumatoid arthritis, which continues throughout their lives.

Many studies since the 1960s have confirmed that rubella vaccine causes **acute arthritis** in both children and adults. Joint pain and arthritis occur in 10 to 40 percent of women after vaccination, and less often in children. One study showed that 25 percent of women in their 20s and 50 percent of those aged 25 to 33 had joint symptoms following rubella vaccination (Swartz *et al.*, 1971). In another study, acute arthritis occurred in 46 percent of women above age 25 years (Weibel *et al.*, 1972). No children involved in these two small studies developed arthritis.

Chronic persistent arthritis occurs following both natural rubella infection and rubella vaccination. Natural rubella has been associated with chronic arthritis, as evidenced in several studies. For example, rubella virus antigen was demonstrated in joint cavities of one-third of patients with juvenile rheumatoid arthritis (Ogra *et al.*, 1975), and the virus was isolated from blood cells or joint fluid in one-third of children with chronic rheumatic disease (Chantler *et al.*, 1985). Many cases of recurrent or persistent arthritis have been reported in the medical literature following rubella vaccination. One study reported 11 children with recurrent arthritis 36 months after vaccination (Thompson *et al.*, 1973). Arthritis persisting for at least 2–7 years has been reported in several women following rubella vaccine injection (Tingle *et al.*, 1984; Tingle *et al.*, 1985). The author has seen a case of rheumatoid arthritis with joint destruction that began after rubella vaccination and has persisted for over 20 years.

One study compared the effects of natural rubella infection in 46 people with the effects of rubella vaccination in a second group of 44 women. In the group with natural rubella, 65 percent had acute arthritis or joint pain. Eighteen months later, 30 percent of the women and 8 percent of the men had joint symptoms. In the vaccinated group, 55 percent had arthritis or joint pain within four weeks, and 5 percent had persistent joint symptoms 18 months later (Tingle *et al.*, 1986). In their analysis of these and other studies, the Vaccine Safety Committee concluded that rubella vaccine causes acute and chronic arthritis (Institute of Medicine, 1991).

Various types of **central and peripheral nervous system disorders** have been frequently reported to follow rubella vaccination. One study examined 299 reported cases of peripheral neuropathies, including 10 children with symptoms that persisted for more than 32 months. That study found an incidence of two cases of neuropathies per 1,000 doses of one vaccine virus strain, and 0.1 per 1,000 doses of a second strain (Schaffner *et al.*, 1974). Other individual cases have been scattered through the literature. These include reports of cases of nerve pain and numbness, carpal tunnel syndrome, two cases of Guillain-Barré syndrome, and three cases of transverse myelitis (Institute of Medicine, 1991).

The following case was reported in the *American Journal of Diseases of Children.*

A 20-month-old white boy was well until ten days after inoculation with the combined mumps-rubella vaccine. Initial com-
plaints were the inability to stand on the left leg and pain in all
extremities. The weakness progressed to include both legs and
ascended to involve all extremities. . . . Examination revealed an
apprehensive child with a complete flaccid paralysis of all extremities and inability to hold his head up. The patient had marked soft
tissue tenderness of all extremities. Neurologic evaluation revealed
no muscle stretch reflexes. . . . Over a three-month period he
completely recovered all motor functions (Gunderman, 1973).

This case is similar to other descriptions of weakness or paralysis of
extremities, loss of sensation, and difficulty walking in other children who reacted to the rubella vaccine (Kilroy, 1970; Gilmartin *et
al.*, 1972).

A 13-year-old boy developed **Guillain-Barré syndrome** three weeks
after he received MMR and booster doses of diphtheria, tetanus, and
oral polio vaccines. Symptoms began with tingling in the feet and
muscular weakness, which progressed for two weeks, when he could
still walk but could not stand up or climb stairs without assistance.
He recovered after a month. Blood tests revealed high levels of rubella
antibody consistent with rubella infection. No other symptoms of
rubella occurred, and his illness was attributed to the rubella vaccination (Mühlebach-Sponer *et al.*, 1994).

A questionnaire administered to mothers of **autistic children**
revealed an alarming connection to vaccines. This time the effects
were apparently passed from mother to infant. Of the 240 mothers
surveyed, 25 had received a rubella vaccine or MMR vaccine during
the postpartum period, and 20 of these women (80 percent) had children with autism. Nine of these children were born just prior to the
vaccination, and it is presumed that transmission occurred through
the mother's breast milk. The rubella vaccine insert states that "lactating postpartum women immunized with rubella live attenuated
vaccine may secrete the virus in breast milk and transmit it to breastfed infants." The author states that "caution should be exercised when
the vaccine is administered to a nursing mother." In ten of the cases the

subsequent child developed autism, suggesting a placental or genetic transmission of factors that could cause the disease (Yazbak, 1999). Seven women in this survey received a rubella, measles, hepatitis B, or MMR during pregnancy. "Six out of the seven children (85%) who resulted from these pregnancies were diagnosed with autism, and the seventh, whose mother received a measles vaccine, exhibits symptoms which suggest autistic spectrum. This child's twin brother was still-born" (Yazbak, 1999a).

Several case reports have indicated an association between rubella and thrombocytopenia, decrease of blood platelets with consequent spontaneous bleeding. Four cases were reported within 10 days to 3 weeks of rubella vaccination. A 26-year-old woman developed thrombocytopenia with bleeding into the skin and mucous membranes, and marked reduction in blood platelets after rubella vaccination (Bartos, 1972). Other cases involved the MMR vaccine, and reactions were impossible to distinguish between measles and rubella.

Rubella Facts

- Rubella is a mild childhood disease that requires no treatment.

- A woman who contracts rubella during the first three months of pregnancy risks abortion, miscarriage, or birth defects in her child.

- Rubella incidence has shifted to older age groups since widespread vaccination.

- Rubella vaccine is associated with significant adverse effects, including arthritis and central nervous system disorders.

A Personal Strategy

Parents have three options: avoid the vaccine entirely; vaccinate their child against rubella; or test girls for antibodies at adolescence or before considering pregnancy, and decide whether to vaccinate then. Since a child's health is not compromised by contracting rubella, there is no advantage to the child from vaccination.

Every adolescent girl and woman of childbearing age should have a blood test for immunity to rubella. If they do not have evidence of immunity, then they should decide whether they wish to have the vaccine. Susceptible women who decline the vaccine should attempt to avoid exposure to children with colds, fevers, and rashes during the first three months of pregnancy. Again, the consideration is whether the possible adverse effects of the vaccine are worth prevention of problems during pregnancy. Avoidance of the vaccine during childhood will eliminate the risk of untoward vaccine reactions in your child.

Women should not receive the rubella vaccine during pregnancy or while breastfeeding.

PERTUSSIS (WHOOPING COUGH)

The vaccine controversy reached an emotional and political zenith with the publicity generated by pertussis vaccine reactions. Public awareness was fueled by media presentations that focused on deaths and nervous system damage suffered by children after pertussis vaccination. The media attention to this issue included television documentaries, books in the popular press (Coulter & Fisher, 1991), and many magazine articles. Children in countries throughout Europe and the United Kingdom stopped receiving the pertussis vaccine. Japan postponed pertussis vaccination until children were two years old. The United States Congress passed the National Childhood Vaccine Injury Act to provide compensation to parents of injured children when vaccine companies threatened to stop producing pertussis vaccine. All in response to this public scrutiny of vaccine reactions.

This heightened interest in the pertussis vaccine was stimulated by consistent reports of dramatic vaccine reactions and permanent damage suffered by children after vaccination. Reactions to the vaccine have included fever, persistent crying, encephalitis, epilepsy, retardation, and death. Other neurologic diseases have been associated with the vaccine as well.

Pertussis is an infectious disease of childhood, associated with a specific bacterium. It can have dramatic and alarming symptoms. The illness usually begins as a mild cold, which lasts for a week. Then the characteristic cough starts, which makes this disease recognizable, especially when it occurs in children. The cough comes in paroxysms and is often preceded by a feeling of apprehension or anxiety and tightness in the chest. The cough itself consists of short explosive expirations in rapid succession followed by a long crowing inspiration. During the coughing spell, the child's face may become red or even blue; the eyes bulge, and the tongue protrudes. A number of such paroxysms are sometimes followed by spitting up a mucous plug and vomiting. This will end the attack, and the child will rest. Many of these attacks may occur in one day, more frequently at night and in a stuffy room. They may be brought on by physical exertion, crying, and often by eating or drinking. Infants, and even older children, do not always have "whooping" with their cough, and in adults the cough may be mild and never diagnosed at all. The disease usually lasts for at least six weeks regardless of treatment. Complications of pertussis may include cerebral hemorrhage, convulsions and brain damage, pneumonia, emphysema, or a collapsed lung. Deaths are usually due to complicating respiratory infections. Pneumonia is the most frequent cause of death in children under three years of age, but fatalities in children over 12 months are rare.

Standard treatment with antibiotics may help reduce the period of contagion to others and prevent complications. It does not change the course of symptoms. Homeopathic treatment has been used extensively in the past, and one study suggests there may be a beneficial effect from homeopathy in pertussis cases (English, 1987b). This survey followed children who received a homeopathic preventive for pertussis, who subsequently did contract the disease and were then treated homeopathically. The results of this survey suggest that the group of children treated with homeopathy experienced relatively mild cases of pertussis, compared to children who received antibiotic treatment. The author of this study acknowledges that the number of children followed was too small to make any definitive conclusions about the efficacy of homeopathy in the treatment of pertussis.

Two different vaccines have been developed for the prevention of whooping cough, the whole-cell vaccine and the acellular vaccine. The first acellular pertussis vaccine was licensed in the United States in 1991 for use as the fourth and fifth doses of the recommended DTP schedule for children ages 16 months through 6 years (Centers for Disease Control, 1992c). In 1997 acellular vaccine was licensed for use in children as young as six weeks of age, combined with diphtheria and tetanus vaccines as DTaP.

INCIDENCE

Pertussis still occurs with regularity as a common childhood disease. Prior to 1940, it was estimated that 95 percent of all individuals had some form of pertussis during their lifetimes. The incidence of pertussis has declined from at least 100 reported cases per 100,000 population during the period 1930–1945 to an average of 1.5 per 100,000 population during 1984–1993. An average of 6,000 cases were reported per year during the period 1990–2000 (CDC, 2001). However, it is estimated that only 10 percent of pertussis cases are reported. Whooping cough is still among us, despite widespread vaccination coverage.

Pertussis has become an increasingly common cause of cough in adolescents and adults. Immunity derived from the vaccine wanes after 5 to 10 years (Bass, 1985), and pertussis vaccine cannot be administered past seven years of age because of severe reactions. Pertussis occurs regularly in older children and adults who have been fully vaccinated (Cherry et al., 1989).

An outbreak that occurred in a middle school is typical. Thirteen eighth-grade students had culture-confirmed pertussis despite full vaccination (Mink et al., 1994). In an evaluation of college students with prolonged cough, 26 percent proved to have pertussis (Morgan et al., 1992). Pertussis is now a typical disease of adults who did not develop permanent immunity from the disease in childhood.

VACCINE EFFICACY

The most reliable studies of vaccine efficacy involve vaccinated children living in a house with someone who has contracted the disease. These studies have shown a variation in whole-cell vaccine efficacy of 63 to 91 percent (Cherry et al., 1988). One study showed an efficacy of 80 percent 3 years after the last dose, 50 percent between 4 and 7 years, and none after 12 years (Lambert, 1965).

Vaccine trials using acellular pertussis have revealed a similarly wide range of effectiveness. In a Swedish study of culture-confirmed pertussis, the observed efficacy of acellular vaccine was 64 percent for one strain and 54 percent for a second (Ad hoc group, 1988). Sweden withdrew an application for licensure of the vaccine on the basis of these tests (License, 1989). Other studies have shown an average of 70–80 percent efficacy (Blackwelder *et al.*, 1991; NIH, 1996).

VACCINE REACTIONS

Whole-Cell Vaccine Reactions

The political cover-up, distortion of facts, and outright disinformation campaign of the vaccine industry are perfectly exemplified in the efforts to exonerate the whole-cell pertussis vaccine. Efforts to vindicate the pertussis vaccine have appeared in countless forms despite the many reports and studies documenting its toxicity. These reports have included official statements to the media, analysis and re-analysis of data, editorials denouncing vaccine critics, and denial in the face of incontrovertible facts.

The most comprehensive pertussis study was conducted in Los Angeles during 1978–1979, at UCLA (Cody *et al.*, 1981). Children who received the DTP vaccine were compared to those who received the DT vaccine, and reactions that occurred during the first 48 hours after vaccine administration were recorded. The most serious criticism of the UCLA study and similar studies is that the vaccine may cause delayed reactions not apparent within the first two days. Delayed reactions are difficult to distinguish from the background occurrence of these problems.

The UCLA study data show that 50 percent of vaccinees developed fever, 34 percent irritability, 35 percent had crying episodes, and 40 percent had localized inflammation. The more significant major reactions included 3 percent of children who had persistent inconsolable crying and screaming, and 31 percent with excessive sleepiness (compared to 14 percent in the DT controls). The authors claimed that the occurrence of seizures could not be statistically verified because of the small numbers of children (16,536 vaccinations in the total study), although 1 in 1,750 doses of DTP caused seizures, or 1 in 333 children suffered seizures within 48 hours of vaccination.

A study with larger numbers also found a significant difference in seizure occurrence when 134,000 children receiving DTP were compared to 133,000 DT recipients. The relative risk of seizures after DTP compared to DT was 5.3 (Pollock & Morris, 1983). The authors of this study also attempted to minimize their findings, this time questioning whether these reactions were overreported by participating physicians because of the adverse publicity concerning the pertussis vaccine.

The occurrence of **encephalopathy** following pertussis vaccine has been reported in hundreds of cases and evaluated in several large studies. Encephalopathy is a vague term that one study defined as a spectrum of characteristics including "altered levels of consciousness, confusion, irritability, changes in behavior, screaming attacks, neck stiffness, convulsions, visual, auditory and speech disturbances, motor and sensory deficit" (Alderslade *et al.*, 1981). Convulsions are the most dramatic and often the most immediate of these symptoms, therefore seizures have been reported most frequently in the literature. An early report in 1948 described 15 cases of encephalopathy following pertussis vaccination at Children's Hospital in Boston. These cases consisted of fever, irritability, convulsions, and coma occurring within 12 hours of pertussis vaccination (Byers & Moll, 1948). Six of these children suffered from permanent cerebral palsy, 6 had seizures and mental retardation, and 2 died of pneumonia.

A later study reviewed 107 cases of neurologic illness occurring within 48 hours of pertussis vaccination (Berg, 1958). Fifty-nine cases of encephalopathy were reported in a study in 1974 from Germany. Seizures occurred in 39, and 11 had abnormal brain scans (Ehrengut, 1974). The same year, another study reported 36 cases of encephalopathy in London that occurred within 24 hours of pertussis vaccination. Most were accompanied by seizures (Kulenkampff *et al.*, 1974). A report of 72 infants who suffered severe adverse reactions was published in 1979. Thirteen of these infants died, and 59 had seizures, shock, persistent screaming, and other severe involvement of the nervous system (Hennessen & Quast, 1979).

Controversy surrounds the issue of permanent **neurologic damage** (injury to the brain and retardation) caused by pertussis vaccine reactions. The typical case involves an initial seizure after the vaccine's administration, followed by recurrent seizures after a few days or weeks. Then mental and motor retardation become apparent over the ensuing months (Cherry *et al.*, 1988). Other cases of neurologic symptoms may include hyperactivity and attention deficit disorder, learning disabilities, and behavior problems. The most reliable research conducted to investigate neurologic disorders after DTP vaccine was carried out in England, Wales, and Scotland during 1976–1979 in the National Childhood Encephalopathy Study (NCES) (Alderslade *et al.*, 1981). This case-control study sought to find a risk factor for vaccine reaction by examining all cases of neurologic disease, and comparing those cases to a control group. Only hospitalized cases were examined. DTP vaccination had occurred significantly more frequently within the previous 72-hour and seven-day periods in the children with neurologic illness than in the controls. The estimated risk of serious neurologic disorder within seven days after DTP was 1:110,000 vaccinations, and the estimated risk of persistent neurologic damage 1 year later was 1:310,000.

A follow-up study in 1993 of permanent neurologic damage suffered by the children in the NCES data confirmed that these children continued to display neurologic abnormalities, thus vindicating the original findings of this study. This study traced over 80 percent of the children who suffered severe acute neurological illness following pertussis vaccine, as well as control children. All surviving children were administered a battery of intelligence and achievement tests; questionnaires on behavior and progress were completed by parents and teachers; and clinical and neurologic exams were performed by physicians. The authors concluded that "Case children were significantly more likely than controls to have died or to have some form of educational, behavioural, neurological, or physical dysfunction a decade after their illness" (Miller *et al.*, 1993).

Two follow-up studies of 16 children with neurologic reactions in the UCLA study showed continuing abnormalities in those children as well. In the follow-up study sponsored by the FDA, 13 children were administered neurologic and educational examinations.

These researchers found normal performance IQ scores (104.3 ± 15.8) and low verbal IQ scores (91.8 ± 18.4). One child had a verbal IQ score of 65 and performance IQ score of 88. Another had a verbal IQ score of 70 and performance IQ score of 106. The authors casually remark that "these lower verbal IQ scores can be explained by the proportion of Hispanic and bilingual children in this sample." If the researchers were not so eager to discount the findings of IQ scores in the mentally retarded range in these vaccine-damaged children, perhaps they might have administered these tests in Spanish. Despite this overall discrepancy between performance and verbal IQ, a criterion for language processing disability, the authors conclude, "there is no evidence that any of these 16 children suffered any serious neurologic damage as a result of either convulsions or hypotonic-hyporesponsive episodes" (Baraff *et al.*, 1988).

Evaluation of these same children by an independent pediatric neurologist who administered IQ tests in Spanish when necessary revealed significant language and learning disabilities. These included significant discrepancies between verbal and performance IQ, as well as language delays, attention deficit disorder, motor abnormalities, borderline low IQ, and mental retardation. His conclusion about these same children was drastically different than the government-sponsored findings. In reporting his evaluations to an Institute of Medicine Committee researching pertussis vaccine reactions, he stated, "Only 4 of the 13 tested were unequivocally normal" (Gabriel, 1990).

Given the controversies surrounding the association of permanent neurologic damage to pertussis vaccine in these two studies, the Institute of Medicine Committee found insufficient evidence to establish a causal relation between these permanent symptoms and the vaccine (Institute of Medicine, 1991).

The relationship of pertussis vaccine to **deaths** is even more controversial. The reports of many deaths following DTP vaccination led investigators to conduct studies on the incidence of SIDS (sudden infant death syndrome) and its relationship to DTP. In 1979, four infants in Tennessee all died within 24 hours of their first DTP vaccination (Hutcheson, 1979). All of these children received the same lot of vaccine. Two sets of twins, aged 5 and 10 months, died within 24 hours of DTP (Roberts, 1987; Werne & Garrow, 1946). And one study summarized case reports of more than 150 deaths following DTP by 37 authors in 12 countries (Torch, 1986).

Three studies have found a temporal association between infant deaths and DTP vaccination (Baraff *et al.*, 1983; Torch 1982; Walker *et al.*, 1987). In Walker's case-control study, the relative risk for SIDS (sudden infant death syndrome) within three days of vaccination was 7.3, a very significant risk (Walker, 1990). The Torch study found an increased incidence of SIDS in the period immediately after vaccination compared to a control period several weeks later. The Baraff study concluded, "The excess of deaths in the 24 hours and one week following immunization and the absence of deaths in the fourth week following immunization were all statistically significant."

At least four other studies found no significant association between SIDS and pertussis vaccination. Two of these studies included large populations of children, and they are most frequently cited as the best evidence that SIDS has no relationship to the vaccine. The largest study included an analysis of 716 cases of SIDS during the period 1978–1979 in a birth population of 350,000 children (Hoffman *et al.*, 1987).

The methods of this study have been assailed in a critique submitted to the Institute of Medicine (Coulter, 1990b). The conclusions of that critique discount the study's findings. "In fact, these results prove nothing at all, and this study is just an exercise in confusion. . . . As the study was done, no meaning can be extracted from it." The manipulation of data in that study clearly attempted to disprove the connection to SIDS, and study methods were biased to ensure that the finding of an association did not occur. The other major study cited as proof that SIDS is unrelated to pertussis vaccination is the notorious Griffin fiasco of 1988. That study's methods were discussed in Part I (page 20) where bias, lack of follow-up, and exclusion of significant findings were revealed as major flaws in this political attempt to exonerate the pertussis vaccine. Not unexpectedly, the American Academy of Pediatrics Task Force on Pertussis concluded that there is no convincing evidence for a causative role for DTP vaccination in SIDS in their review of these seven studies (Cherry *et al.*, 1988). The Institute of Medicine committee formed to review adverse consequences of pertussis vaccine reached the same conclusion (Institute of Medicine, 1991).

Anaphylaxis, sudden onset of a life-threatening allergic reaction and systemic collapse, has been recognized as a consequence of many vaccines including pertussis. In one report of DTP reactions, seven infants had severe shock with loss of consciousness or swelling of the larynx (Osvath *et al.*, 1979). Another study reported eight children with anaphylaxis or collapse within 24 hours of DTP vaccination, for a rate of six cases per 100,000 children vaccinated (Pollock & Morris, 1983). Other individual cases of anaphylactic reactions have been reported as well (Leung, 1985; Ovens, 1986; Cody *et al.*, 1981; Galazka *et al.*, 1972).

Hemolytic anemia, the destruction of red blood cells that could be caused by toxic agents or antibody responses to vaccines (Facktor *et al.*, 1973), has been associated with the DTP vaccine. One report cited three cases of hemolytic anemia in infants after DTP. These occurred in a 4-month-old boy four days after vaccination, a 6-month-old girl hospitalized with anemia three weeks after vaccination, and a boy aged 10 months who had been sick for weeks following his DTP vaccination at six months (Haneberg *et al.*, 1978). Another case of acute hemolytic anemia following vaccination was discovered in a review of 44 children with autoimmune hemolytic anemia (Zupanska *et al.*, 1976). A 2.5-year-old boy developed hemolytic anemia six days after his fourth dose of DTP and then again six days after his fifth dose (Coulter & Fisher, 1991).

These severe reactions led to the search for a safer vaccine, but the acellular vaccine has been plagued with the same types of adverse events as the whole-cell vaccine.

Acellular Vaccine Reactions

A review of acellular pertussis vaccine reports to VAERS was conducted for the first two years of vaccine use, including the period

January 1995 through June 1998. "Agitation" was the most commonly reported adverse event (26 percent of reports), and prolonged crying longer than three hours occurred in 14 percent of DtaP reports. Encephalitis was cited in eight reports, meningitis in 11 reports. There were 82 reports of convulsions. Of these, 34 were determined possibly linked to the vaccine because the convulsions occurred within one week of vaccination. The rate of convulsions for the acellular vaccine was equivalent to the rate for the whole-cell vaccine during this period (Braun *et al.*, 2000).

This vaccine seems to cause fewer of the mild-type reactions than the older whole-cell vaccine. In Japan, the replacement of whole-cell with acellular vaccine resulted in a 60 percent reduction of "mild" reactions, particularly febrile seizures. But the rate of severe reactions did not differ significantly between the acellular and whole-cell vaccine (Noble *et al.*, 1987).

A study in Sweden also revealed that the acellular vaccine caused less of the mild-type reactions than the whole-cell vaccine. But **encephalitis** reactions did occur with the acellular vaccine. A total of 212 infants received the acellular vaccine. Two serious reactions occurred. These reactions are identical to those following the whole-cell vaccine. The case descriptions are quoted here at length.

- A girl who had received two doses of the acellular vaccine as primary vaccination started to cry persistently seven hours after the booster injection. The parents had never heard such a cry before. She cried for 1.5 to 2 hours, and then went to bed and slept normally. The following morning she was found in bed pale, hypotonic, and unresponsive.

- A boy who had received three doses of the acellular vaccine as primary vaccination became fretful and tired, and refused to eat 2 to 3 hours after the booster injection. The unusual behavior of the child continued, and he was hospitalized the following day. These symptoms recurred periodically during the four days of hospitalization. Clinical and laboratory examinations yielded no signs of infection or hypoglycemia. The boy recovered fully. Two EEGs [studies of brain waves] showed pathologic activity. The diagnosis was focal encephalitis of unknown origin (Blennow and Granstrom, 1989).

These limited studies of the acellular vaccine reveal that children vaccinated during infancy have serious vaccine reactions. In the Swedish study the rate of serious reactions was 1 in 100 vaccinated children. The limited scope of this study does not allow us to draw conclusions about frequency of severe reactions, but this rate is much *higher* than that reported for the whole-cell vaccine.

Another Swedish study observed 2,800 infants who received acellular pertussis vaccine in a double-blind placebo-controlled experiment with the vaccine. Four of the children died within two weeks to five months of vaccination. Two cases are summarized here.

- A previously healthy 10-month-old girl developed *H. influenzae* meningitis 9 days after her second dose of acellular pertussis vaccine and she was hospitalized that day. Five days later she died. Autopsy revealed severe brain damage.

- A 15-month-old boy began having symptoms 10 weeks after his second vaccination. He cried during the night, and then had convulsions at 4:00 AM. He was found dead 5 hours later.

(Storsaeter *et al.*, 1988).

The reports of the two fatalities that were possibly related to the acellular pertussis vaccine contributed to the decision of Swedish authorities to recommend withdrawal of the application for vaccine licensure. They said, "The Division of Drugs judges that the efficacy of the vaccine may be lower than that of whole-cell vaccines. The uncertainty about a possible association with deaths due to serious bacterial infections, which occurred among vaccinated children, has also contributed to the recommendation" (License, 1989).

A PERSONAL STRATEGY

Pertussis vaccine is one of the most reactive vaccines ever developed. The acellular vaccine has been plagued by the same problems as the previous whole-cell vaccine. Parents who choose to give the pertussis vaccine risk seizures and brain damage in their children. Although other vaccines have taken the spotlight in recent years, pertussis still remains the classic toxic vaccine. The measles/autism phenomenon has caused droves of parents to avoid MMR. The meningococcal vaccine reactions in England caused worldwide shock. And the hepatitis scandal forced the vaccine industry to answer for their conflicts of interest in front of congressional committees. But no other vaccine has approached the cumulative damage inflicted by the pertussis vaccine. The vaccine industry's denials of pertussis vaccine reactions is unforgivable. Parents should never forget the tragedies associated with this vaccine. Fortunately, homeopathy is able to provide treatment for whooping cough when it occurs (English, 1987b), and parents have an alternative to the vaccine.

POLIO

At its worst, poliomyelitis is a disease that invades the nervous system and produces weakness and flaccid paralysis of the muscles supplied by affected nerves. Polio has probably existed for centuries, but no major epidemics occurred until the end of the nineteenth century. During the period 1900–1930, 80 to 90 percent of those afflicted with diagnosed polio were under five years of age, and the disease received its name of "infantile paralysis." No epidemics have occurred in the United States since 1954.

In underdeveloped countries where sanitation is poor, polioviruses are widespread. Almost 100 percent of children develop antibodies due to infection in infancy. Paralytic cases are few, the great majority being minor illnesses, and epidemics are unknown. As standards of living change, epidemics can be predicted to occur within a few years. This may be due to lack of general exposure to the virus and subsequent greater susceptibility in large numbers of people when virulent strains appear later. Immunization campaigns have also been associated with dramatic increases in polio cases in developing countries.

The polio virus enters the body through the nose or mouth, and multiplies in the digestive tract. From there it can enter the bloodstream and may then infect nerve cells. Most cases (90 to 98 percent) of illness associated with poliovirus remain either inapparent or characterized by sore throat, headache, nausea, and abdominal pain. It is usually diagnosed as a cold or flu. Only one percent of infections results in paralytic disease. Only a small percentage of these cases have residual paralysis.

Paralytic polio begins with a minor illness followed by a few days of well-being. Then more severe symptoms occur with stiffness of the back and neck, and muscle pain. Paralysis of the arms and/or legs soon follows. Rarely, paralysis of the muscles of respiration occurs. Return of muscle power begins after a period of days or weeks, and usually reaches its limit in 18 months. After that, any residual paralysis is permanent. Fatalities occur in 5 to 10 percent of the cases of paralytic polio, usually from respiratory paralysis.

There is no effective specific orthodox treatment for paralytic polio. Homeopaths have treated cases of paralytic polio with reported success, though no studies of treatment effectiveness have been conducted.

INCIDENCE

Wild polio does not exist in the United States or the Western Hemisphere at this time. One case of paralytic poliomyelitis was reported in Peru in 1991 (Centers for Disease Control, 1991a). Since that time the Americas have been polio-free. The goal of the World Health Organization since 1988 has been global eradication of polio (Centers for Disease Control, 1994b). All cases of paralytic polio in this country since 1979 were either caused by the oral vaccine or contracted in a foreign country during travel. The risk of acquiring wild polio in the United States is zero.

VACCINE EFFICACY

Two forms of vaccine are available. The inactivated or killed-virus vaccine, IPV, is given by injection. It works by producing circulating antibodies only. Booster doses are required as antibody levels decline. The oral live-virus vaccine, OPV, produces both intestinal and circulating antibodies, which apparently persist at high levels for years. The oral live-virus vaccine (OPV) replaced the killed vaccine (IPV) in 1962. The oral vaccine was favored because it was easier to administer and had less adverse effects. It was expected to produce longer-lasting and more complete immunity, and to also produce immunity in unvaccinated contacts of vaccine recipients who spread the virus to others after vaccination.

Experience with the killed and live vaccines subsequent to that time has proven the contrary. Live vaccine actually causes paralytic polio. The killed vaccine works just as well, and killed vaccine is claimed to reduce the spread of naturally occurring viruses in the community (Salk & Drucker, 1988). In 1991 a phased program of reintroduction of the killed vaccine IPV was begun, and in 1999 the CDC announced that in January 2000 IPV would be the only polio vaccine recommended (CDC, 2000c). Four doses of IPV beginning at two months of age are necessary to boost antibody levels for long-term protection.

A great deal of controversy exists concerning the effectiveness of the polio vaccines. Proponents claim the vaccine was responsible for the dramatic decline in polio cases subsequent to the mass immunization campaigns of the late 1950s. Critics suggest that the epidemic just lost its steam. In Great Britain the incidence of death from polio was at its height in 1950. By 1956, when the vaccine campaign was begun, it had already declined by 82 percent. Walene James, in her book *Immunization: The Reality Behind the Myth,* accuses the medical profession of distorting statistics to prove the vaccine's efficacy.

Dr. Bernard Greenberg, a biostatistics expert, was chairman of the Committee on Evaluation and Standards of the American Public Health Association during the 1950s. He testified at a panel discussion that was used as evidence for the congressional hearings on polio vaccine in 1962. During these hearings he elaborated on the problems associated with polio statistics, and disputed claims for the vaccine's effectiveness. He attributed the dramatic decline in polio cases to a change in reporting practices by physicians. Fewer cases were identified as polio after the vaccination for very specific reasons. This discussion has relevance to other vaccine experiences as well, and his remarks are therefore quoted at length.

> Prior to 1954 any physician who reported paralytic poliomyelitis was doing his patient a service by way of subsidizing the cost of hospitalization and was being community-minded in reporting a communicable disease. The criterion of diagnosis at that time in most health departments followed the World Health Organization definition: 'Spinal paralytic poliomyelitis: signs

and symptoms of nonparalytic poliomyelitis with the addition of partial or complete paralysis of one or more muscle groups, detected on two examinations at least 24 hours apart.'

Note that 'two examinations at least 24 hours apart' was all that was required. Laboratory confirmation and presence of residual paralysis was not required. In 1955 the criteria were changed to conform more closely to the definition used in the 1954 field trials: residual paralysis was determined 10 to 20 days after onset of illness and again 50 to 70 days after onset. . . .

This change in definition meant that in 1955 we started reporting a new disease, namely, paralytic poliomyelitis with a longer-lasting paralysis. Furthermore, diagnostic procedures have continued to be refined. Coxsackie virus infections and aseptic meningitis have been distinguished from paralytic poliomyelitis. Prior to 1954 large numbers of these cases undoubtedly were mislabeled as paralytic poliomyelitis. Thus, simply by changes in diagnostic criteria, the number of paralytic cases was predetermined to decrease in 1955–1957, whether or not any vaccine was used. . . .

There is still another reason for the decrease in the reported paralytic poliomyelitis cases in 1955–57. As a result of the publicity given the Salk vaccine, the public questioned the possibility of a vaccinated child developing paralytic poliomyelitis. Whenever such an event occurred, every effort was made to ascertain whether or not the disease was truly paralytic poliomyelitis. . . . We have been conditioned today to screen out false positive cases in a way that was not even imagined prior to 1954.

As a result of these changes in both diagnosis and diagnostic methods, the rates of paralytic poliomyelitis plummeted from the early 1950s to a low in 1957 (Intensive Immunization Programs, Hearings, 1962; pp. 96–97).

These factors called into question the claims for polio vaccine efficacy and the polio vaccine campaign in general. Nonetheless the polio vaccines, both OPV and IPV, have been credited with the elimination of polio from many countries throughout the world, including the United States.

Despite the goals for global eradication of polio, outbreaks continue to occur in vaccinated populations. These outbreaks cast doubts on the claims for polio vaccine effectiveness. A widespread outbreak of type 1 polio occurred in Oman during 1988 and 1989. A total of 118 cases occurred, primarily in children younger than 2 years old, despite a universal vaccination program and full coverage (at least 3 doses of OPV) for 87 percent of children by the age of 12 months. The high rate of paralytic polio in this population means that thousands of fully vaccinated children became infected during the outbreak. More than 25 percent of fully vaccinated children may have been infected in the areas affected by the outbreak. The authors of the published report from the Centers for Disease Control question the effectiveness of existing polio vaccines and the present dosage schedules (Sutter *et al.*, 1991).

An even larger epidemic of 305 polio cases in 1- to 7-year-old children occurred in The Gambia, western Africa, in 1986, in a vaccinated population. The effectiveness of three doses of OPV was only 72 percent in this population. In other African countries the presence of protective levels of polio antibodies after appropriate vaccination was correspondingly low—36 percent in Ghana, 48 percent in Nigeria, and 55–74 percent in Kenya. The authors of the Gambian polio epidemic study concluded, "protection was not achieved by a well-established vaccination program that had fully vaccinated an estimated 64 percent of the age group with the highest attack rate. . . . Therefore, we doubt that substantially higher efficacy will be achieved in other African countries using the same trivalent oral polio vaccine formulation and vaccination schedule" (Deming *et al.*, 1992).

In Taiwan an outbreak of 1,031 paralytic polio cases occurred in 1982, in a population with an 80 percent vaccination level of infants. Although the polio cases occurred predominantly in unvaccinated children, spread of polio in such high numbers implies that many thousands of children were infected. An interesting finding in this study was the attribution of polio cases to contaminated water sources.

Children were 5 times more likely to contract polio if they received water from non-municipal rather than municipal sources (Kim-Farley *et al.,* 1984). This epidemic provides evidence that the level of sanitation rather than the vaccination level in a community contributes significantly to the incidence of paralytic polio.

VACCINE REACTIONS

Oral Polio Vaccine (OPV) Reactions

The oral live-virus polio vaccine (OPV) is capable of causing paralytic polio in the vaccine recipient and close contacts. The CDC case definition of **vaccine-associated paralytic poliomyelitis (VAPP)** includes the onset of disease symptoms within 7 to 30 days postvaccination, or the onset of disease in a contact of a vaccine recipient within 7 to 60 days. The attack rate of VAPP is much higher for individuals receiving their first dose of live vaccine compared to subsequent doses. The risk of acquiring polio from the oral live vaccine is estimated to be 1 case per 520,000 first doses distributed (Nkowane *et al.,* 1987). The risk to household contacts is estimated at about 1 per 6 million vaccinees, and 1 per 23 million for community contacts (Nightingale, 1977).

The statistics of VAPP frequency could be disputed because of the strict guidelines for the definition of vaccine-associated paralytic polio cases. VAPP may occur with greater frequency than vaccine researchers claim. For example, in a World Health Organization review of VAPP in Latin America, 33 percent of 6,000 cases of acute flaccid paralysis were eliminated from consideration as VAPP because it was not possible to determine the presence of neurologic sequelae 60 days after paralysis onset (Andrus *et al.,* 1995). These cases were apparently lost to follow-up. If a case was diagnosed as Guillain-Barré syndrome (GBS) or aseptic meningitis it was also eliminated from consideration, even though these symptoms could have been caused by the vaccine also. Of the 125 cases of acute flaccid paralysis that met the criterion of onset of symptoms within 4 to 40 days postvaccine and persistent documented paralysis longer than 60 days, 65 percent of the cases were eliminated from the final statistics because they were labeled GBS or meningitis. These kinds of statistical trimming procedures are notorious for reducing the apparent adverse effects reported for vaccines.

In Romania the incidence of VAPP in infants was found to be exceedingly high compared to other countries. For the period 1984 to 1992, the risk of VAPP following receipt of the first dose of oral vaccine was 1 case per 85,000 doses distributed (Strebel *et al.*, 1994) compared to 1:520,000 in the United States. The authors also concluded that the true level of risk could be even higher because they did not adjust for wastage of vaccine. A follow-up study suggested that the higher rate of VAPP reactions in Romania could have been caused by the frequency of intramuscular injections of other drugs such as antibiotics in vaccine recipients in that country compared to other nations (Strebel, 1995). This ability of injections to provoke paralytic polio had previously been noted for wild-type polio as well. An injection given during the incubation period of wild-type poliovirus in infected persons may increase the risk of paralytic disease (Wyatt, 1985; Sutter *et al.*, 1992).

Guillain-Barré syndrome (GBS), characterized by progressive muscle weakness and destruction of the myelin sheath of nerves, is a well recognized adverse effect of oral polio vaccine. A mass polio vaccination campaign in Finland during February and March 1985 resulted in a higher incidence of GBS cases in the first two quarters of 1985 (16 total cases) compared to a mean incidence of GBS in the population of 3 cases per quarter during a six-year surveillance period, 1981–1986. Ten of these cases (ages 15 to 73 years) were diagnosed with GBS within 10 weeks after vaccination with OPV (Kinnunen *et al.*, 1989). A second research group in Finland identified a cluster of 10 GBS cases in children ages 0.4 to 14 years old during 1985. This cluster of GBS cases also coincided with the OPV campaign (Uhari *et al.*, 1989).

The Vaccine Safety Committee has acknowledged that OPV causes both paralytic polio and Guillain-Barré syndrome (Institute of Medicine, 1994).

Killed or inactivated polio vaccine (IPV) reactions

A review of VAERS reports following IPV administration examined all adverse events reported during the years 1991 through 1998. A total of 800 reports were reviewed for infants 1-6 months of age, which included 83 deaths. The most commonly reported conditions were neurologic, including convulsions, apnea, hypotonia, screaming, and agitation. Other serious adverse reactions were allergic reactions (asthma, hives), gastrointestinal symptoms, and fever (Wattigney *et al.*, 2001). No anaphylaxis reactions to IPV have been reported (Institute of Medicine, 1994).

A review of Guillain-Barré syndrome during the years 1949–1966 revealed five cases associated with IPV, but few details were described (Leneman, 1966).

In 1955 a preparation of IPV produced by Cutter Biological contained active virus that caused 260 cases of poliomyelitis in vaccine recipients (Nathanson & Langmuir, 1963). It was determined that bottles of tissue culture fluid containing the virus had been stored prior to inactivation with formaldehyde, and tissues that settled to the bottom of containers protected the virus particles from the formaldehyde treatment (Klein, 1972). Since the introduction of new manufacturing safety requirements stimulated by the Cutter incident, no similar cases have been reported.

During the period 1954 to 1963 when IPV was used exclusively, a monkey virus known as SV40 was transmitted in the polio vaccine, exposing an estimated 98 million Americans (Fisher *et al.*, 1999). An increased incidence of brain tumors was later found among persons who had received the contaminated vaccine (Geissler, 1990). And a study of more than 58,000 women who had received IPV during the years that SV40 contaminated the vaccine showed a thirteenfold increased risk of brain tumors in their children (Rosa *et al.*, 1988).

Later research confirmed the association between the SV40 virus transmitted through polio vaccine and cancers. SV40 does cause cancer when injected into laboratory animals. Now, more than 60 scientific studies have found SV40 in human brain, bone and lung-related cancers, the same kinds of tumors the virus causes in laboratory animals. Researchers also determined that SV40 viral strains can infect humans, and that the authentic SV40 present in monkeys is associated with brain tumors in early childhood (Butel *et al.*, 1998). A study conducted in China confirmed that SV40 was present in a majority of brain tumors tested, and that the SV40 involved was actively expressing proteins and stimulating tumor production (Zhen *et al.*, 1999). When vaccine from 1955 was tested, the vials were found to contain SV40 genetically identical to the strains found in human bone and brain tumors and in monkeys (Bookchin and Schumacher, 2000). Humans have continued to transmit the SV40 monkey virus acquired from the polio vaccine over a period of at least 40 years, probably through blood transfusions, breastfeeding, and sexual contact, and the virus continues to cause cancers. For a full discussion of contaminated polio vaccines, see page 58.

POLIO FACTS

- No cases of wild polio have occurred in the United States since 1979. The risk of a child acquiring polio in the United States is zero, except from the vaccine itself.
- The vaccines have questionable effectiveness.
- Oral, live-virus vaccine (OPV) does cause polio in vaccine recipients and contacts. It has caused Guillain-Barré syndrome (GBS) in recipients. It also may contain live monkey viruses that have been associated with human diseases.
- Killed polio vaccine (IPV) has also caused significant adverse effects, including cancers from a contaminated vaccine, but it does not cause polio in recipients.

A PERSONAL STRATEGY

Since the risk of acquiring polio is near zero if a child is not vaccinated, it seems unjustifiable to risk adverse effects from the polio vaccine. Since the live oral vaccine is no longer in use, there is no risk of acquiring polio from previously vaccinated children.

SMALLPOX

Smallpox (or variola) has an infamous history as a dreaded contagious disease, and a deadly weapon of war. Unfortunately, the smallpox vaccine has a similar history. Smallpox arose from a relatively harmless rodent virus that became deadly when it jumped the species barrier to humans thousands of years ago. The oldest reference to the disease is in Egyptian records of 3700 B.C. Since that time, smallpox has killed hundreds of millions of people. The disease is especially devastating to cultures that have not been previously exposed. The native populations of North and South America were decimated by smallpox and war, reducing their numbers from 72 million when Columbus landed in 1492 to 600,000 by 1800 (Thornton, 1987).

The last outbreaks of smallpox occurred in the 1970s. During the period of smallpox epidemics, modern medicine had no effective treatment for this deadly virus. The fatality rate was about 30 percent in epidemics. The death rate was highest among those never vaccinated. In one review of 680 smallpox cases in Europe during the period 1950–1971, vaccination over 20 years prior to exposure reduced the death rate to 11 percent compared to about 50 percent in the unvaccinated (Mack, 1972). It is estimated that the fatality rate would be dramatically reduced by the use of modern antiviral drugs and other pharmaceutical approaches.

Smallpox was declared officially eliminated from the planet in 1980. Subsequently, the virus was maintained in government storage facilities, and developed as a weapon of war.

The only possible causes of smallpox disease now would be laboratory accidents, a mass release during wartime, or through terrorist acts. No one knows what a modern epidemic would be like because today's weapons-grade smallpox virus is designed to be lethal, and because the United States stopped routine smallpox vaccination in 1971.

Another similar pox virus does cause disease and deaths, termed human monkeypox when it was discovered in 1970 because the virus resembled a pox virus found in captive monkeys in 1958 (Mukinda et al., 1996). Monkeypox exists in rainforest villages of central and western Africa, where it is transferred through person-to-person contact. It causes the same symptoms as smallpox, and differs from smallpox virus only in its nucleotide sequences. Several outbreaks have occurred. In 1996, 71 cases were reported in the Katako-Kombe area in Zaire with four deaths. In one small village of 346 inhabitants, 42 cases were reported, including three deaths (WHO, 1996). By December of 1997 more than 500 cases of monkeypox were reported in Zaire. It is possible that smallpox has already made a comeback in this remote part of the world.

SMALLPOX SYMPTOMS

Twelve days after exposure, smallpox begins with fever, tiredness, vomiting, and severe back pain. Within three days a rash develops on the face, then spreads to the trunk, arms, and legs. The victim is potentially contagious from the onset of symptoms until all eruptions have healed. The hardy virus is spread through droplets from the nose or mouth, which can even travel through ventilation systems to infect others. The skin lesions themselves are also contagious. Once the rash appears, the flat red eruptions develop into hardened pustules over the course of a week. These lesions can be felt as lumps under the skin. Thousands of these pustules may occur over the body, with swelling and generalized redness of the skin, and severe, fiery itching. The swollen face is often completely covered with lesions. On the eighth day of the eruption a dark spot appears on the pustule and then it opens, discharging pus, forming a scab, and then leaving a depressed scar, which is often permanent. Complete recovery usually occurs within three weeks.

However, in severe cases of the disease, fever begins again on day 11 with a rampant worsening of symptoms. Infections of the eye can cause blindness, fluids collect in the airways resulting in suffocation, sores and abscesses develop, and the body bloats and swells. An especially vicious form of smallpox results in bleeding from the skin lesions and internal organs, and frequently these patients die. It is during the second week that most deaths from smallpox occur.

Biological Warfare

Smallpox is a potent weapon of war. The British purposefully inflicted smallpox on Native Americans during the French and Indian War in Canada (1754–1767), and on the Continental army during the American Revolution. A Confederate doctor deliberately sold clothes contaminated with smallpox to Union soldiers during the American Civil War, and Japanese doctors exposed Chinese prisoners of war to aerosolized virus in germ warfare experiments during World War II (Tucker, 2001).

It was the Soviets, however, who developed secret stocks of lethal smallpox for use in war. The Soviets established their first smallpox bioweapons laboratory in 1947 near Moscow. By the 1970s they maintained an annual stockpile of twenty tons of virulent, weapons-grade smallpox (Alibek, 1999). This was enough to blanket 4,000 square miles of enemy territory. The Soviets utilized gene-splicing techniques, adding toxins to the virus that could induce systemic hemorrhage, neurologic disease, and brain damage. The smallpox designer weapon also resulted in a shortened incubation period of a few days rather than the usual two-week period of the natural disease. Several countries, including Iraq and North Korea, also possess smallpox virus for use as a biowarfare weapon. The question remains whether Russian or Iraqi scientists would supply smallpox vaccine to terrorists knowing the devastating consequences to their own populations of a worldwide epidemic.

Unlike anthrax, dispersing smallpox through a terrorist act is relatively simple. Spray the infectious live virus in a public place and a widespread epidemic is nearly guaranteed. The terrorists themselves would face no risk of disease if they were previously vaccinated; however, the ensuing worldwide epidemic would certainly return to affect their own families and comrades.

Smallpox Vaccine

People who contract smallpox through their skin are much less likely to die of the disease. This discovery led to the practice in India (around 1000 B.C.) of making incisions in the skin of healthy people and inoculating them with pus from a smallpox lesion. The fatality rate was thereby reduced from 30 percent to one percent. The practice spread to Tibet and to China by 1000 A.D., but it did not reach Europe until 1718, when the first western child was inoculated through the skin, a process that came to be known as variolation.

The practice of variolation spread to America and throughout Europe during the eighteenth century, accompanied by severe opposition. Although variolation did result in immunity to smallpox, the non-sterile technique also served to spread other diseases, such as syphilis and tetanus. The discovery that milkmaids who contracted cowpox from the udders of cows were rendered immune to human smallpox led to the development of a vaccine (from the Latin vacca for cow). By the early 1800s, vaccination with cowpox replaced variolation with smallpox.

The vaccination procedure involves piercing the skin and inserting the live cowpox virus into the lesion. Eventually the cowpox virus in the vaccine became altered through many years of culture and was assigned a new name, vaccinia virus. Otherwise smallpox vaccination has remained relatively unchanged over the past 200 years.

Vaccine Efficacy

Over 95 percent of those receiving smallpox vaccine for the first time will develop antibodies at a titer of 1:10 or greater; however, the level of antibody that protects against smallpox infection is not known (CDC, 1991d).

Smallpox vaccination is certainly not a guarantee against contracting the disease. During an epidemic in India (in 1953) 80 percent of people with smallpox had a history of at least one vaccination and 50 percent had been vaccinated two or three times (Kempe, 1960). As a result of that experience the author recommended yearly smallpox vaccinations during periods of epidemics.

During the nineteenth and early twentieth centuries, when smallpox epidemics ran rampant, vaccination had a terrible reputation, and seemed quite ineffective in preventing disease. A disastrous smallpox epidemic occurred in England during the period 1871–1873 at a time when a compulsory smallpox vaccination law had resulted in nearly universal coverage. A Royal Commission was appointed in 1889 to investigate the history of vaccination in the United Kingdom. Evidence mounted that smallpox epidemics increased dramatically after 1854, the year the compulsory vaccination law went into effect. In the London epidemic of 1857–1859, there were more than 14,000 deaths; in the 1863–1865 outbreak 20,000 deaths; and from 1871 to 1873 all of Europe was swept by the worst smallpox epidemic in recorded history. In England and Wales alone, 45,000 people died of smallpox at a time when, according to official estimates, 97 percent of the population had been vaccinated. Their investigation led to the repeal of England's compulsory smallpox vaccination law.

When Japan started compulsory vaccination against smallpox in 1872 the disease steadily increased each year. In 1892 more than 165,000 cases occurred with 30,000 deaths in a completely vaccinated population. During the same time period Australia had no compulsory vaccination laws, and only three deaths occurred from smallpox over a 15-year period.

In the Philippines between 1917 and 1919, the US government staged a compulsory vaccination campaign, which brought on the worst epidemic of smallpox in the country's history with over 160,000 cases and over 70,000 deaths in a completely vaccinated population. The entire population of the Philippines at the time was only 11 million.

Current smallpox vaccination differs very little from the vaccine used in the nineteenth century, and no one knows whether the vaccine will be similarly ineffective if a modern epidemic were to occur. Most important, however, is the complete uncertainty whether the current vaccine would have any protective effect against a weaponized smallpox virus used in a terrorist attack.

Vaccine Strategy

Two different strategies exist to contain an outbreak of smallpox through vaccination. One is to vaccinate the entire population. This is expensive, in financial terms, and in human life, because the vaccine would undoubtedly cause significant damage and deaths. A universal vaccination campaign such as this might be instituted in an uncontrolled and widespread epidemic. The second strategy is to isolate and contain the outbreak. Locate every person who had face-to-face contact with the victim, and vaccinate them. Then find everyone who came into contact with those people and vaccinate them too. That creates a ring of safety around the index case. This method works for smallpox because the vaccine will have some protective effect if given within four days of exposure. The method is not foolproof, vaccination is not always protective, and vaccine given within four days of exposure still results in a 10–40 percent incidence of smallpox (Kempe, 1960).

The US government retained only 15 million doses of smallpox vaccine after the disease was declared eliminated in 1980. In response to the terrorist attack on September 11, 2001 and the use of anthrax as a bioweapon in the following months, the United States arranged to purchase 300 million doses of live smallpox vaccine from Acambis, a British vaccine manufacturer, for a total of $850 million. Subsequent to the placement of this order, a French vaccine manufacturer, Aventis Pasteur, discovered a previously unknown stockpile of 85 million doses of smallpox vaccine in a freezer. The vaccine maker donated this supply of 40-year-old vaccine to the United States. Additionally, a study published in April 2002 showed that the vaccine supply could probably be greatly extended. Patients in that study received a vaccination with either the full strength smallpox vaccine or a 1:5 or 1:10 dilution of the vaccine. No significant difference was noted in the response to the vaccine in any of the three groups (Frey, et al., 2002). This suggests that the supply of vaccine could potentially be multiplied by a factor of ten. Calls have also gone out from Congress for development of a safer, killed vaccine.

The simple practice of vaccination applied on a worldwide scale eventually eliminated smallpox disease from the planet, but not without a price.

Vaccine Reactions

The usual response to vaccination in an individual is the development of a half-inch pustule and inflammation at the site that persists for two to three weeks then crusts over, leaving a scar. Mild fever and illness with a rash and swollen lymph nodes often occur, but severe adverse reactions are not uncommon. The death rate from smallpox vaccine is at least one to two deaths per million vaccinations, making smallpox the most toxic vaccine ever invented. Vaccinating the entire US population would result in at least 300 to 600 deaths.

Other adverse effects of vaccination are more common. A severe form of **eczema** with inflamed skin, high temperature, and swollen lymph nodes occurs in as many as one in 26,000 vaccinations (Lane, 1970). The result is sometimes fatal. **Encephalitis**, or inflammation of the brain, is the other severe adverse reaction. It occurs in as many as one in 80,000 people vaccinated. Symptoms include fever, convulsions, partial paralysis, and death in approximately 25 percent of people with this reaction. Those who recover usually suffer some permanent mental impairment and paralysis. Statistics on the rate of complications vary depending on the type of survey. They are lower for voluntary reports and higher when physicians are polled for their experience. No controlled studies have ever been published. Rates are probably much higher than reported.

Infants and children under twelve months have a significantly higher risk of serious adverse reactions compared to older children and adults. The rate of brain inflammation is as high as one in 24,000 vaccinations in children under twelve months (Lane, 1970).

It is possible to spread the vaccinia virus from an inoculation to other sites on the body or to other people within the period 2–5 days following vaccination. This form of transmission will cause eczema vaccinatum in 30 percent of those contacts affected, a condition which may be fatal.

Because of the significant risk of adverse reactions, no one with a history of eczema or those with household contacts with a history of eczema should receive the smallpox vaccine. Pregnant women should never receive the vaccine because of the risk of fetal infection, which results in stillbirth or death of the infant after delivery. Individuals with immune deficiency disease, immunosuppression, and HIV infection should not be vaccinated (CDC, 1991d).

Treatment of the complications that occur after smallpox vaccination consists of vaccinia immune globulin (VIG). This is a sterile solution of the immune globulin from plasma of individuals previously vaccinated for smallpox. VIG has been effective in the treatment of eczema and vaccinia caused by the smallpox vaccine. It is not effective for post-vaccine encephalitis (CDC, 1991d).

In the late nineteenth century, a British homeopathic physician, Dr. J. Compton Burnett, published a treatise that asserted smallpox vaccination caused a chronic nervous system and skin disease. He named this chronic disease "vaccinosis," distinguishing it from the immediate adverse reactions to vaccination. Symptoms were characterized by nerve pain and various skin ailments such as acne and psoriasis that began soon after a smallpox vaccination and persisted. Burnett discovered that a homeopathic medicine, Thuja occidentalis, cured the vaccinosis disease, and Thuja became the routine medicine prescribed in homeopathic practice for smallpox vaccine reactions (Burnett, 1892).

Opposition to smallpox vaccination has been vocal and vehement since the first Anti-Compulsory Vaccination League was formed in England in 1866. Newspapers during the early twentieth century were filled with accounts of disease and death following vaccination. The anti-compulsory associations doubted the safety of vaccination and often asserted that vaccination caused more brain damage and deaths than smallpox itself. They were especially opposed to forced vaccination. Accounts were circulated of vaccine squads who forcibly vaccinated citizens, literally holding them down while a health worker administered the inoculation. In 1907 Britain passed a law allowing conscientious objection to enforced vaccination. By contrast, in 1905 the US Supreme Court ruled that the state could pass laws requiring vaccination to protect the public in the case of a dangerous communicable disease.

It is conceivable that a safer vaccine than the current live-virus inoculation could be produced, and proposed manufacturing processes do exist for a killed vaccine, but several factors make development of a safe vaccine difficult (Rosenthal, 2001). First, there is no animal model to use in researching smallpox. Second, in the absence of naturally occurring smallpox disease, there is no way to establish whether a new vaccine would work. And third, research on a new vaccine takes five to ten years. In the meantime, we are stuck with the two-hundred-year-old vaccine and all its shortcomings.

Smallpox Facts

- Smallpox disease was declared eradicated from the world in 1980. The only threat of infection is from a terrorist attack or biowarfare.

- The effectiveness of vaccination during historic epidemics is questionable.

- Antibody levels induced by vaccination begin to diminish after one year, although even more than 20 years later there is some reduction in incidence of death among those previously vaccinated.

- Vaccination administered within four days after exposure reduces the incidence of smallpox, the severity of disease, and the fatality rate.

- Smallpox is deadly, but so is the vaccine.

- The smallpox vaccine may not be effective against the genetically engineered virus designed as a bioweapon.

A Personal Strategy

In June 2002 the CDC recommended the smallpox vaccine only for those professionals who would actively manage the care of people who fell victim to a terrorist release of the virus. Members of "smallpox response teams" in each state (doctors, nurses, police, and investigators) should receive the vaccine, according to the recommendations. In addition, staff at pre-designated hospitals that would handle patients should also be vaccinated. The CDC advisory panel declined to recommend the vaccine to the general public because of concerns about side effects,

If an outbreak of smallpox occurs, the vaccine may be recommended for some portion of the population, or for those people with a possible history of exposure to the virus. Assess the likelihood of your exposure based on the location of index cases. For example, if you live in rural Oregon you are less likely to encounter the virus than in a large metropolitan area such as Chicago or Los Angeles. Remember that the vaccine reduces the severity of illness and risk of death when given within four days of exposure to someone with the disease. Individuals with a history of eczema should not be vaccinated because of the increased risk of skin reactions and death. If anyone in a household has eczema, then no one in the household should be vaccinated.

If you decide to receive the vaccination, make sure your doctor has access to vaccinia immune globulin (VIG) to treat adverse reactions, which has been in short supply. If you decide not to receive the vaccine, then consider discussing your situation with a homeopathic practitioner for alternative approaches. Homeopaths have been treating smallpox and epidemic diseases for two hundred years.

FURTHER READING

Tucker, Jonathan B. Scourge: The Once and Future Threat of Smallpox, Atlantic Monthly Press, New York, 2001.

www.vaccinewebsite.com contains many historical articles about smallpox and the anti-compulsory vaccination campaign.

www.vaccines.org is a searchable database of scientific and CDC vaccine articles.

TETANUS

The disease that everyone worries about most is tetanus. Unlike the other diseases discussed in this book, tetanus is caused by a microorganism that enters the skin through a wound. Tetanus is potentially fatal, and it strikes otherwise healthy individuals. The repeated exposure of young children to cuts, scrapes, and dirt provides a continual source of anxiety for parents of unvaccinated children. The organism responsible for tetanus is found in soil and the intestinal tracts of animals. Tetanus can be found in the feces of 10–20 percent of horses, and 25–30 percent of dogs (Kerrin, 1929). Any manure-treated soil may be infectious.

The symptoms of tetanus begin with stiffness of muscles; the muscles of the jaw and neck are the first to be involved. In the 24 to 48 hours after onset of the disease, muscle rigidity may be fully developed and involve the trunk and extremities. The neck and back become stiff and arched, and the abdomen board-like. Painful spasms can be produced by the slightest stimulant (noise, touch, light), and it is spasms of the respiratory muscles that cause asphyxia and death.

The incubation period for tetanus varies from one day to three weeks, although the usual range is one to two weeks. There is no sign of tetanus in the wound itself, and usually no symptoms until the muscle stiffness begins. Fever is generally low-grade or absent, and the senses remain clear.

Treatment for tetanus is drastic. Muscle relaxants, sedatives, antibiotics, immune globulin, and antitoxins are administered. The person is put in a low-stimulus environment and often fed through a stomach tube, and an artificial airway may be required during treatment. There is no effective alternative treatment.

INCIDENCE

The following statistics will help to put the tetanus problem into perspective. Between 1991 and 2000 there were 40–50 cases of tetanus per year in the United States (CDC, 2001). The majority of these cases are people over age 60 and intravenous drug users. Tetanus is now recognized as primarily a disease of older adults in the US. On average 5 percent or less of tetanus cases occur in individuals less than 20 years of age. In 1999 only two cases of tetanus occurred in children. During 1995–1997 half of all reported cases occurred as a result of puncture wounds. Other causes included self-body piercing, and surgeries. Those cases not associated with injuries accompanied intravenous drug use (18 percent of all cases) or predisposing chronic medical conditions such as cancer. The total case-fatality ratio is approximately 11 percent (CDC, 1998c).

The higher distribution of tetanus cases among the elderly is generally attributed to the low rate of tetanus vaccination among this group. Eighty-seven percent of children at two years old have received a primary series of tetanus vaccine injections (Centers for Disease Control, 1994a). By contrast, serosurveys indicate that one-half to two-thirds of persons 60 or older lack protective levels of circulating antitoxin antibody against tetanus (Centers for Disease Control, 1985). The high percentage of vaccinated children is at least partially responsible for the low incidence of tetanus in this age group. Just prior to the era of widespread vaccination, there were approximately 500 cases of tetanus each year.

To summarize this data, young people do not tend to get tetanus, and fatalities are extremely rare. Older people get tetanus more, and the case-fatality rate is higher (18 percent in people over 60). Less than 60 cases of tetanus each year is a very low incidence, especially if a large percentage of the older population has no immunity. Tetanus has been almost completely eliminated from the United States, primarily because of good hygiene and proper wound management. Unlike the contagious diseases, the use of vaccines in some of the population will not help to protect those who are not vaccinated.

Vaccine Administration

The primary series of tetanus toxoid vaccination consists of four injections. The first three doses are given at two-month intervals (though the intervals may be longer without forfeiting immunity) and the fourth dose about one year after the third dose. Boosters are recommended at five years old and every ten years thereafter. If a child has had the initial series of shots and recommended boosters, he or she does not need any further shots after injuries. Tetanus toxoid is often combined with other vaccines (e.g. diphtheria and pertussis in DT and DTaP), though it can be given alone.

Protection from tetanus following adequate vaccination lasts for at least twelve years. In people who have had at least two doses of tetanus toxoid at any time in their lives, response to a booster injection of toxoid is rapid and adequate to prevent tetanus if given within 72 hours after an injury.

For individuals who have had less than two previous injections of tetanus toxoid, an injection of Tetanus Immune Globulin, Human (TIG) is administered for serious wounds. This vaccine introduces antibodies directly into the body to fight tetanus bacteria. This process is known as passive immunization; the body does not develop its own antibodies. The antibody levels achieved with TIG are sufficient to protect against tetanus if the injection is given within 72 hours after the injury.

VACCINE EFFICACY

There is no question that a series of tetanus toxoid injections is highly effective at preventing tetanus (Edsall, 1959). This has been documented in several large studies during World War II, and with studies of large groups of horses. The fact that nearly all recent tetanus cases in the United States occurred in individuals who had not received the recommended schedule of vaccinations provides further evidence that active immunization is extremely effective.

Tetanus disease in those fully vaccinated has occurred, though failure of vaccination is rare. For example, a 34-year-old construction worker was hospitalized after having a reported epileptic fit and experiencing flu-like symptoms. Any attempts to speak or get up resulted in attacks of severe muscle spasms. The patient recovered, and a review of his medical history revealed a complete tetanus vaccination history with booster shots five and two years before being hospitalized (Shimoni *et al.*, 1999). In another report, three patients with recent tetanus vaccination and high antibody titers nonetheless acquired severe tetanus disease (Crone and Reder, 1992).

The effectiveness of Tetanus Immune Globulin (TIG) in protecting previously unvaccinated individuals at the time of injury is more difficult to document. It is not possible to conduct controlled studies in humans. Evaluating the efficacy of TIG in the prevention of tetanus must be accomplished by measuring antibody responses after injection and by clinical experience. TIG raises antibodies in previously non-immune individuals to levels that indicate adequate protection from tetanus for at least 28 days (McComb & Dwyer, 1963). In addition, the record of tetanus immune globulin in the prevention of fatalities from tetanus is also extremely good. Clinical experience with TIG has led to a high level of confidence in the immune globulin's ability to prevent tetanus and death from tetanus when used in adequate doses within the prescribed interval following injury. A recent study evaluating two tetanus immunoglobulin preparations in 134 adults presenting to a hospital with tetanus-prone wounds confirmed adequate antibody responses and no cases of tetanus in recipients (Lang *et al.*, 2000). There have been rare cases of fatalities in individuals who received tetanus immune globulin soon after injury (Johnson, 1969), but it is generally assumed that one dose of TIG will provide protection from tetanus when administered soon after an injury.

VACCINE REACTIONS

Tetanus toxoid is generally considered safe, yet even this vaccine causes occasional severe reactions. It has been associated with an overall reaction incidence of 3 to 13 percent (White, W.G. *et al.*, 1983; Relihan, 1969). Most adverse reactions include swelling and abscesses at the injection site (Church & Richards, 1985) or mild fever and illness; however, severe allergic and nervous system reactions have been reported. Two deaths following tetanus injections given alone were reported, one in 1933 (Regamey, 1965) and one in 1973 (Staak &

Wirth, 1973). These were attributed to anaphylactic reactions, severe systemic allergic responses resulting in shock and collapse within four hours of injection. Thirteen cases of life-threatening allergic reactions meeting this definition have been reported in the literature (Institute of Medicine, 1994). Since tetanus toxoid is frequently administered in combination with diphtheria toxoid to both children and adults, adverse reactions to the two vaccines become difficult to distinguish in modern practice.

Many cases of **central nervous system disease** following tetanus toxoid injection have been reported in the medical literature. These cases include demyelinating diseases, Guillain-Barré syndrome (a demyelinating inflammatory disease of the peripheral nervous system with rapid onset of motor weakness and loss of sensation), neuropathies, and encephalopathies. They are often accompanied by severe, debilitating symptoms and hospitalization. A few of these cases are summarized below.

- A 50-year-old man received a dose of tetanus toxoid after suffering a wound to his foot. Ten days later he developed muscle aching, lethargy, fatigue, and headache. Two days after that he was admitted to the hospital with flaccid paralysis of the legs, no reflexes, loss of sensation, back pain, and inability to urinate. One month later his symptoms remained unchanged (Read *et al.*, 1992).

- An 11-year-old girl received a routine tetanus booster dose and three days later developed blindness in the right eye and light perception only in the left eye. Her optic discs were swollen on exam. Two days later she had partial paralysis of her legs and loss of bladder control, then more widespread sensory loss including a lack of vibrational and positional senses. Seven weeks later she still had some vision loss and decreased muscle power. Within one year she recovered (Topaloglu *et al.*, 1992).

- A 21-year-old man developed coma on two separate occasions (2.5 years apart) within eight days of tetanus toxoid injections (Schwarz *et al.*, 1988).

- A 36-year-old woman developed lethargy, slurred speech, and decreased sensation five days after receiving a tetanus booster. She recovered over the next year (Schlenska, 1977).

- A 42-year-old man received tetanus toxoid on three separate occasions over a period of 13 years. Following each vaccination he developed acute polyneuropathy diagnosed as Guillain-Barré syndrome (Pollard & Selby, 1978). A nerve biopsy revealed demyelination. Following his last injection he continued to experience multiple recurrences, and continued to show sensory findings on examination as of 1993 (Pollard, 1993).

Arthritis, or joint inflammation and swelling, has occurred following both tetanus toxoid given alone and in combination with diphtheria toxoid. For example, a 34-year-old woman received two doses of tetanus toxoid one month apart, and one week after the second dose she developed persistent inflammation in several joints. Laboratory tests confirmed that her condition was rheumatoid arthritis, a chronic and usually permanent disease (Jawad & Scott, 1989). In a review of 100 million doses of tetanus toxoid given over 15 years in Germany, 13 cases of "swelling and inflammatory changes of joints" were reported (Korger *et al.,* 1986). Ninety-nine cases of joint inflammation following tetanus and diphtheria vaccine (Td) were reported to the Monitoring System of Adverse Events Following Immunization (MSAEFI) operated by the CDC during the period 1979 to 1990. Of 39 patients available for follow-up, 12 had not recovered (Institute of Medicine, 1994).

The long-term adverse effects of tetanus toxoid are unknown.

Tetanus immune globulin (human) has not been associated with reactions. Since it is a product made from human serum, it may contain infectious material, though this possibility is highly unlikely. All globulin products are tested for contamination by known pathogens such as hepatitis and HIV viruses. The alcohol fractionation process used in the production of TIG is a further safeguard, since this process destroys such contaminating microorganisms.

Tetanus Facts

- Tetanus is a potentially life-threatening disease.

- Infection occurs through wounds.

- Incidence of tetanus is approximately 50 cases per year for the past 10 years; less than 10 of these cases are under 30 years old, and these cases are rarely fatal.

- A series of tetanus toxoid injections does provide protection from tetanus for at least 10 years. Tetanus immune globulin protects unvaccinated individuals if they receive an injection soon after injury.

- Immediate vaccine reactions are usually mild, though many severe reactions have been reported, some of them causing permanent disability and a few fatalities. Long-term adverse effects are unknown.

A Personal Strategy

Consumers need to decide whether the low risk from possible tetanus exposure warrants giving the vaccine. This is primarily an issue of comfort level and likelihood of exposure. People who live on farms or work with horses are more likely to be exposed than those who live in urban or suburban areas. Anxiety about tetanus may be high in parents because the disease progresses rapidly and can attack healthy children. However, tetanus is rarely fatal in children. Each parent must make the difficult decision about the tetanus vaccine.

If a child has a high likelihood of exposure or is traveling to a foreign country where sanitation is poor and the incidence of tetanus is higher than the United States, then tetanus vaccine administration should be seriously considered. Workers exposed to frequent injuries may also choose to receive regular tetanus boosters rather than worry about each individual injury.

Some tetanus vaccine issues are clear. There is no reason to vaccinate infants because they are extremely unlikely to injure themselves. Delaying the vaccine until children are older may prevent adverse effects. A child does not need any protection from tetanus until he or she is old enough to play outdoors and get scrapes and cuts. Children under two years old are not at risk of contracting tetanus.

Some individuals may feel that the tetanus vaccine is necessary even if they have decided against giving other vaccines. Tetanus toxoid is available as a single vaccine, or combined with diphtheria toxoid, or combined with diphtheria and pertussis. Anyone can therefore choose to give the tetanus vaccine alone.

Do not allow your child to receive any vaccine you do not want. Parents can decide to do one of two things:

1. Give the series of tetanus toxoid injections (preferably after 12 months of age). After the primary series, a child only needs boosters every 10 years, regardless of injuries sustained.

2. Avoid the routine series and give TIG (Tetanus Immune Globulin, human) only if a child has a serious wound or a deep puncture.

Anyone with a serious wound should receive tetanus immune globulin (TIG) if they have had less than two previous injections of tetanus toxoid. The human immune globulin (TIG) contains tetanus antibodies that will directly attack circulating tetanus bacteria. This will help prevent the multiplication of bacteria and developing infection if it is given within a few days of injury. TIG will not confer lasting immunity to tetanus. By contrast, tetanus toxoid will not provide adequate protection in previously unvaccinated people until the second dose of the series is given 1 to 2 months after the first. This is too long a period of time to protect a person from a wound that has already occurred.

All wounds should be adequately cleansed. This subject was discussed in an article by Drs. Skudder and McCarrol in the *Journal of the American Medical Association* in the 1960s, when physician encounters with unvaccinated people were more common than today. Their statements and recommendations help to establish guidelines for the treatment of wounds:

> Good wound care is probably the single most important factor in the prevention of tetanus in fresh wounds. This implies thorough cleansing of the wound and removal of all foreign bodies and devitalized [dead] tissue. This is important since the tetanus bacillus is an anaerobic organism and can grow only in necrotic tissue which has no blood supply.
>
> For adequate prophylaxis of tetanus, wounds must be divided arbitrarily into those considered tetanus prone and non-prone. . . . Any wound containing foreign material or devitalized tissue must be considered tetanus prone, as well as crushing injuries, deep second and third degree burns, [and] any infected wound. . . .
>
> The severity of a wound is not a reliable guide to the likelihood of tetanus developing since the disease may arise from minor or even unnoticed injuries. Many tetanus prone wounds, however, can be converted to non-prone wounds by proper cleansing and debridement (Skudder & McCarroll, 1964).

Children who are not vaccinated should have all wounds carefully cleansed at home or by a qualified health professional. If a serious wound occurs, or if there is a question about the need for tetanus protection, then the advice of a qualified physician should be sought and the administration of tetanus immune globulin (TIG) should be considered.

TRAVEL

Here is the simple formula for vaccine decisions prior to international travel.

- First, gather information about current disease incidence in the city, province, or specific area of a country on your itinerary.

- Second, decide if the risks from vaccines for this disease outweigh your risk of exposure and significant illness.

- Third, determine whether the vaccine's efficacy is high enough to warrant risking its side effects.

- Your decision is made.

Vaccines prior to travel fall into three general categories:

- *routine vaccines* normally given in childhood that may have lapsed or you never received

- *exotic vaccines* recommended for travel to specific countries

- *required vaccines* for entry into specific countries (Yellow fever is the only vaccine currently in this category.)

Information about international disease incidence and recommended vaccines for travel can be obtained at the following websites:

- *www.cdc.gov* This is the official website of the CDC that contains an extensive section for travelers' health. Information includes disease incidence by region, recommended vaccines, and extensive information about the vaccines.

- *www.tripprep.com* A private company, Shoreland, Inc., maintains this site of health conditions and recommendations, country by country.

- For questions about disease incidence in specific areas you are visiting, call the CDC Traveler's Health Hotline: 404-332-4559.

No vaccine is currently available in the US for cholera because of the limited duration of effectiveness produced by the vaccine.

HEPATITIS A

Hepatitis A exists in many areas of the world where sanitation standards are relatively low. Transmission occurs through water contaminated with sewage. Travelers to North America (except Mexico), Japan, Australia, New Zealand, and developed countries in Europe are at no greater risk of infection than in the United States. But travelers to developing countries including the continents of South America, Africa, and Asia are at risk of contracting hepatitis A from contaminated water sources and raw foods. Traveling to rural areas and eating in settings with poor sanitation will increase the risk of contracting hepatitis A.

Three strategies exist for the prevention of hepatitis A.

First, avoid exposure. Do not drink the water, except safe, bottled water or boiled water. This includes brushing your teeth and ice in drinks. Peel all fruit, and do not eat salads or other raw foods. Do not buy food from street vendors. Do not swim in potentially polluted bodies of water.

Second, consider prevention with immune globulin (IG). This shot will provide protection against hepatitis A for up to 4–6 months. IG carries significantly less risk than the vaccine, and is probably more effective, though the duration of protection is limited. Protection also begins immediately following the injection. IG will provide more types of antibodies than those stimulated by the vaccines. IG can be used in infants. The vaccine, by contrast, cannot be used in anyone less than two years old.

Third, consider the hepatitis A vaccine. A single injection of vaccine will result in protective antibody titers *after four weeks* that persist for six months to one year. It is estimated that 95 to 100 percent of young, healthy adults develop protective levels of antibodies one month after vaccination. A booster dose 6–12 months later will produce protection that persists for up to ten years. In older adults the vaccine is less effective. In one study, only 70 percent of vaccine recipients aged 40 to 65 years developed adequate antibody responses compared to 91 percent of recipients 18 to 39 years old after a single dose of vaccine (Reuman *et al.*, 1997). If travel is scheduled less than four weeks following vaccination, protection may not be adequate to prevent infection. No studies have been published that evaluate protection in travelers vaccinated less than two weeks prior to travel.

Serious adverse event reports for hepatitis A vaccine include anaphylaxis, Guillain-Barré syndrome, brachial plexus neuropathy, transverse myelitis, multiple sclerosis, encephalopathy, and erythema multiforme. For a more complete discussion of adverse reactions, see page 165.

Hepatitis A Facts

- Avoidance of contaminated water and food is the best preventive.

- One dose of Immune Globulin will prevent hepatitis A with minimal side effects.

- Hepatitis A vaccine is associated with significant serious adverse effects.

TYPHOID

Typhoid fever is caused by the bacterium *Salmonella typhi,* which is contracted from water contaminated with sewage. It is passed through the fecal-oral route. The same precautions should be observed as those for hepatitis A. In the United States, about 400 cases occur each year, and 70 percent of these are contracted while traveling internationally. Typhoid is most commonly acquired during travel to Asia, Africa, and Latin America.

The disease causes a sustained fever of 103° or higher accompanied by weakness, stomach pains, headache, or loss of appetite. Antibiotics can successfully treat typhoid, and deaths from typhoid are extremely rare.

Oral live typhoid vaccine is taken as a capsule or liquid suspension in four doses. The most common side effects are abdominal pain, diarrhea, and vomiting. Serious adverse reactions have not been recorded, even in large population-based trials. However, studies of vaccine efficacy have not fared so well. Studies have shown an average efficacy of about 70 percent (Lin *et al.*, 2001). The oral vaccine is licensed only for adults and children over six years of age since the vaccine is ineffective in young children. In controlled field trials conducted among schoolchildren in Chile, three doses of the oral vaccine reduced infection by 66 percent over a period of 5 years (Levine *et al.*, 1987; Levine *et al.*, 1989), but in a subsequent trial vaccine efficacy was only 33 percent (Levine *et al.*, 1990).

An inactivated polysaccharide vaccine given by injection has a similarly low effectiveness, averaging 60 to 70 percent (Jong, 1999). In a trial in Nepal among persons 5–44 years of age, vaccine recipients had 74 percent fewer cases of typhoid than occurred with controls (Acharya *et al.*, 1987). In a trial involving schoolchildren in South Africa who were 5–15 years of age, one dose of the inactivated vaccine resulted in 55 percent fewer cases of typhoid fever over a period of three years than occurred with controls. (Klugman *et al.*, 1987).

Killed, whole-cell vaccines given by injection are more effective, but have an unacceptably high rate of serious adverse reactions including shock, multiple sclerosis, autoimmune reactions, and kidney disease. Newer vaccines are also being investigated.

Typhoid Fever Facts

- Avoidance of contaminated water and food is the best preventive.

- Oral typhoid vaccine in a four-dose schedule and inactivated vaccine in a single injection are only 60–70 percent effective in preventing disease.

Yellow Fever

Yellow fever occurs in tropical areas of Africa and South America. It is a viral disease transmitted between humans, or from monkeys to humans, by mosquitoes in those areas of the world. Most cases occur in forestry and agricultural workers exposed in jungle locations, but sporadic epidemics occur, sometimes involving more than 30 percent of the population (Monath, 1999). Yellow fever is very rare in travelers.

The disease is characterized by three stages. The first includes a fever and flu-like stage with vomiting, nosebleeds, and a rash. This is followed by a period of calm, and then the onset of agitation, prostration, jaundice, bleeding from multiple sites, kidney failure, and death. In an epidemic during 1969 in Nigeria, 45 percent of hospitalized patients died (Jones *et al.*, 1972). Overall case fatality rates in epidemics are about 20 percent (Wilson, 2001). Modern medicine has no effective treatment, but homeopathy developed an exceptional reputation for treating yellow fever during the nineteenth century epidemics. In 1878 a devastating yellow fever epidemic occurred in New Orleans and the Mississippi valley. During the epidemic the overall case fatality rate was at least 16 percent (Coulter, 1982). Homeopathically treated cases had a mortality rate of 5.6 percent in New Orleans and 7.7 percent throughout the South (American Institute of Homeopathy, 1880).

Live attenuated yellow fever vaccines have been in use since 1927. Most studies of vaccine effectiveness were conducted in the 1930s. In one study of 60,000 people the vaccine proved to be 95 percent effective in producing antibodies (Smith *et al.*, 1938). In the period 1938–1942 in Colombia, only one case of yellow fever occurred in a population where 127,000 vaccinations were given annually (Bugher & Gast-Galvis, 1944). However, a more recent study showed that only 75 percent of vaccinated children in Brazil developed adequate antibodies (Guerra *et al.*, 1997).

Vaccine Reactions

Severe reactions to the vaccine sometimes occur, especially in children and elderly travelers who receive the vaccine. These reactions are typically characterized by encephalitis. Most cases of vaccine-associated encephalitis have occurred in infants. Prior to 1956 there were 15 cases of encephalitis published in the world literature (Stuart, 1956). A mass vaccination campaign for yellow fever in Senegal during 1965 resulted in 248 cases of vaccine-associated encephalitis. Children under 12 years of age constituted 90 percent of cases. A total of 67 percent had convulsions, 34 percent suffered coma, and 23 cases died (Collomb *et al.*, 1966). Between 1965 and 1991 six cases of encephalitis were reported. Then during the period 1996–2001 five people aged 56–79 years (four US residents and one Australian) and two Brazilians aged 5 and 22 years became ill after receiving yellow fever vaccine. Six of the seven died (CDC, 2001d).

Requirements for Travel

More than 100 countries require evidence of yellow fever vaccination for entry. Many countries in Africa and French Guiana in South America require a yellow fever vaccination certificate for entry by anyone. Other countries in Africa, South America, Asia, Europe, the Caribbean, the South Pacific, and the Middle East require a yellow fever certificate for travelers arriving from areas where yellow fever is endemic. For a complete list of the current requirements, see the CDC website at *www.cdc.gov/travel/yelfever.htm* or contact your state health department.

Vaccine is obtained from Yellow Fever Vaccine Centers designated by state health departments. The vaccine's protection is presumed to persist for at least 10 years, and a yellow fever certificate is also valid for 10 years.

Those who cannot receive the vaccine for medical reasons can obtain a medical waiver. A valid medical reason includes allergy to eggs, or any immunocompromised condition. The CDC recommends obtaining written waivers from consular or embassy officials before departure.

Yellow Fever Facts

- Yellow fever is present in tropical areas of Africa and South America.

- It is transmitted by mosquito bites.

- Severe reactions to the vaccine have occurred.

- More than 100 countries require vaccination for entry for some travelers, but a medical exemption is available.

CONCLUSION

More Vaccines

The medical profession and drug manufacturers continually develop new vaccines for childhood and adult illnesses. Research studies are performed. Then cost analyses determine whether the price of the vaccine is less than the cost in health care dollars for treatment of the disease. Debate on this subject occurs, and the FDA eventually decides to license the new vaccine for widespread use at the behest of drug companies, as long as prelicensure studies show adequate antibody responses to the vaccine and not too many adverse effects. Only then will the millions of dollars invested by drug companies in research and development be recouped many times over in the form of profits. Vaccines are rushed to market with minimal studies of safety. Embarrassing scandals inevitably occur, sometimes forcing the vaccine's withdrawal. The rotavirus vaccine was withdrawn six months after approval, the Lyme disease vaccine was withdrawn three years after its approval, and debate has continued to rage around the dangers and advisability of routine hepatitis vaccination for children.

After a period of time during which large numbers of children are vaccinated, the adverse effects of each vaccine begin to appear. Hundreds of thousands of children must be vaccinated before these adverse effects appear, because vaccine reactions often go unreported, and it is often difficult to attribute delayed effects to a vaccine. The use of new vaccines is an experiment conducted on healthy children.

No research is done on the long-term effects of vaccines before licensure, because drug companies must market their product as quickly as possible. They cannot wait for a thirty-year study. Furthermore, they have little motivation to discover adverse effects or generate negative data about their vaccines. Studies to monitor the adverse effects of vaccines are unpopular, and researchers find it difficult to obtain funding for such projects.

The impetus to discover adverse effects comes from parents of vaccine-injured children and journalists sympathetic to their stories. The medical profession is quick to adopt new vaccines, and is generally disinterested in their problems. Denial of problems with vaccines and suppression of information are the typical official responses by the medical profession when questions of vaccine safety arise.

When parents began suing drug companies for the damages inflicted on children by vaccines, the United States Government was compelled to step in and protect vaccine manufacturers from the ruinous lawsuits. Drug companies would otherwise stop producing vaccines. Financial investments of drug companies and the vaccine industry dictate the direction of research on vaccination policy. Their interests lie in promotion of vaccines, not investigation of vaccine reactions.

Simply put, vaccine manufacturers do not have your interests in mind. They are concerned with their own profit margins and the welfare of stockholders. They influence government officials as much as they can, lobbying for their product and placing their paid consultants on government vaccine advisory committees. They also pay for state legislation that forces citizens to use their product.

Public health officials are concerned with eliminating diseases from populations and saving health care dollars. If vaccines cause some injuries or deaths, the calculated savings and benefits for the population may be worth the risk. These policies may conflict with your family's best interests if the risk of contracting a disease is significantly low. You are the only one concerned about your own health and your child's well-being. Make your own decisions for your individual health needs. You are the best person to assess your need for a specific vaccine.

The vaccine industry continues unabated in the quest for more vaccines. Children already routinely receive 11 or more different vaccines, but many more are currently in development. Vaccines for HIV, rotavirus diarrhea, sexually transmitted disease, cancer, malaria, and even tooth decay are all just a few years away. New technologies include nucleic acid vaccines, DNA priming techniques prior to vaccination, delivery of vaccines through nasal sprays, and vaccines that trigger white blood cell responses rather than antibody production. All of these experimental techniques will be tested on your children.

YOUR INFORMED CHOICE

Most parents take the issue of vaccinations for granted. The pediatrician says children need them, so parents comply. Parents may have misgivings and they may not like the idea, but they often have no support for these feelings. The pediatrician has a powerful influence on parents, and most pediatricians are committed to the campaign for universal vaccination. Questions about vaccination remain unanswered. The issues of vaccine efficacy, risks of toxicity, and long-term adverse effects are troubling issues for vaccine researchers.

Some parents are philosophically opposed to the concept of vaccinating their children. They are more horrified by the idea of injecting poisonous substances into their child than they are concerned about the remote future possibility of the diseases. For these parents, the vaccines represent a dangerous form of Russian roulette they are unwilling to play.

Other parents may be anxious about the effects of vaccines on their child, but they are concerned that if enough people avoid the shots then the diseases will begin to reappear: "The vaccines may cause bad reactions, but if I avoid them for my child, then the vaccine campaign will not work for the general population." This is a sacrificial philosophy, and your child is the sacrifice. The stakes of this game may be exceedingly high since vaccines are capable of causing immune system damage that potentially affects the entire population. If that is true, then we are simply trading acute diseases for chronic autoimmune disease and brain damage.

Most readers of this book are concerned about the adverse effects of vaccines. Most people are also anxious about some of the diseases discussed here. At least for parents, the impetus to give vaccines is primarily based on anxiety: "What if one of these diseases should happen to my unvaccinated child?" The potential guilt factor is tremendous. Never mind that some of the vaccines themselves have very questionable efficacy. If parents do vaccinate, at least they eliminate the guilt if a child contracts a disease. So one of the main tasks for parents to accomplish when they choose not to vaccinate is overcoming anxiety and guilt.

Anxiety about disease is a serious issue for parents. Tetanus is the best example. Parents who choose not to get tetanus shots for their children often think about cuts and puncture wounds. When little Josh climbs up the slide, they wonder about tetanus bacteria in the fertilized soil of the playground. This is enough to distract a parent from enjoying playtime.

Exposure to other children may also cause anxiety for parents of unvaccinated children. You may worry that your child could be exposed to children who bring diseases from other countries. Parents especially worry about polio and whooping cough. Parents should keep in mind the figures cited in the polio section of this book. No cases of polio—except those contracted from the vaccine itself—have occurred in the United States since 1979. This includes immigrants, aliens, and visitors from other countries.

Your child cannot contract a disease unless he or she is exposed to one. Other diseases, such as measles, mumps, and chickenpox, do exist in the United States, but exposure to them may be beneficial to your child, providing lifelong immunity. The pertussis vaccine carries a significant risk of toxic reactions for any child, and parents need to carefully evaluate their child's risk of exposure to the disease.

The only way for parents of unvaccinated children to feel secure is to remember the original reasons for their decision. Parents often need booster doses of vaccine education. They should keep in mind four points of information:

1. Vaccines cause immediate, sometimes drastic, adverse reactions.

2. Vaccines have unknown long-term adverse effects, which may include persisting autoimmune disease and nervous system damage.

3. Vaccine efficacy may decrease over time, making children susceptible to diseases as adults, when complications are more common.

4. Many vaccines are questionably effective.

Parents of unvaccinated children experience continual harassment and reproaches about their child's "immunization status." Kindred friends may offer support, but the concerns and pressure of family members can be almost overwhelming. Their well-intentioned comments or their accusations should be politely ignored. At best, parents can offer books like this one to troubled family members.

If two spouses disagree about vaccination and reach an impasse, then I recommend that the spouse opposed to the vaccines firmly hold his or her ground. There is no more tenacious an animal than a mother protecting her child from harm. If you are convinced that vaccines present a significant threat to your child's health, then do not allow them. No one can inject vaccines without your consent. Withhold your consent if you have serious doubts about their safety and advisability, and seek legal advice if your rights as a parent to refuse vaccines are threatened.

Schools may provide a continual source of difficulty to parents of unvaccinated children. Again, parents should simply hold firm in their resolve. Seek out a medical provider who is willing to sign a medical release. School-district personnel in states that offer a religious or philosophical exemption may need to be educated about this option. Provide them with information about your state's laws governing immunization exemptions. You will be paving the way for another parent in your position. Colleges and universities also require vaccinations, and the same rules apply as for other schools. No child should be vaccinated against a parent's better judgment. Legal protection is available against forced vaccination.

The final frontier in communicating your decision about vaccinations is the pediatrician or family physician. These doctors care for your child, medically and emotionally. They should be a source of support for you and your child. They may disagree with your decision and voice their own concerns, but they should respect your opinions and judgments. Talk with them about your misgivings, and show them that you are knowledgeable about vaccine reactions and disease incidence. Share this book with them. Do your part in communicating. They will benefit from your insights. If you meet with hostility or terminal resistance, then you may want to seek another medical provider who is more receptive and understanding. Do not give up, and do not be intimidated. Your physician is working for you, as part of a team that cares for your child. And you are the manager of that team.

You will not convince your pediatrician that the vaccine industry is wrong. No professional likes to think that their entire training and literature is biased and manipulated for profits by corporations with little concern for altruistic issues. Most pediatricians have the best interests of children at heart. They are convinced that vaccines have saved countless children's lives. They have been trained to accept and praise vaccinations as the most successful preventive intervention in the history of medicine. They are dedicated to continuing this proud tradition of preventive medicine for children.

If you have made an educated and informed decision not to vaccinate your child, then you can be proud of your choice. If you have doubts at any point, you can stop giving the vaccines. Remember that vaccines often cause severe reactions after the third or fourth shot, even if the first two caused no apparent problems.

Stay informed about vaccine issues. Subscribe to newsletters such as the one produced by NVIC (*www.909shot.com*) and this author *www.cure-guide.com*. Stay in touch with the community of concerned consumers. Vaccine laws change, new vaccines are recommended, and adverse reaction reports alter the landscape of vaccine advisability. The more you know about vaccines, the more confidence you will maintain in your informed choices.

APPENDICES

A: Vaccination Schedule and Checklist

The schedule for vaccination on the following page is included so that parents will know what to expect from health providers who recommend the vaccines. Vaccinations can be delayed and given at any time parents prefer. Parents can choose to give some vaccines and not others. If you decide to give the vaccines, the tetanus, diphtheria, pertussis, or polio vaccines should be given as a series, in order to achieve recommended antibody levels. Interruption of a series does not require starting the series again. The interval between vaccines is not crucial to their effectiveness. Most of the vaccines that occur in combined shots can also be given individually.

A vaccination checklist is provided so that parents can keep track of which vaccines they choose to give and when.

VACCINATION CHECKLIST

	Infancy	Later	Never
Chickenpox (Varicella)			
Diphtheria			
Hepatitis A			
Hepatitis B			
Meningitis Vaccines			
Haemophilus Influenzae Type B (Hib)			
Pneumococcus			
Meningococcus			
MMR			
Measles			
Mumps			
Rubella			
Pertussis (Whooping Cough)			
Polio			
Tetanus			

Age ▶ Vaccine ▼	Birth	1 mo	2 mos	4 mos	6 mos	12 mos	15 mos	18 mos	24 mos	4–6 yrs	11–12 yrs	14–16 yrs
Hepatitis B	Hep B #1		Hep B #2			Hep B #3					(Hep B)	
Diphtheria, Tetanus, Pertussis			DTaP	DTaP	DTaP		DTaP			DTaP	Td	
H. influenzae type b			Hib	Hib	Hib	Hib						
Inactivated Polio			IPV	IPV		IPV				IPV		
Pneumococcus Conjugate			PCV	PCV	PCV	PCV						
Measles, Mumps, Rubella						MMR				MMR	(MMR)	
Varicella						Var					(Var)	
										Hep A—in selected areas		

Ovals indicate vaccines to be given if previously recommended doses were missing.

B: Resources

ORGANIZATIONS

National Vaccine Information Center (NVIC)
512 W. Maple Avenue, #206, Vienna, VA 22180,
800-909-SHOT, 703-938-DPT3, FAX 703-938-5768
www.909shot.com

An organization of concerned lay people and professionals that promotes information about vaccines, promotes legislation relating to safe vaccinations and free choice, and assists parents in their legal battles to obtain compensation for vaccine injury, and to avoid vaccination in situations where legal pressures are applied. Members receive a regular newsletter. They publish a law-firm directory, as well as booklets on the vaccine-injury compensation system, and instructions for filing claims.

Centers for Disease Control
National Immunization Program, Information Services
Office, Mail Stop E-06, Atlanta, GA 30333-4018,
800-232-SHOT
International Travelers Hotline, 404-332-4559
www.cdc.gov

Provides information to the public on vaccination policies, standards, and recommendations, as well as international travel and disease outbreaks around the world.

National Center for Homeopathy
801 North Fairfax St., Suite 306, Alexandria, VA 22314,
703-548-7790
www.homeopathic.org

Information resource center for homeopathic medicine. They publish a national directory of homeopathic practitioners.

Council for Homeopathic Certification
www.homeopathicdirectory.com

A certification board that tests practitioners in classical homeopathy through a written and oral examination. The website contains a searchable directory of certificate holders.

Homeopathic Educational Services
2124 Kittredge St., Berkeley, CA 94704, 800-359-9051
(orders), 510-649-0294, FAX 510-649-1955
www.homeopathic.com

A distributor and mail-order supplier of homeopathic books, medicines, audiotapes, and summaries of homeopathic research. Online and printed catalogs are available.

Vaccine Adverse Event Reporting System
P.O. Box 1100, Rockville, MD 20849-1100, 800-822-7967
www.fda.gov/cber/vaers/vaers.htm

The surveillance system established by the National Childhood Vaccine Injury Act to collect reports of adverse reactions following vaccination. Health care providers are obligated to report specific adverse events following particular vaccines. Parents, other relatives, or anyone aware of the occurrence of an adverse event may also file a report. Call or check online for reporting forms.

BOOKS

Cave, Stephanie, *What Your Doctor May Not Tell You about Children's Vaccinations,* Warner Books, 2001.

> Pros and cons of childhood vaccines with brief discussions of each and an alternative vaccine schedule.

Coulter, H.L. & Fisher, B.L. *A Shot in the Dark,* Garden City, New York: Avery Publishing Group, Inc., 1991.

> Documentation of the devastating effects of the pertussis vaccine, including vivid case examples and an exposé of the campaign for mandatory immunization of children regardless of the risks.

Coulter, H.L. *Vaccination, Social Violence, and Criminality: The Medical Assault on the American Brain,* North Atlantic Books, Berkeley, California, 1990.

> Describes childhood vaccines as a possible cause of encephalitis characterized by learning problems, developmental delays, behavior disorders, and autism.

Cummings, S. & Ullman, D. *Everybody's Guide to Homeopathic Medicines,* New York: Jeremy P Tarcher/Putnam, 1997.

An introduction to homeopathic principles, and the use of homeopathic medicines to treat common acute illnesses of children and adults.

James, W. *Immunization: The Reality Behind the Myth,* Bergin & Garvey Publishers, Granberry, Massachusetts, 1995.

A description of the problems with immunization statistics and a proposal for parents to build a strong immune system in their children without using vaccines.

Mendelsohn, R. *How to Raise a Healthy Child . . . In Spite of Your Doctor,* Contemporary Books, Chicago, 1990.

A practical and common-sense guide advising parents to avoid overtreatment, immunizations, and other hazards encountered in the pediatrician's office.

Miller, N. *Vaccines: Are They Really Safe and Effective?* New Atlantean Press, Santa Fe, 1992; and *Immunization: Theory vs. Reality,* New Atlantean Press, Santa Fe, 1996.

Both books take a hard-hitting critical approach to vaccinations. Vaccines presents the issues surrounding each vaccine in summary form. Immunization provides detailed descriptions of the vaccine industry's tactics: threats, evasion, denial, and genocidal policies.

Murphy, J. *What Every Parent Should Know about Childhood Immunization,* Earth Healing Products, Boston, 1993.

A thorough and easily understandable critique of vaccination based on arguments about toxicity, low efficacy, and failure to establish true immunity to disease.

Palmer, Michael, *Fatal,* New York: Bantam Books, 2002.

A novel that exposes the corruption within the vaccine industry, where lives are sacrificed for profit and political gain. A medical thriller filled with rip-roaring action.

Rozario, D. *The Immunization Resource Guide,* Patter Publications, P.O. Box 204, Burlington, IA 52601

The most complete single resource for books, organizations, information services, publishers, and government offices that have anything to do with vaccines, both pro and con. Extensive annotated bibliography, address lists, book reviews, and organization descriptions. The complete directory on vaccination for the consumer.

Seroussi, K. *Unraveling the Mystery of Autism and Pervasive Developmental Disorder,* Broadway Books, New York, 2002.

A guide to the dietary treatment of autism spectrum disorders.

Shaw, William. *Biological Treatments for Autism and PDD.*, Great Plains Laboratory Inc., 2002.

Appropriate laboratory tests for evaluating children with autism, and the treatment programs that correspond to different clinical and laboratory findings.

WEBSITES

CONSUMER-ORIENTED SITES THAT QUESTION VACCINATION AND VACCINE POLICY

www.cure-guide.com

This author's website that includes updates to *The Vaccine Guide* and many articles on natural health care for children.

http://home.san.rr.com/via/

Vaccine Information & Awareness (VIA) contains links to most other websites and newsgroups with vaccine information, including both pro-vaccine and pro-choice sites. This site has many articles about vaccines and diseases, legal requirements, and links all over the Internet.

www.909shot.com

Website for the National Vaccine Information Center, a parent-sponsored group that lobbies for safer vaccines and freedom of choice legislation. The site includes their newsletter, referral information, special reports, and the ability to order books and materials from their extensive catalog. An email news service is available.

www.whale.to

This is a huge site of articles that question the advisability of vaccinations, a truly comprehensive and searchable database of information and links across the Internet. You could spend days at this site plumbing the depths of these source materials.

www.thinktwice.com

This site contains ordering information for books on vaccines and other health-related topics. The site also contains articles about vaccines and an inclusive list of worldwide vaccination support groups and information services.

www.vaccineinfo.net

Updates on vaccine topics in the media and legal issues pertaining to vaccines. This site is operated by a Texas-based consumer group, Parents Requesting Open Vaccine Education (PROVE). An email news service is available.

GOVERNMENT AND VACCINE INDUSTRY SITES

www.cdc.gov

This is the official US government site with current vaccine recommendations and updates on diseases, travel advisories, and suggestions published by the Centers for Disease Control.

www.vaccines.org

Provides consumers and professionals with data on diseases and vaccines, current research, official international vaccine websites, contacts for medical journals, medical associations, and research centers.

PRACTITIONER DIRECTORIES

www.homeopathicdirectory.com

Qualified homeopathic practitioners who have passed a national certification exam in classical homeopathy.

www.aaom.org

American Association of Oriental Medicine members

www.csomaonline.org

Members of the California State Oriental Medical Association

www.naturopathic.org

Directory of naturopathic physicians

LEGAL RESOURCES

IMMUNIZATION HOTLINE
James Filenbaum
2 Executive Blvd. #201-P
Suffern, NY 10901
Phone: 800-753-LAWS, 914-357-0020

A law firm specializing in vaccination law and exemptions. They assist parents in securing religious exemptions based on individual religious belief. Representation for parents seeking compensation for vaccine damage.

THE RUTHERFORD INSTITUTE
PO Box 7482
Charlottesville, VA 22906
Phone: 434-978-3888

Advocates of religious freedom. Provide legal assistance regarding religious liberty.

SHOEMAKER & HORN
9711 Meadowlark Road
Vienna, VA 22182
Phone: 703-281-6395
Fax: 703-281-5807
Email: shoehorn@bellatlantic.net

Law firm that represents individuals damaged by vaccines.

CONWAY CROWLEY & HOMER
332 Congress Street
Boston, MA 02210-1217
Phone: 617-695-1990
Fax: 617-695-0880

Law firm that represents individuals damaged by vaccines.

ALTOM M. MAGLIO, P.A.
22 S. Tuttle Ave #4
Sarasota, FL 34237
Phone: 941-952-5242
Fax: 941-952-5042
Email: assistance@sarasotalaw.com

Lawyer who represents individuals damaged by vaccines.

GAGE & MOXLEY
PO Box 1223
Cheyenne, WY 82003-1223
Email: vaccinelaw@aol.com

Lawyers who practice in the Childhood Vaccine Injury Program, and represent parents who are being denied religious exemption.

DAVID E. LEWIS, ESQ.
2828 Donald Douglas Loop North
Santa Monica, CA 90405
Phone: 310-314-1140
Fax: 310-314-1136

Lawyer who represents individuals damaged by vaccines.

BARTON, BENEDETTO, & BISHOP
Bruce A. Barton
180 W. Michigan Ave., Harris Bldg., 6th Floor
Jackson, MI 49201
Phone: 517-787-6532

Law firm that represents vaccine-damaged children.

TONI BLAKE
2632 B Street
San Diego, CA 92102
Phone: 619-234-8664

Lawyer who specializes in helping parents who have been accused of Shaken Baby Syndrome after their child died following a vaccine.

ELAINE WHITFIELD SHARP
196 Atlantic Avenue
Marblehead, MA 01945
Phone: 781-639-1862
Fax: 781-639-1771

Lawyer who specializes in vaccine law, including Shaken Baby Syndrome.

ANDREW DODD
21525 Hawthorne Bl Pav A
Torrance, CA 90503

Attorney for a safe vaccine.

ART BOYER
>   20 N. Clark #808
>   Chicago, IL 60602
>   Phone: 312-443-1998

Attorney for vaccine-damaged children.

MICHAEL SKOW
>   Phone: 916-929-6000

Attorney for vaccine-damaged children

C: Glossary

acellular pertussis vaccine—A vaccine prepared from one or more antigens derived from the active components of the *B pertussis* bacterium, particularly pertussis toxin. Developed in an attempt to reduce the adverse effects associated with the whole-cell pertussis vaccine.

acupuncture—A technique involving the insertion of fine stainless steel needles into points on the surface of the body that trigger healing responses. Administered in accordance with the theories and principles of Chinese medicine.

adjuvant—A chemical, such as aluminum, added to vaccines to promote antibody response and increase the effectiveness of vaccines.

adsorb—To bind one substance, through a chemical process, to the surface molecule of another in order to promote or increase its effectiveness.

AIDS—Acquired Immunodeficiency Syndrome, a disease characterized by failure of the immune system and accompanied by opportunistic infections (e.g. pneumonia and fungal infections), skin cancers, wasting, and death.

anaphylaxis—An acute, often explosive, systemic reaction characterized by skin eruptions including hives and rashes, respiratory distress, and cardiac collapse that may prove fatal. It occurs in a previously sensitized person who again receives the sensitizing antigen.

antigen—Allergen; any material (protein, toxoid, microorganism) that can induce a state of sensitivity or resistance in the body to that material when it is encountered again.

antibody—Any body substance manufactured in response to the stimulus of an antigen introduced into the body, that reacts specifically with that antigen. Many antibodies fight infection and indicate immunity to specific diseases.

arthropathy—Any joint disease, often associated with joint swelling and pain.

autism—A developmental delay that includes symptoms such as speech difficulties, lack of eye contact, isolation, and no fear of danger.

autoimmune response—An antibody response developed by the body against its own tissues or cells.

carcinogenic—Having the ability, as a chemical or substance, to cause cancer.

case-control study—A controlled observational study that starts with the identification of persons with a disease or condition (adverse event) of interest and a suitable control group of persons without the disease. The relation of an attribute (e.g. vaccination) to the disease is examined by comparing the diseased and nondiseased groups with regard to how fre quently the attribute is present.

chronic fatigue syndrome—A condition characterized by persistent tiredness and other symptoms which may include fevers, poor concentration, joint and muscle pain, sore throat, swollen lymph nodes, and headaches, following a sudden onset of symptoms, often flu-like in nature, but continuing into a persistent or relapsing state.

CNS—Central nervous system; the brain and spinal cord.

conjugate—To bind a vaccine to a protein carrier, thereby increasing its efficacy.

dementia—Loss of brain functions that can manifest as loss of memory, learning ability, and motor control.

demyelination—A process in which the myelin sheath, which acts like an insulator on some nerves, is destroyed, resulting in faulty nerve and brain function.

diabetes—Specifically Insulin-Dependent Diabetes Mellitus (IDDM), characterized by an insufficiency of insulin secretion by the pancreas and an inability to metabolize sugars. Diabetes is thought to arise in response to both genetic and environmental factors.

double-blind study—A clinical experiment in which neither the subjects nor the experimenters know which individual subjects receive the active treatment or intervention and which subjects receive a placebo or non-medicinal treatment.

DTP (or DPT)—Diphtheria toxoid, tetanus toxoid, and pertussis vaccine.

EEG—Electroencephalogram; measurement of brainwaves (changes in electrical potential) by means of electrodes attached to the skull, used to diagnose epilepsy and localize brain lesions.

E-IPV—Enhanced Inactivated Polio Vaccine. Produced in human cells rather than monkey cells, this vaccine has a higher antigenic content and can be used in fewer doses than conventional IPV.

encephalitis—An inflammatory response within the brain.

encephalopathy—A clinical condition with a spectrum of characteristics including altered levels of consciousness, confusion, irritability, changes in behavior, screaming attacks, neck stiffness, convulsions, visual, auditory and speech disturbances, and motor and sensory deficit.

epithelial cell—The surface layer covering the skin, mucous membranes, glands, and body cavities.

GBS (Guillain-Barré Syndrome)—A demyelinating inflammatory disease of the peripheral nervous system with rapid onset of motor weakness and loss of sensation.

HBV—Hepatitis B vaccine.

hemolytic anemia—An abnormally low number of red blood cells caused by their destruction.

homeopathy—The practice of prescribing natural substances (plant, mineral, or animal) according to the principle that such a substance can cure the same symptoms that it can cause. When used medicinally, these substances are usually prepared through a process of serial dilution that enhances their ability to stimulate healing responses in the body.

HIV—Human Immunodeficiency Virus; a retrovirus associated with AIDS. HIV-1 is associated with AIDS cases in Europe and the Americas, HIV-2 with African cases.

HTLV—Human T-Lymphotropic Virus; a group of retroviruses that infect humans and cause leukemia and cancer of lymph nodes.

IDDM Insulin-Dependent Diabetes Mellitus—see diabetes.

IgE antibody—One of the immunoglobulins within the blood that denotes allergy to specific antigens. For example, the presence of IgE antibody to milk within a person's blood shows that an individual has allergic responses to milk.

IPV—Inactivated Polio Vaccine (killed vaccine or Salk vaccine); a sterile suspension of three types of polioviruses used as an injection to vaccinate against polio.

leukemia—A disease characterized by an abnormal continuing increase in white blood cells.

lymphocyte—A white blood cell responsible for providing protection against infection and disease.

meningitis—Inflammation of the membranes of the brain or spinal cord.

MMR—Measles, mumps, and rubella vaccine.

MSAEFI—Monitoring System for Adverse Events Following Immunization; a passive-surveillance system designed and monitored by the Centers for Disease Control for the purpose of collecting nationwide data on adverse events associated with vaccination.

multiple sclerosis—A chronic central nervous system demyelinating disease in which the nerve lesions occur in multiple locations.

myelin—The sheath, on the surface of a nerve, made of fats and protein that acts as an insulator.

neurologic—Pertaining to the nervous system.

optic neuritis—A central demyelinating disease of the optic nerve, affecting vision.

OPV—Oral Polio Vaccine; a live-virus vaccine prepared from three types of poliovirus given as an oral dose.

passive surveillance—The collection of voluntary reports from health care providers and the public that describe adverse vaccine reactions.

potency—The strength of a homeopathic medicine corresponding to the number of times it has been diluted and shaken in the pharmaceutical preparation process. These numbers are typically recorded as 12x, 30x, 30c, 200c, 1M, etc., signifying whether the dilutions occurred 1/10 (x) or 1/100 (c), and the number of dilutions performed.

PRP—The early polysaccharide capsular *Haemophilus influenzae* type b vaccine, which is no longer used. The name "PRP" corresponds to the polysaccharide itself, a repeating polymer of ribose and ribitol linked by a phosphate group.

purpura—Bleeding into the skin, mucous membranes, and internal organs.

relative risk—The ratio of the risk of disease or other outcome among the exposed compared to the risk among the unexposed.

SIDS—Sudden Infant Death Syndrome; the unexpected and unexplained death of an apparently well infant.

SIV—Simian Immunodeficiency Virus; a group of retroviruses found in monkeys that are associated with Simian Acquired Immunodeficiency (simian AIDS).

squamous cells—Cells in the form of scales that are spread like a pavement over the superficial layer of body cavities or surface membranes.

SSPE—See subacute sclerosing panencephalitis.

Stealth virus—A virus that fails to evoke an inflammatory reaction in the patient from whom it was isolated because the virus lacks target antigens for recognition by the body's cellular immune system

STLV—Simian T-Lymphotropic Virus; a group of retroviruses that infect monkeys.

Subacute sclerosing panencephalitis—A form of brain inflammation characterized by insidious onset of a progressive cerebral dysfunction occurring over the course of weeks or months. Symptoms include jerking motions, spasticity, difficulty swallowing, and progressive loss of vision. The average patient dies within 2 years after a persistent coma.

SV40—The fortieth simian virus discovered.

thrombocytopenia—A decrease in blood platelets responsible for blood clotting with accompanying spontaneous bleeding.

toxoid—The toxin of a microorganism that has been treated (commonly with formaldehyde) to diminish its toxic effects, but which still has the power to stimulate antibody production.

Traditional Chinese Medicine—The science of using herbs, acupuncture, and related practices based on principles of healing developed in China over the past 5,000 years.

transverse myelitis—A set of symptoms, including lack of motor control and sensation in isolated parts of the body, suggesting a lesion at one level of the spinal cord.

VAERS—Vaccine Adverse Event Reporting System; a passive surveillance system intended to collect reports of reactions to vaccines operated by the Centers for Disease Control and the U.S. Food and Drug Administration.

VAPP—Vaccine Associated Paralytic Poliomyelitis; polio caused by the vaccine rather than a natural infection.

REFERENCES

AAP News, Vaccine brochures: AAP proposes changes. June 1989, p. 2.

Aberer, W. Vaccination despite thimerosal sensitivity. *Contact Dermatitis* 1991; 24:6–10.

Abernathy, R.S., Spink, W.W. Increased susceptibility of mice to bacterial endotoxins induced by pertussis vaccine. Fed Proc 1956; 15:580.

Abramova, F., Grinberg, L., Yampolskaya, O., Walker, D. Pathology of inhalational anthrax in forty-two cases from the Sverdlovsk outbreak of 1979. *Proceedings National Academy Sciences USA* 1993; 90:2291–4.

ACHA (American College Health Association). Position statement on immunization policy. *Journal of American College Health* 1983; 32:7–8.

Acharya, I.L., Lowe, C.U., Thapa, R. *et al.* Prevention of typhoid fever in Nepal with the Vi capsular polysaccharide of Salmonella typhi. *New England Journal Medicine* 1987; 317:1101–4.

Acheson, E.D., Barnes, H.R., Gardner, M.J. *et al.* Formaldehyde in the British chemical industry. An occupational cohort study. *Lancet* 1984; 1(8377):611–616.

Ad hoc group for the study of pertussis vaccines. Placebo-controlled trial of two acellular pertussis vaccines in Sweden—Protective efficacy and adverse events. *Lancet* 1988; I:955–960.

Adler, J.B., Mazzotta, S.A., Barkin, J.S. Pancreatitis caused by measles, mumps, and rubella vaccine. *Pancreas* 1991; 6:489–490.

Agy, M.B., Frumkin, L.R., Corey, L. *et al.* Infection of Macaca nemestrina by human immunodeficiency virus type 1. *Science* 1992; 257:103–106.

Albert, R.E., Sellakumar, A.R., Laskin, S. *et al.* Gaseous formaldehyde and hydrogen chloride induction of nasal cancer in the rat. *Journal of the National Cancer Institute* 1982; 68(4):597–603.

Albrecht, P., Ennis, F.A., Saltzman, E.J., Krugman, S. Persistence of maternal antibody in infants beyond 12 months: mechanisms of measles vaccine failure. *Journal of Pediatrics* 1977; 91:715–718.

Alderslade, R., Bellman, M.H., Rawson, N.S. *et al.* The National Childhood Encephalopathy Study, in Whooping Cough: Reports from the Committee on Safety of Medicines and the Joint Committee on Vaccination and Immunisation.

London, Department of Health and Social Security, Her Majesty's Stationery Office, 1981, pp 79–154.

Alfrey, A.C. *et al.* Syndrome of dyspraxia and multifocal seizures associated with chronic hemodialysis. *Transactions of the American Society of Artificial Internal Organs* 1972; 18:257.

Alfrey, A.C. *et al.* The dialysis encephalopathy syndrome, possible aluminum intoxication. *New England Journal of Medicine* 1976; 94:184.

Alibek, K. *Biohazard.* New York: Dell Publishing, 1999.

Alter, M.J., Hadler, S.C., Margolis, H.S., Alexander J. *et al.* The changing epidemiology of hepatitis B in the United States. *Journal of the American Medical Association* 1990; 263:1218–1222.

American Institute of Homeopathy. Special Report of the Homeopathic Yellow Fever Commission Ordered by the AIH for Presentation to Congress. Philadelphia and New York: Boericke and Tafel, 1880.

Andrus, J.K., Strebel, P.M., de Quadros, C.A., Olivé, J.M. Risk of vaccine-associated paralytic poliomyelitis in Latin America, 1989–91. *Bulletin of the World Health Organization* 1995; 73:33–40.

Arbeter, A.M., Starr, S.E., Plotkin, S.A. Varicella vaccine studies in healthy children and adults. *Pediatrics* 1986; 78 (suppl):748–756.

Asa, P.B., Cao, Y., Garry, R.F. Antibodies to squalene in Gulf War syndrome. *Exp Mol Pathol* 2000; 68:55–64

Ascherio, A., Zhang, S.M. *et al.* Hepatitis B vaccination and the risk of multiple sclerosis. *New England Journal of Medicine* 2001; 344(5):327–32.

Aukrust, L., Almeland, T.L., Refsum, D., Aas, K. Severe hypersensitivity or intolerance reactions to measles vaccine in six children: clinical and immunological studies. *Allergy* 1980; 35:581–587.

Austrian, R. *Review Infectious Disease* 1981; 3 (suppl):S1–S17.

Auwaerter, P.G. et al. Changes within T cell receptor V beta subsets in infants following measles vaccination. *Clinical Immunology and Immunopathology* 1996; 79(2):163–7.

Backon, J. Prolonged breast feeding as a prophylaxis for recurrent otitis media: relevance of prostaglandins. *Medical Hypotheses* 1984, 13:161.

Bakir, F., Damluji, S.F., Amin-Zaki, L. *et al.* Methylmercury poisoning in Iraq. *Science* 1973; 181:230–241.

Balfour, H.H., Kelly, J.M., Suarez, C.S. *et al.* Acyclovir treatment of varicella in otherwise healthy children. *Journal of Pediatrics* 1990; 116:633–639.

Ballinger, A.B., Clark, M.L. Severe acute hepatitis B infection after vaccination. *Lancet* 1994; 344:1292–1293.

Bannister, B., & Corbel, M.J. The effect of Schick testing on diphtheria antitoxin status. *Journal of Infection* 1991; 22:11–15.

Baraff, L.J., Ablon, W.J., Weiss, R.C. Possible temporal association between diphtheria-tetanus toxoid-pertussis vaccination and sudden infant death syndrome. *Pediatric Infectious Diseases* 1983; 2:7–11.

Baraff, L.J., Shields, D., Beckwith, L. *et al.* Infants and children with convulsions and hypotonic-hyporesponsive episodes following diphtheria-tetanus-pertussis immunization: follow-up evaluation. *Pediatrics* 1988; 81:789–794.

Baraff, L.J., Lee, S.I., Schriger, D.L. Outcomes of bacterial meningitis in children: a meta-analysis. *Pediatric Infectious Disease Journal* 1993; 12:389–94.

Barr, M., Glenny, A.T., Randall, K.J. Concentration of diphtheria antitoxin in cord blood. *Lancet* 1949; ii: 324–326.

Barrett, L.J. *et al.* Dialysis-associated dementia. *Australian and New Zealand Journal of Medicine* 1975; 5:62.

Bart, K.J., Orenstein, W.A., Preblud, S.R., Hinman, A.R. Universal immunization to interrupt rubella. *Review of Infectious Diseases* 1985; 7 (suppl 1):S177–184.

Bartos, H.R. Thrombocytopenia asociated with rubella vaccination. *New York State Journal of Medicine* 1972; 72:499.

Bass, J.W. Pertussis: current status of prevention and treatment. *Pediatric Infectious Diseases* 1985; 4:614–619.

Beale, A.J. Measles vaccines. *Proceedings of the Royal Society of Medicine* 1974; 67:1116–1119.

Beall, J.R., Ulsamer, A.G. Formaldehyde and hepatotoxicity: a review. *Journal of Toxicology and Environmental Health* 1984; 14(1):1–21.

Beasley R.P., Hwang, L-Y. Epidemiology of hepatocellular carcinoma. In: Vyas, G.N., Dienstag, J.L., Hoofnagle, J.H., eds. *Viral hepatitis and liver disease.* New York: Grune & Stratton, 1984:209–224.

Belshe, R.B., Mendelman, P.M., Treanor, J.J. *et al.* The efficacy of live attenuated, cold-adapted, trivalent, intranasal influenzavirus vaccine in children. *New England Journal of Medicine* 1998; 338:1405–12.

Benveniste, E.N. Inflammatory cytokines within the central nervous system: sources, function, and mechanism of action. *American Journal of Physiology* 1992; 263:C1–C16.

Berg, J.M. Neurological complications of pertussis immunization. *British Medical Journal* 1958; 2:24–27.

Berkowitz, C.D., Ward, J.I., Meier, K. *et al.* Persistence of antibody (AB) to Haemophilus influenzae type b (Hib) and response to PRP and PRP-D booster immunization in children initially immunized with either vaccine at 15 to 24 months (Abstract no. 889). *Pediatric Research* 1987; 21:321A.

Bernstein, H.H., Rothstein, E.P., Pichichero, M.E. *et al.* Clinical reactions and immunogenicity of the BIKEN acellular diphtheria and tetanus toxoids and pertussis vaccine in 4- through 6-year old US children. *American Journal of Diseases of Children* 1992; 146:556–559.

Bisgard, K.M., Kao, A., Leake, J. *et al.* Haemophilus influenzae invasive disease in the United States 1994–1995: Near disappearance of a vaccine-preventable childhood disease. *Emerging Infectious Diseases* 1998; 4(2):229–37.

Black, S., Shinefield, H., Hiatt, R.A. *et al.* b-CAPSA 1 *Haemophilus influenzae* type b capsular polysaccharide vaccine safety. *Pediatrics* 1987; 79:321–325.

Black, S., Shinefield, H., Hiatt, R.A. *et al.* Efficacy of *Haemophilus influenzae* type b capsular polysaccharide vaccine. *Pediatric Infectious Disease Journal* 1988; 7:149–156.

Black, S., Shinefield, H., Fireman, B., Hiatt, R. *et al.* Efficacy in infancy of oligosaccharide conjugate *Haemophilus influenzae* type b (HbOC) vaccine in a United States population of 61,080 children. *Pediatric Infectious Disease Journal* 1991; 10:97–104.

Black, S.B., Cherry, J.D., Shinefield, H.R. *et al.* Apparent decreased risk of invasive bacterial disease after heterologous childhood immunization. *American Journal of Diseases of Children* 1991(a); 145:746–749.

Black, S., Shinefield, H., Fireman, B. *et al.* Efficacy, safety and immunogenicity of heptavalent pneumococcal conjugate vaccine in children. *Pediatric Infectious Disease Journal* 2000; 19:187–95.

Blackwelder, W.C., Storsaeter, J., Olin, P., Hallander, H.O. Acellular pertussis vaccines efficacy and evaluation of clinical case definitions. *American Journal of Diseases of Children* 1991; 145:1285–9.

Blair, A., Stewart, P., O'Berg, M., *et al.* Mortality among industrial workers exposed to formaldehyde. *Journal of the National Cancer Institute*, 1986; 76(6):1071–1084.

Blair, A., Saracci, R., Stewart, P.A. *et al.* Epidemiologic evidence on the relationship between formaldehyde exposure and cancer. *Scandinavian Journal of Work, Environment and Health* 1990; 16(6):381–393.

Blennow, M., Granstrom, M. Adverse reactions and serologic response to a booster dose of acellular pertussis vaccine in children immunized with acellular or whole-cell vaccine as infants. *Pediatrics* 1989; 84:62–67.

Bluestone, C.D., Klein, J.O. *Otitis Media in Infants and Children.* Philadelphia: W.B. Saunders Company, 1988.

Bohannon, R.C., Donehower, L.A., Ford, R.J. Isolation of a Type D retrovirus from B-cell lymphomas of a patient with AIDS. *Journal of Virology* 1991; 65:5663–5672.

Bookchin, D., Schumacher, J. The virus and the vaccine. *Atlantic Monthly* 2000; 285(2):68.

Bottiger, M., Christenson, B., Romanus, V. *et al.* Swedish experience of two dose vaccination programme aiming at eliminating measles, mumps, and rubella. *British Medical Journal* 1987; 295:1264–1267.

Bowie, C. Lessons from the pertussis vaccine court trial. *Lancet* 1990; 335:397–399.

Brachman, P.S. Inhalation anthrax. *Annals New York Academy Science* 1980; 353:83–93.

Bradford, T.L. *The Logic of Figures or Comparative Results of Homeopathic and Other Treatments*. Philadelphia: Boericke and Tafel, 1900.

Braun, M.M., Mootrey, G.T., Salive, M.E. *et al.* Infant immunization with acellular pertussis vaccines in the United States: Assessment of the first two years' data from the Vaccine Adverse Event Reporting System (VAERS). *Pediatrics* 2000; 106(4):e51.

Breiman, R.F., Butler, J.C., Tenover, F.C. *et al.* Emergence of drug-resistant pneumococcal infections in the United States. *JAMA* 1994; 271:1831.

Brodsky, L., Stanievich, J. Sensorineural hearing loss following live measles virus vaccination. *International Journal of Pediatric Otorhinolaryngology* 1985; 10:159–163.

Broome, C.V. Epidemiology of *Haemophilus influenzae* type b infections in the United States. *Pediatric Infectious Disease Journal* 1987; 6:779–782.

Brunell, P.A. Varicella vaccine—Where are we? *Pediatrics* 1986; 78 (suppl):721–722.

Brunell, P.A., Novelli, V.M., Lipton, S.V., Pollock, B. Combined vaccine against measles, mumps, rubella, and varicella. *Pediatrics* 1988; 81:779–784.

Brunell, P.A. Chickenpox—examining our options. *New England Journal of Medicine* 1991; 325:1577–1579.

Bugher, J.C., Gast-Galvis, A. The efficacy of vaccination in the prevention of yellow fever in Colombia. *American Journal of Hygiene* 1944; 39:58–66.

Burnett, J.C. *Vaccinosis and its Cure by Thuja*. 1892, published in *Best of Burnett*. New Delhi, India: B. Jain, 1992.

Burton, D. Instant recall on any vaccine going into our children that has mercury in it. House of Representatives, May 15, 2001; Page H2174.

Butel, J.S., Jafar, S., Stewart, A.R., Lednicky, J.A. Detection of authentic SV 40 DNA sequences in human brain and bone tumours. *Dev Biol Stand* 1998; 94:23–32.

Byers, R.K., Moll, F.C. Encephalopathies following prophylactic pertussis vaccination. *Pediatrics* 1948; 1:437–457.

California Department of Health Services. Measles in Southeast Asian children in the San Joaquin Valley. *California Morbidity* 1990; 51/52.

California Department of Health Services. DTP Vaccine: Truth and consequences, a two-part series. *California Morbidity* 1994; 1.

California Medical Association. Amicus curiae brief of California Medical Association. People of the State of California v. Donna Shalala *et al.* No. 93–15700 in the United States Court of Appeals for the Ninth Circuit. 1993.

Calman, K.C. Measles vaccination as a risk factor for inflammatory bowel disease (letter). *Lancet* 1995; 345:1362.

Candy, J.M., Oakley, A.E., Klinowski, J. *et al.* Aluminosilicates and senile plaque formation in Alzheimer's disease. *Lancet* 1986; I:354–357.

Castro, D., Nogueira, G.G. Use of the nosode Meningococcinum as a preventive against meningitis. *Journal of the American Institute of Homeopathy* 1975; 68:211–219.

Center for Law and the Public's Health at Georgetown and Johns Hopkins Universities for the Centers for Disease Control. *Model State Emergency Health Powers Act: A draft for discussion*, December 21, 2001.

Centers for Disease Control. Mumps Surveillance. *MMWR (Morbidity and Mortality Weekly Report)* 1972; No. 2.

Centers for Disease Control. Tetanus in a child with improper medical exemption from immunization—Florida. *MMWR (Morbidity and Mortality Weekly Report)* 1985; 34:550–552.

Centers for Disease Control. Tetanus—United States, 1982–1985. *MMWR (Morbidity and Mortality Weekly Report)* 1985; 34:602, 607–611.

Centers for Disease Control. International notes: Imported paralytic poliomyelitis—United States, 1986. *MMWR (Morbidity and Mortality Weekly Report)* 1986; 35:671–674.

Centers for Disease Control. Tetanus—United States, 1982–1986. *MMWR (Morbidity and Mortality Weekly Report)* 1987; 36:477–481.

Centers for Disease Control. Prevention of *Haemophilus influenzae* type b disease. *MMWR (Morbidity and Mortality Weekly Report)* 1988; 37:13–16.

Centers for Disease Control. Measles—Quebec. *MMWR (Morbidity and Mortality Weekly Report)* 1989(a); 38:329–330.

Centers for Disease Control. ACIP: General recommendation on immunization. *MMWR (Morbidity and Mortality Weekly Report)* 1989(b); 38:205–227.

Centers for Disease Control. Measles—Los Angeles County, California, 1988. *MMWR (Morbidity and Mortality Weekly Report)* 1989(c); 38:49–57.

Centers for Disease Control. ACIP: Measles prevention: supplementary statement. *MMWR (Morbidity and Mortality Weekly Report)* 1989(d); 38:11–14.

Centers for Disease Control. Mumps—United States, 1985–1988. *MMWR (Morbidity and Mortality Weekly Report)* 1989(e); 38:101–105.

Centers for Disease Control. Rubella and congenital rubella syndrome—United States, 1985–1988. *MMWR (Morbidity and Mortality Weekly Report)* 1989(f) 38:173–178.

Centers for Disease Control. Mumps prevention. *MMWR (Morbidity and Mortality Weekly Report)* 1989(g) 38:388–400.

Centers for Disease Control. Pneumococcal polysaccharide vaccine. *MMWR (Morbidity and Mortality Weekly Report)* 1989(h); 38:64–76.

Centers for Disease Control. Measles prevention: recommendation of the Advisory Committee on Immunization Practices (ACIP). *MMWR (Morbidity and Mortality Weekly Report)* 1989(i); 38:(No. S-9).

Centers for Disease Control. Pertussis surveillance—United States, 1986–1988. *MMWR (Morbidity and Mortality Weekly Report)* 1990; 39:57–66.

Centers for Disease Control. Measles—United States, 1990. *MMWR (Morbidity and Mortality Weekly Report)* 1991; 40:369–372.

Centers for Disease Control. Update: Eradication of paralytic poliomyelitis in the Americas. *MMWR (Morbidity and Mortality Weekly Report)* 1991(a); 41:681–683.

Centers for Disease Control. Hepatitis B virus: a comprehensive strategy for eliminating transmission in the United States through universal childhood vaccination. Recommendations of the Advisory Committee on Immunization Practices (ACIP). *MMWR (Morbidity and Mortality Weekly Report)*, 1991(c); 40, No. RR-13.

Centers for Disease Control. Vaccinia (smallpox) vaccine: Recommendations of the Advisory Committee on Immunization Practices (ACIP). *MMWR* 1991(d); 40(RR14):1–10.

Centers for Disease Control. Asthma—United States, 1980–1990. *MMWR (Morbidity and Mortality Weekly Report)* 1992, 41:733–735.

Centers for Disease Control. Measles surveillance—United States, 1991. *MMWR (Morbidity and Mortality Weekly Report)* 1992(b), 41 (No. SS-6):1–13.

Centers for Disease Control. Pertussis vaccination: acellular pertussis vaccine for reinforcing and booster use—Recommendations of the Advisory Committee on Immunization Practices (ACIP). *MMWR (Morbidity and Mortality Weekly Report)* 1992(c), 41 (No. RR-1):1–10.

Centers for Disease Control. Recommendations for use of Haemophilus b conjugate vaccines and a combined diphtheria, tetanus, pertussis, and Haemophilus b vaccine; Recommendations of the Advisory Committee on Immunization Practices (ACIP). *MMWR (Morbidity and Mortality Weekly Report)*, 1993, 42: No. RR-13.

Centers for Disease Control. Summary of notifiable diseases, United States, 1993. *MMWR (Morbidity and Mortality Weekly Report)* 1994, 42: No. 53.

Centers for Disease Control. Vaccination coverage of 2-year-old children—United States, 1992–1993. *MMWR (Morbidity and Mortality Weekly Report)* 1994(a); 43:282–283.

Centers for Disease Control. Progress toward global eradication of poliomyelitis, 1988–1993. *MMWR (Morbidity and Mortality Weekly Report)* 1994(b); 43:499–503.

Centers for Disease Control. Hepatitis surveillance report no. 56. Atlanta, GA: US Department of Health Services, Public Health Service, 1996.

Centers for Disease Control. Prevention of pneumococcal disease: Recommendations of the Advisory Committee on Immunization Practices (ACIP). *MMWR* 1997; 46:1.

Centers for Disease Control. Varicella-related deaths among adults – United States, 1997. *MMWR* 1998; 46(19):409–12.

Centers for Disease Control. Varicella-related deaths among children – United States, 1997. *MMWR* 1998(b); 47(18):365–8.

Centers for Disease Control. Tetanus Surveillance – United States, 1995–1997. *MMWR* 1998(c); 47(No. SS-2):1–14.

Centers for Disease Control. Varicella-related deaths – Florida, 1998. *MMWR* 1999; 48(18):379–81.

Centers for Disease Control. Prevention of hepatitis A through active or passive immunization: Recommendations of the Advisory Committee on Immunization Practices (ACIP). *MMWR* 1999(b); 48(No. RR-12).

Centers for Disease Control. Surveillance for adverse events associated with anthrax vaccination – US Department of Defense, 1998–2000. *MMWR* 2000; 49:341–45.

Centers for Disease Control. Prevention and control of meningococcal disease: Recommendations of the Advisory Committee on Immunization Practices (ACIP). *MMWR* 2000; 49(No. RR-07):1–10.

Centers for Disease Control. Preventing pneumococcal disease among infants and young children: Recommendations of the Advisory Committee on Immunization Practices (ACIP). *MMWR* 2000(b); 49(No. RR-09):1–38.

Centers for Disease Control. Poliomyelitis prevention in the United States: Updated Recommendations of the Advisory Committee on Immunization Practices (ACIP). *MMWR* 2000(c); 49(No. RR-05):1–22.

Centers for Disease Control. Summary of Notifiable Diseases, United States. *MMWR* 2001; 48(53):1–104.

Centers for Disease Control. Prevention and control of influenza: Recommendations of the Advisory Committee on Immunization Practices (ACIP). *MMWR* 2001(b); 50(RR04):1–46.

Centers for Disease Control. Update: Investigation of bioterrorism-related inhalational anthrax – Connecticut, 2001 *MMWR* 2001(c); 50(47):1049–51.

Centers for Disease Control. Notice to Readers: Fever, jaundice, and multiple organ system failure associated with 17D-derived yellow fever vaccination, 1996–2001. *MMWR* 2001(d); 50(30):643–5.

Chaffin, D., Dinman, B., Miller, J. *et al.* An evaluation of the effects of chronic mercury exposure on EMG and psychomotor functions. *U.S. Department of Health and Human Services, National Institute of Occupational Safety and Health.* Document no. HSM-099-71-62. Washington, DC, 1973.

Chandra, R.K. Immunological aspects of human milk. *Nutrition Review* 1978; 36:265.

Chantler, J.K., Tingle, A.J., Petty, R.E. Persistent rubella virus infection associated with chronic arthritis in children. *New England Journal of Medicine* 1985; 313:1117.

Chavanon, P. *La Diptherie.* Paris: 1932.

Cherry, J.D. 'Pertussis vaccine encephalopathy': It is time to recognize it as the myth that it is. *Journal of the American Medical Association* 1990; 263:1679–1680.

Cherry, J.D., Feigin, R.D., Lobes, L.A., Shackelford, P.G. Atypical measles in children previously immunized with attenuated measles virus vaccines. *Pediatrics* 1972; 50:712.

Cherry, J.D., Brunell, P.A., Golden, G.S., Karzon, D.T. Report of the task force on pertussis and pertussis immunization—1988. *Pediatrics* 1988; 81 (suppl):939–984.

Cherry, J.D., Baraff, L.J., Hewlett, E. The past, present, and future of pertussis: the role of adults in epidemiology and future control (Specialty Conference). *Western Journal of Medicine* 1989; 150:319–328.

Christopher, G.W., Cieslak, T.J., Pavlin, J.A., Eitzen, E.M. Biological warfare: a historical perspective. *JAMA* 1997; 278:412–417.

Church, J.A, Richards, W. Recurrent abscess formation following DTP immunizations: association with hypersensitivity to tetanus toxoid. *Pediatrics* 1985; 75:899–900.

Cizman, M., Mozetic, M., Radescek-Rakar, R. *et al.* Aseptic meningitis after vaccination against measles and mumps. *Pediatric Infectious Disease Journal* 1989; 8:302–308.

Clarke, J.H. *A Dictionary of Practical Materia Medica.* Sussex, England: Health Science Press, 1967.

Classen, J.B. Childhood immunization and diabetes mellitus. *New Zealand Medical Journal* 1996; 109:195.

Classen, D.C. Diabetes and vaccines. October 17, 1996(a), email communication.

Classen, D.C., Classen, J.B. The timing of pediatric immunization and the risk of insulin-dependent diabetes mellitus. *Infectious Diseases in Clinical Practice* 1997; 6:449–54.

Classen, J.B., Classen, D.C. Haemophilus vaccine and increased IDDM, causal relationship likely. *British Medical Journal* 1999: email letter.

Clemens, J.D., Ferreccio, C., Levine, M.M. *et al.* Impact of Haemophilus influenzae type b polysaccharide-tetanus protein conjugate vaccine on responses to concurrently administered diphtheria-tetanus-pertussis vaccine. *Journal of the American Medical Association* 1992; 267:673–8.

Clement International Corporation. Toxicological profile for mercury. *U.S. Department of Health and Human Services, Public Health Service, Agency for Toxic Substances and Disease Registry.* Washington, DC, 1992.

Cochi, S.L., Fleming, E.W., Hightower, A.W. *et al.* Primary invasive Haemophilus influenzae type b disease: a population-based assessment of risk factors. *Journal of Pediatrics* 1986; 108:887–896.

Cochi, S.L., Preblud, S.R., Orenstein, W.A. Perspectives on the relative resurgence of mumps in the United States. *American Journal of Diseases of Children* 1988; 142:499–507.

Cody, C.L., Baraff, L.J., Cherry, J.D. *et al.* Nature and rates of adverse reactions associated with DTP and DT immunizations in infants and children. *Pediatrics* 1981; 68:650–660.

Cohen, A.D., Shoenfeld, Y. Vaccine-induced autoimmunity. *Journal of Autoimmunity* 1996; 9(6):699–703.

Collier, L.H., Polakoff, S., Mortimer, J. Reactions and antibody responses to reinforcing doses of adsorbed and plain tetanus vaccines. *Lancet* 1979; 1:1364.

Collomb, H., Rey, M., Dumas, M. *et al.* Syndromes neurophychiques au cours des encephalitis postvaccinales (vaccination antimalile). *Bull. Soc. Med. D'Afrique Noire Lang. Franc.* 1966; 11:575–86.

Colville, A., Pugh, S. Mumps meningitis and measles, mumps, and rubella vaccine. *Lancet* 1992; 340:786.

Committee on Government Reform, US House of Representatives. Conflict of interest in vaccine policy making, majority staff report, June 15, 2000.

Committee on Infectious Diseases, American Academy of Pediatrics. Recommendations for using pneumococcal vaccine in children. *Pediatrics* 1985; 75:1153–1158.

Committee on Infectious Diseases, American Academy of Pediatrics. Recommendations for the use of live attenuated varicella vaccine. *Pediatrics* 1995; 95:791–796.

Confavreux, C., Suissa, S. *et al.* Vaccinations and the risk of relapse in multiple sclerosis. *New England Journal of Medicine* 2001; 344(5):319–26.

Conflict of interest in pertussis vaccine study. *The Doctor's People* 1990; 3:4.

Corrigan, F.M., Reynolds, G.P., Ward, N.I. Aluminium and Alzheimer's disease (letter). *Lancet* 1989; 339:268.

Coulter, H.L. *Divided Legacy: A History of the Schism in Medical Thought, Volume 3, The Conflict Between Homoeopathy and the American Medical Association: 1800–1914.* Berkeley, CA: North Atlantic Books, 1982.

Coulter, H.L. *Vaccination, Social Violence, and Criminality: The Medical Assault on the American Brain.* Berkeley, CA: North Atlantic Books, 1990.

Coulter, H.L. Review of Marie R. Griffin DTP study. Unpublished, 1990(a).

Coulter, H.L. Contribution to the discussion of connection between childhood vaccinations and neurologic disease. Submitted to the Institute of Medicine's Committee to review the adverse consequences of pertussis and rubella vaccines, 1990(b).

Coulter, H.L., Fisher, B.L. *A Shot in the Dark.* Garden City, New York: Avery Publishing Group, Inc., 1991.

Coulter, H.L., personal communication, 1995.

Coulter, H. Childhood vaccination and juvenile onset (type-1) diabetes. Testimony before the Congress of the United States, House of Representatives, Committee on Appropriations. *International Vaccination Newsletter* September 1997:3–9.

Crapper-McLachlan, D.R., Kruck, T.P., Lukiw, W.J., Krishnan, S.S. Would decreased aluminum ingestion reduce the incidence of Alzheimer's disease? *Canadian Medical Association Journal* 1991; 145:793–804.

Croke, C.L., Munson, E.L., Lovrich, S.D. *et al.* Occurrence of severe destructive lyme arthritis in hamsters vaccinated with outer surface protein A and challenged with Borrelia burgdorferi. *Infection and Immunity* 2000; 68(2):658–63.

Crone, N.E., Reder, A.T. Severe tetanus in immunized patients with high anti-tetanus titers *Neurology* 1992; 42:761–764.

Crowder, M., Higgins, H.L., Frost, J.J. Rubella susceptibility in young women of rural east Texas: 1980 and 1985. *Texas Medicine* 1987; 83:43–47.

Cummings, S., Ullman, D. *Everybody's Guide to Homeopathic Medicines.* Los Angeles: Jeremy P Tarcher, Inc., 1997.

Curtis, T. The origin of AIDS: a startling new theory attempts to answer the question "Was it an act of God or man?" *Rolling Stone* March 19, 1992.

D'Cruz, O.F., Shapiro, E.D., Spiegelman, K.N., Leicher, C.R. *et al.* Acute inflammatory demyelinating polyradiculoneuropathy (Guillain-Barré syndrome) after immunization with *Haemophilus influenzae* type b conjugate vaccine. *Journal of Pediatrics* 1989; 115:743–746.

Dacou-Voutetakis, C., Constantinidis, M., Moschos, S. *et al.* Diabetes mellitus following mumps: insulin reserve. *American Journal of Diseases of Children* 1974; 127:890–891.

Daum, R.S., Sood, S.K., Osterholm, M.T. *et al.* Decline in serum antibody to the capsule of *Haemophilus influenzae* type b in the immediate postimmunization period. *Journal of Pediatrics* 1989; 1114:742–747.

Davidson, M., Letson, G.W., Ward. J.I. *et al.* DTP immunization and susceptibility to infectious diseases: Is there a relationship? *American Journal of Diseases of Children* 1991; 145:750–754.

Davis, L.E., Wands, J.R., Weiss, S.A. *et al.* Central nervous system intoxication from mercurous chloride laxatives—quantitative, histochemical and ultrastructure studies. *Archives of Neurology* 1974; 30:428–431.

Deming, M.S., Jaiteh, K.O., Otten, M.W., Flagg, E.W. Epidemic poliomyelitis in The Gambia following the control of poliomyelitis as an endemic disease; II. Clinical efficacy of trivalent oral polio vaccine. *American Journal of Epidemiology* 1992; 135:393.

Desrosiers, R.C. HIV-1 origins: A finger on the missing link. *Nature* 1990; 345:288–289.

Developments with respect to the manufacture of live polio vaccine and results of utilization of killed polio vaccine. Hearing before subcommittee of the Committee on Interstate and Foreign Commerce House of Representatives (87th Congress, first session). Washington, DC: US Government Printing Office, 1961: 317–325.

Diamandopoulos, G.T. Leukemia, lymphoma, and osteosarcoma induced in the Syrian golden hamster by simian virus 40. *Science* 1972; 176:173–5.

Dieter, M.P., Luster, M.I., Boorman, G.A. *et al.* Immunological and biochemical responses in mice treated with mercuric chloride. *Toxicology and Applied Pharmacology* 1983; 68:218–228.

Dodge, P.R., Davis, H., Feigin, R.D. *et al.* Prospective evaluation of hearing impairment as a sequelae of acute bacterial meningitis. *New England Journal of Medicine* 1984; 311:869–874.

Dokheel, T.M. An epidemic of childhood diabetes in the United States? Evidence from Allegheny County, Pennsylvania. Pittsburgh Diabetes Epidemiology Research Group. *Diabetes Care* 1993; 16(12):1606–11.

Dollinger, H.C., Zumkey, H., Spieker, C. *et al.* Aluminum in antacids shown to accumulate in brain and bone tissue. *Gastroenterol Obs* 1986; 5:478.

Druet, P., Druet, E., Potdevin, F. *et al.* Immune type glomerulonephritis induced by HgCl2 in the Brown Norway rat. *Annals of Immunology* 1978; 129C:777–792.

Dudley, S.F., May, P.M., O'Flynn, J.A. *Medical Research Council, Special Report Series, No. 195.* UK, 1934.

Duncan, B., Ey, J., Holberg, C.J., Wright, A.L. *et al.* Exclusive breast-feeding for at least 4 months protects against otitis media. *Pediatrics* 1993, 91:867–872.

Dunkle, L.M., Arvin, A.M., Whitley, R.J. *et al.* A controlled trial of acyclovir for chickenpox in normal children. *New England Journal of Medicine* 1991; 325:1539–1544.

Durbaca, S., Stoean, C. Investigations concerning the possibility to replace the Schick test by the passive hemagglutination reaction for evaluating the diphtheria immunity level in population. *Roumanian Archives of Microbiology and Immunology* 1992; 51:141–146.

Dyken, P.R., Cunningham, S.C., Ward, L.C. Changing character of subacute sclerosing panencephalitis in the United States. *Pediatric Neurology* 1989; 5:339–341.

Eaton, C.W. The Facts about Variolinum. *Transactions of the American Institute of Homeopathy* 1907:547–567.

Edsall, G. Specific prophylaxis of tetanus. *Journal of American Medical Association* 1959; 171:417–427.

Edsall, G., Altman, J.S., Gaspar, A.J. Combined tetanus-diphtheria immunization of adults: use of small doses of diphtheria toxoid. *American Journal of Public Health* 1954; 44:1537–1545.

Ehrengut, W. Konvulsive Reaktionen nach Pertussis-Schutzimpfung. [Convulsive reactions after pertussis immunization.] *Deutsche Medizinische Wochenschrift* 1974; 99:2273–2279.

Eichhorn, G.L. In Katzman, R., Terry, R.D., Bick, K.L., eds. *Alzheimer's Disease: Senile Dementia and Related Disorders.* New York: Raven Press, 1978.

Eichhorn, G.L. Aging, genetics and the environment: Potential of errors introduced into genetic information transfer by metal ions. *Mech Ageing Dev* 1979; 9:291–301.

Eichhorn, G.L. Is there any relationship between aluminum and Alzheimer's disease? *Experimental Gerontology* 1993; 28:493–498.

Eisfelder, H.W. Poliomyelitis immunization—a final report. *Journal of the American Institute of Homeopathy* 1961; 54:166–167.

Elswood, B.F., Stricker, R.B. Polio vaccines and the origin of AIDS. *Research in Virology* 1993; 144:175–177.

Elswood, B.F., Stricker, R.B. Polio vaccines and the origin of AIDS. *Medical Hypotheses* 1994; 42:347–354.

English, J.M. (a) Pertussin 30—preventive for whooping cough? A pilot study. *British Homeopathic Journal* 1987; 76:61–65.

English, J.M. (b) Symptoms and treatment of whooping cough, 1980–1982. *British Homeopathic Journal* 1987; 76:66–68.

Eskola, J., Peltola, H., Takala, A.K. *et al.* Efficacy of *Haemophilus influenzae* type b polysaccharide-diphtheria toxoid conjugate vaccine in infancy. *New England Journal of Medicine* 1987; 317:717–722.

Eskola, J., Peltola, H., Takala, A.K. *et al.* Protective efficacy of the *Haemophilus influenzae* type b conjugate vaccine HbOC in Finnish infants [Abstract #60]. *Thirtieth Interscience Conference on Antimicrobial Agents and Chemotherapy*, Atlanta, Georgia, October 1990.

Essex, M., Kanki, P. The origins of the AIDS virus. *Scientific American* 1988; 259:64–71.

Experts question need for proposed HBV requirements. *Hospital Infection Control* 1990; 17:17–28.

Facktor, M., Bernstein, R.A., Fireman, P. Hypersensitivity to tetanus toxoid. *Journal of Allergy and Clinical Immunology* 1973; 52:1–12.

Faculty review of Asian influenza. *Homeopathy* 1958; 8:115–124.

Feldman, H.M., Michaels, R.H. Academic achievement in children ten to 12 years after *Haemophilus influenzae* meningitis. *Pediatrics* 1988; 81:339–344.

Fenichel, G.M. Neurological complications of immunization. *Annals of Neurology* 1982; 12:119–128.

Ferencei, M., Masar, I., Sonak, R. Comparison of the Schick test and the haemagglutination test for detection of the level of diphtheria antitoxin in the serum. *Journal of Hygiene, Epidemiology, Microbiology, and Immunology* 1969; 13: 141–148.

Fescharek, R., Quast, U., Maass, G. *et al.* Measles-mumps vaccination in the FRG: an empirical analysis after 14 years of use. II. Tolerability and analysis of spontaneously reported side effects. *Vaccine* 1990; 8:446–456.

Fine, M.J., Smith, M.A., Carson, C.A., et al. Efficacy of pneumococcal vaccination in adults. A meta-analysis of randomized controlled trials. *Archives of Internal Medicine* 1994; 154:2666.

Finn, T. *Dangers of Compulsory Immunizations: How to Avoid Them Legally.* New Port Richey, FL: Family Fitness Press, 1983.

Fisher, S.G., Weber, L., Carbone, M. Cancer risk associated with simian virus 40 contaminated polio vaccine. *Anticancer Research* 1999; 19(3B):2173–80.

Fleming, D.W., Leibenhaut, M.D., Albanes, D. *et al.* Secondary *Haemophilus influenzae* type b in day-care facilities; risk factors and prevention. *Journal of the American Medical Association* 1985; 254:509–514.

Flewett, T.H., Hoult, J.G. Influenzal encephalopathy and postinfluenzal encephalitis. *Lancet* 1958; 2:11–5.

Forrester, H.L., Jahnigen, D.W., LaForce, F.M. Inefficacy of pneumococcal vaccine in a high-risk population. *American Journal of Medicine* 1987; 83:425–430.

Förström, L., Hannuksela, M., Kousa, M., Kehmuskallio, E. Merthiolate hypersensitivity and vaccination. *Contact Dermatitis* 1980; 6:241–245.

Frecker, M.F. Dementia in Newfoundland: identification of a geographical isolate? In Crapper-McLachlan, D.R., Kruck, T.P., Lukiw, W.J., Krishnan, S.S. Would decreased aluminum ingestion reduce the incidence of Alzheimer's disease? *Canadian Medical Association Journal* 1991; 145:793–804.

Freed, G.L., Bordley, W.C., Clark, S.J., Konrad, T.R. Reactions of pediatricians to a new Centers for Disease Control recommendation for universal immunization of infants with hepatitis B vaccine. *Pediatrics* 1993; 91:699–702.

Freed, G.L., Bordley, W.C., Clark, S.J., Konrad, T.R. Family physician acceptance of universal hepatitis B immunization of infants. *Journal of Family Practice* 1993(a); 36:153–157.

Frei, H., Thurneysen, A. Homeopathy in acute otitis media in children: treatment effect or spontaneous resolution? *British Homeopathic Journal* 2001; 90(4):180–2

Frey, S.E., Couch, R.B., Tacket, C.O. *et al.* Clinical response to undiluted and diluted smallpox vaccine. *New England Journal of Medicine* 2002; 346(17).

Fukuda, K., Nisenbaum, R., Stewart, G. *et al.* Chronic multi-symptom illness affecting air force veterans of the Gulf War. *JAMA* 1998; 280:981–88.

Fulginiti, V.A. Controversies in current immunization policies and practices. *Current Problems in Pediatrics* 1976; 6:6–16.

Fulginiti, V.A. A pertussis vaccine myth dies. *American Journal of Diseases of Children* 1990; 144:860–861.

Gabriel, R. Testimony before the Committee to Review the Adverse Consequences of Pertussis and Rubella Vaccines, Institute of Medicine, May, 1990; In Coulter, H.L. & Fisher, B.L. *A Shot in the Dark*. Garden City, New York: Avery Publishing Group, Inc., 1991.

Galazka, A., Andrzejczak-Kardymowicz, B. Complication and reactions after vaccination against pertussis. *Epidemiological Review* 1972; 26:411–424.

Gale, J.L., Thapa, P.B., Bobo, J.R. *et al.* Acute neurological illness and DTP: report of a case-control study in Washington and Oregon. In Manclark, C.R., ed. Sixth International Symposium on Pertussis, Abstracts. Bethesda, Maryland: Department of Health and Human Services, 1990:228–9 (DHSS publication No. (FDA) 90–1162).

Galil, K., Singleton, R., Levine, O.S. *et al.* Reemergence of invasive Haemophilus influenzae type b disease in a well-vaccinated population in remote Alaska. *Journal of Infectious Diseases* 1999; 179:101–6.

Ganiats, T.G., Bowersox, M.T., Ralph, L.P. Universal neonatal hepatitis B immunization—Are we jumping on the bandwagon too early? *Journal of Family Practice* 1993; 36:147–149.

Gao, F., Hue, L., White, A.T. *et al.* Human infection by genetically diverse SIVsm-related HIV-2 in West Africa. *Nature* 1992; 358:495–499.

GAO (The U.S. General Accounting Office). Gulf War Illnesses: Questions about the Presence of Squalene Antibodies in Veterans Can be Resolved 1999 (GAO/NSIAD-99-5).

Garrett, A.J., Dunham, A., Wood, D.J. Retroviruses and poliovaccines. *Lancet* 1993; 342:932–933.

Geissler, E. SV40 and human brain tumors. *Progress in Medical Virology* 1990; 37:211–222.

Gelb, L.D., Huang, J.J., Wellinghoff, W.J. Varicella-zoster virus transformation of hamster embryo cells. *Journal Gen Virology* 1980; 51:171–177.

Gellin, B.G., Greenberg, R.N., Hart, R.H. *et al.* Immunogenicity of two doses of yeast recombinant hepatitis B vaccine in healthy older adults. *Journal of Infectious Disease* 1997; 175:1494.

Gershon, A.A., Steinberg, S., Galasso, G. *et al.* Live attenuated varicella vaccine in children with leukemia in remission. *Biken Journal* 1984; 27:77.

Gershon, A.A., Steinberg, S.P., Gelb, L. Live attenuated varicella vaccine use in immunocompromised children and adults. *Pediatrics* 1986; 78 (suppl):757–762.

Gershon, A.A. Live attenuated varicella vaccine. *Annals and Reviews of Medicine* 1987; 38:41–50.

Gervaix, M., Caflisch, S., Suter, A.M., Haenggeli, C.A. Guillain-Barré syndrome following immunization with *Haemophilus influenzae* type b conjugate vaccine. *European Journal of Pediatrics* 1993; 152:613–614.

Gilmartin, R.C., Jabbour, J.T., Duenas, D.A. Rubella vaccine myeloradiculoneuritis. *Journal of Pediatrics* 1972; 80:406–412.

Glikson, M., Galun, E., Oren, R. *et al.* Relapsing hepatitis A. Review of 14 cases and literature survey. *Medicine* 1992; 71:14–23.

Goffin, E., Horsmans, Y., Cornu, C. *et al.* Acute hepatitis B infection after vaccination (letter). *Lancet* 1995; 345:263.

Golden, I. A possible mechanism of homeopathic prophylaxis. *Journal of the American Institute of Homeopathy* 1989; 82: 69–76.

Golden, I. *Vaccination? A Review of Risks and Alternatives.* Aurum Healing Centre, P.O. Box 155, Daylesford, Vic. 3460, Australia, 1998.

Goldman, A.S. *et al.* Immunologic factors in human milk during the first year of lactation. *Journal of Pediatrics* 1982; 100:563.

Goto, N., Akama, K. Histopathological studies of reactions in mice injected with aluminium-adsorbed tetanus toxoid. *Microbiological Immunology* 1982; 26:1121.

Gorter, E. Postvaccinal encephalitis. *JAMA* 1933;101(24):1871–1874.

Goss Gilroy, Inc. Health study of Canadian forces personnel involved in the 1991 conflict in the Persian Gulf. Prepared for Gulf War Illness Advisory Committee. Department of Defence. 1998 (*www.forces.ca/menu/press/Reports/Health/health_study_e_vol1_TOC.htm*)

Grandjean, P., Budtz-Jorgensen, E., White, R.F. *et al.* Methylmercury exposure biomarkers as indicators of neurotoxicity in children aged 7 years. *American Journal of Epidemiology* 1999; 150(3):301–5.

Granoff, D.M., Pandey, J.P., Boies, E. *et al.* Response to immunization with *Haemophilus influenzae* type b polysaccharide-pertussis vaccine and risk of haemophilus meningitis in children with the km(1) immunoglobulin allotype. *Journal of Clinical Investigation* 1984; 74:1708–1714.

Granoff, D.M., Gupta, R.K., Belshe, R.B. et al. Induction of immunologic refreactoriness in adults by meningococcal C polysaccharide vaccination. *Journal of Infectious Disease* 1998; 178:870–4.

Graves, A.B., White, E., Koepsell, T.D. *et al.* The association between aluminum-containing products and Alzheimer's disease. *Journal of Clinical Epidemiology* 1990; 43:35–44.

Greenberg, M., Abrahamson, H., Cooper, H.M., Solomon, H.E. The relation between recent injections and paralytic poliomyelitis in children. *American Journal of Public Health* 1952; 42:142–152.

Griffin, M.R., Ray, W.A., Mortimer, E.A. *et al.* Risk of seizures and encephalopathy after immunization with the Diphtheria-Tetanus-Pertussis vaccine. *Journal of the American Medical Association* 1990, 263:1641–1645.

Grimmer, A.H. Polio prevention. *The Layman Speaks* 1952; 5(3):173–4.

Grose, C., Spigland, I. Guillain-Barré syndrome following administration of live measles vaccine. *American Journal of Medicine* 1976; 60:441–443.

Gross, K., Combe, C., Krüger, K., Schattenkirchner, M. Arthritis after hepatitis vaccination: report of three cases. *Scandinavian Journal Rheumatology* 1995; 24:50–52.

Gross, D.M., Forsthuber, T., Tary-Lehmann, M. *et al.* Identification of LFA-1 as a candidate autoantigen in treatment-resistant Lyme arthritis. *Science* 1998; 281(5377):703–6.

Guardian, The. Vaccine-free French healthier than allies. Feb. 13, 2002.

Guerra, H.L., Sardinha, T.M., da Rosa, A.P., Lima e Costa, M.F. Effectiveness of the yellow fever vaccine 17D: an epidemiologic evaluation in health services. *Rev Panam Salud Publica* 1997; 2(2):115–20.

Guess, H.A., Broughton, D.D., Melton, L.J., Kurland, L.T. Population-based studies of varicella complications. *Pediatrics* 1986; 78 (suppl):723–727.

Gunderman, J.R. Guillain-Barré syndrome: Occurrence following combined mumps-rubella vaccine. *American Journal Diseases of Children* 1973; 125:834–835.

Gupta, R.K., Relyveld, E.H. Adverse reactions after injection of adsorbed diphtheria-pertussis-tetanus (DPT) vaccine are not due only to pertussis organisms or pertussis components in the vaccine. *Vaccine* 1991; 9:699–702.

Gustafson, T.L., Lievens, A.W., Brunell, P.A. *et al.* Measles outbreak in a fully immunized secondary-school population. *New England Journal of Medicine* 1987; 316:771–774.

Hachulla, E., Houvenagel, E., Mingui, A., Vincent, G., Laine, A. Reactive arthritis after hepatitis B vaccination. *Journal of Rheumatology* 1990; 17:1250–1251.

Hadler, S.C., Francis, D.P., Maynard, J.E. *et al.* Long-term immunogenicity and efficacy of hepatitis B vaccine in homosexual men. *New England Journal of Medicine* 1986; 315:209–214.

Hahnemann, S. *The Cure and Prevention of Scarlet Fever.* Gotha: Becker Publ., 1801.

Hahnemann, S. *Organon of Medicine.* Los Angeles: J.P. Tarcher, Inc. 1982.

Hall, A.J. Hepatitis B vaccination: protection for how long and against what? Booster injections are not indicated. *British Medical Journal* 1993; 307:276–277.

Hall, C.B., Halsey, N.A. Control of hepatitis B: to be or not to be? *Pediatrics* 1992; 90:274–277.

Halperin, S.A., Barreto, L., Friesen, B., Meekison, W. Immunogenicity of a five-component acellular pertussis vaccine in infants and young children. *Archives of Pediatric and Adolescent Medicine* 1994; 148:495–502.

Haneberg, B., Matre, R., Winsnes, R. *et al.* Acute hemolytic anemia related to diphtheria-pertussis-tetanus vaccination. *Acta Paediatrica Scandinavica* 1978; 67:345–350.

Hanson, L.A., Ahlestedt, S., Andersson, B. *et al.* Protective factors in milk and the development of the immune system. *Pediatrics* 1985; 75(suppl.):172–176.

Harris, G. After vaccine's recall, regulators begin to look for holes in safety net. *Wall Street Journal*, October 18, 1999.

Harrison, L.H., Broome, C.V., Hightower, M.S. *et al.* A -based study of the efficacy of *Haemophilus influenzae* type b polysaccharide vaccine. *Journal of the American Medical Association* 1988; 260: 1413–1418.

Harrison, L.H., Broome, C.V., Hightower, M.S. *Haemophilus influenzae* type b polysaccharide vaccine: an efficacy study. *Pediatrics* 1989; 84:255–261.

Hassan, W., Oldham, R. Reiter's syndrome and reactive arthritis in health care workers after vaccination. *British Medical Journal* 1994; 309:94.

Hayes, R.B., Raatgever, J.W., de Bruyn, A., Gerin, M. Cancer of the nasal cavity and paranasal sinuses, and formaldehyde exposure. *International Journal of Cancer* 1986; 37(4):487–492.

Hayflick, L., Plotkin, S.A., Norton, T.W., Koprowski, H. Preparation of poliovirus vaccines in a human fetal diploid cell strain. *American Journal of Hygiene* 1962; 75:240–258.

Hedenskog, S., Björksten, B., Blennow, M., Granström, G., Granström, M. Immunoglobulin E response to pertussis toxin in whooping cough and after immunization with a whole-cell and acellular pertussis vaccine. *International Archives of Allergy and Applied Immunology* 1989; 89:156.

Heinonen, O.P., Shapiro, S., Monson, R.R. *et al.* Immunization during pregnancy against poliomyelitis and influenza in relation to childhood malignancy. *International Journal of Epidemiology* 1973; 2:229–35.

Helmke, K., Otten, A., Willems, W.R. *et al.* Islet cell antibodies and the development of diabetes mellitus in relation to mumps infection and mumps vaccination. *Diabetologia* 1986; 29:30–33.

Hennessen, W., Quast, U. Adverse reactions after pertussis vaccination. International Symposium on Immunization: Benefit vs. Risk Factors, Brussels. *Developments in Biological Standardization* 1979; 43:95–100.

Herroelen, L., DeKeyser, J., Ebinger, G. Central-nervous-system demyelination after immunisation with recombinant hepatitis B vaccine. *Lancet* 1991; 338:1174–1175.

Hersh, B.S., Markowitz, L.E., Hoffman, R.E. *et al.* A measles outbreak at a college with a prematriculation immunization requirement. *American Journal of Public Health* 1991; 81:360–363.

Hill, A.B., Knowelden, J. Inoculation and poliomyelitis: A statistical investigation in England and Wales in 1949. *British Medical Journal* 1950; 2:1–6.

Hinman, A.R., Koplan, J.P. Pertussis and pertussis vaccine: reanalysis of benefits, risks, and costs. *Journal of the American Medical Association* 1984; 251:3109–3113.

Hirayama, M. Measles vaccines used in Japan. *Reviews of Infectious Diseases* 1983; 5:495–503.

Hirsch, F., Kuhn, J., Ventura, M. *et al.* Autoimmunity induced by HgCl2 in Brown-Norway rats—part I: Production of monoclonal antibodies. *Journal of Immunology* 1986; 136:3272–3276.

Hirsch, R.L., Mokhtarian, F., Griffin, D.E. *et al.* Measles virus vaccination of measles seropositive individuals suppresses lymphocyte proliferation and chemotactic factor production. *Clinical Immunology and Immunopathology* 1981; 21:341–350.

Hirszel, P., Michaelson, J.H., Dodge, K. *et al.* Mercury-induced autoimmune glomerulonephritis in inbred rats—part II. Immunohistopathology, histopathology and effects of prostaglandin administration. *Survey Synth Pathological Research* 1985; 4:412–422.

Hoffman, H.J., Hunter, J.C., Damus, K. *et al.* Diphtheria-tetanus-pertussis immunization and sudden infant death: results of the National Institute of Child Health and Human Development Cooperative Epidemiological Study of Sudden Infant Death Syndrome Risk Factors. *Pediatrics* 1987; 79:598–611.

Hooper, E., *The River: A Journey to the Source of HIV and AIDS*. Little, Brown and Co., New York, 1999.

Horner, F.A. Neurologic disorders after Asian influenza. *New England Journal of Medicine* 1958; 258:983–5.

Hough, J.C. *et al.* Rubella seroconversion following immunization in a rural practice. *Journal of Family Practice* 1979; 9:587–589.

Howie, P.W. *et al*. Protective effect of breast feeding against infection. *British Medical Journal* 1990; 300:11–16.

Huang, X., Yuan, J., Goddard, A. *et al*. Interferon expression in pancreases of patients with type 1 diabetes. *Diabetes* 1995; 44:658–64.

Huet, T., Cheynier, R., Meyerhans, A. *et al*. Genetic organization of a chimpanzee lentivirus related to HIV-1. *Nature* 1990; 345:356–358.

Hulbert, T.V., Larsen, R.A., Davis, C.L., Holtom, P.D. Bilateral hearing loss after measles and rubella vaccination in an adult. *New England Journal of Medicine* 1991; 325:134.

Hull, H.F., Montes, J.M., Hays, P.C., Lucero, R.L. Risk factors for measles vaccine failure among immunized students. *Pediatrics* 1985; 76:518–523.

Hurwitz, E.L., Morgenstern, H. Effects of diphtheria-tetanus-pertussis or tetanus vaccination on allergies and allergy-related respiratory symptoms among children and adolescents in the US. *Journal of Manipulative and Physiological Therapeutics* 2000; 318(7192):1173–6.

Hussey, G.D. *et al*. The effect of Edmonston-Zagreb and Schwarz measles vaccines on immune response in infants. *Journal of Infectious Disease* 1996; 173(6):1320–6.

Hutcheson, R. DTP immunization and sudden infant death—Tennessee. *Morbidity and Mortality Weekly Report* 1979; 28:131–135.

Imani, F. and Kehoe, K.E. Infection of human B lymphocytes with MMR vaccine induce IgE class switching. *Clinical Immunology* 2001; 100(3):355–61.

Inglesby, T.V. *et al*. Consensus Statement: Anthrax as a Biological Weapon. *JAMA* 1999; 281:1735–1745.

Institute of Medicine. *An Evaluation of Poliomyelitis Vaccine Policy Options*. IOM publication 88–04, Washington, DC: National Academy of Sciences, 1988.

Institute of Medicine. *Adverse Effects of Pertussis and Rubella Vaccines*. Washington, DC: National Academy Press, 1991.

Institute of Medicine. *Adverse Events Associated with Childhood Vaccines: Evidence Bearing on Causality*. Washington, DC: National Academy Press, 1994.

Institute of Medicine. *Immunization Safety Review: Measles-Mumps-Rubella Vaccine and Autism*. Washington, DC: National Academy Press, 2001.

Intensive Immunization Programs. *Hearings before the Committee on Interstate and Foreign Commerce, House of Representatives, 87th Congress, 2nd Session on H.R. 10541*. Washington, DC: US Government Printing Office, 1962.

Istre, G.R., Conner, J.S., Broome, C.V. *et al*. Risk factors for primary invasive *Haemophilus influenzae* disease: Increased risk from day-care attendance in school-age household members. *Journal of Pediatrics* 1985; 106:190–195.

Ivins, B.E., Welkos, S.L. Recent advances in the development of an improved, human anthrax vaccine. *European Journal of Epidemiology* 1998; 4:12–19.

Jaber, L., Shohat, M., Mimouni, M. Infectious episodes following diphtheria-pertussis-tetanus vaccination: a preliminary observation in infants. *Clinical Pediatrics* 1988; 27:491–494.

Jabbour, J.T., Duenas, D.A., Sever, J.L., Krebs, H.M. *et al.* Epidemiology of subacute sclerosing panencephalitis (SSPE). *Journal of the American Medical Association* 1972; 220:959–962.

Jacobs, J., Jimenez, L.M., Gloyd, S.S., Gale, J.L., Crothers, D. Treatment of acute childhood diarrhea with homeopathic medicine: A randomized clinical trial in Nicaragua. *Pediatrics* 1994; 93:719.

Jacobs, J., Springer, D.A., Crothers, D. Homeopathic treatment of acute otitis media in children: a preliminary randomized placebo-controlled trial. *Pediatric Infectious Disease Journal* 2001; 20(2):177–83.

Jacobson v. Commonwealth of Massachusetts, 197 U.S. 11 (1905).

James, W. *Immunization: The Reality Behind the Myth*. Granberry, Massachusetts: Bergin & Garvey Publishers, 1988.

Jawad, A.S., Scott, D.G. Immunisation triggering rheumatoid arthritis? *Annals of Rheumatic Disease* 1989; 48:174.

Jernigan, J.A., Stephens, D.S., Ashford, D.A. *et al.* Bioterrorism-related inhalational anthrax: The first 10 cases reported in the United States. *Centers for Disease Control, Emerging Infectious Diseases* 2001; 7(6).

Johnson, D.M. Fatal tetanus after prophylaxis with human tetanus immune globulin. *Journal of the American Medical Association* 1969; 207:1519.

Jones, E.M.M., Wilson, D.C. Clinical features of yellow fever cases at Vom Christian Hospital during the 1969 epidemic on the Jos Plateau, Nigeria. *Bulletin WHO* 1972; 46:653–7.

Jong, E.C. Travel immunizations. *Medical Clinics of North America* 1999; 83(4):903–922.

Kadlec, R.P., Zelicoff, A.P., Vrtis, A.M. Biological weapons: Control, prospects and implications for the future. *JAMA* 1997; 278:351.

Kanki, P.J., McLane, M.F., King, N.W. *et al.* Serologic identification and characterization of a macaque T-lymphotropic retrovirus closely related to HTLV-II. *Science* 1985; 228:1199–1201.

Kaplan, S.L., Fishman, M.A. Update on bacterial meningitis. *Journal of Child Neurology* 1988; 3:82–93.

Karma, P., Luotonen, J., Timonen, M. *et al.* Efficacy of pneumococcal vaccination against recurrent otitis media. Preliminary results of a field trial in Finland. *Annals of Otology, Rhinology, and Laryngology* 1980; 89:357–362.

Karvonen, M., Zygimantas, C., Tuomilehto, J. Association between type 1 diabetes and Haemophilus influenzae type b vaccination: birth cohort study. *British Medical Journal* 1999; 318:1169–72.

Kawashima, H., Mori, T., Kashiqagi, Y. *et al*. Detection and sequencing of measles virus from peripheral mononuclear cells from patients with inflammatory bowel disease and autism. *Digestive Dis Sci* 2000; 45(4):723–9.

Kazarian, E.L., Gager, W.E. Optic neuritis complicating measles, mumps, and rubella vaccination. *American Journal of Ophthalmology* 1978; 86:544–547.

Keefer, M., Graham, B.S., McElrath, M.J. *et al*. Safety and immunogenicity of Env 2-3, a human immunodeficiency virus type 1 candidate vaccine, in combination with a novel adjuvant MTP-PE/MF-59. *AIDS Research Human Retroviruses* 1996; 12:683–93.

Kemp, T., Pearce, N., Fitzharris, P. *et al*. Is infant immunization a risk factor for childhood asthma or allergy? *Epidemiology* 1997; 8:678.

Kempe, C.H. Studies on smallpox and complications of smallpox vaccination. *Pediatrics* 1960; 26:176–189.

Kerns, W.D., Pavkov, K.L., Donofrio, D.J. *et al*. Carcinogenicity of formaldehyde in rats and mice after long-term inhalation exposure. *Cancer Research* 1983; 43(9):4382–4392.

Kerrin, J.C. The distribution of *B. tetani* in the intestine of animals. *British Journal of Pathology* 1929; 10:370–3.

Keutek, W., Couch, R., Bond, N. *et al*. Pilot evaluation of influenza virus (IVV) combined with adjuvant. *Vaccine* 1993; 11:909–13.

Khabbaz, R.F., Rowe, T., Murphey-Corb, M. *et al*. Simian immunodeficiency virus needlestick accident in a laboratory worker. *Lancet* 1992; 340:271–273.

Kilpi, T., Jokinen, J., Herra, E. et al. Effect of heptavalent pneumococcal conjugate vaccine (PNCCRM) on pneumococcal acute otitis media (AOM) by serotype [Abstract O20]. *2nd International Symposium on Pneumococci and Pneumococcal Diseases,* Sun City, South Africa, 2000.

Kilroy, A.W. Two syndromes following rubella immunization. *Journal of the American Medical Association* 1970; 214:2287–2292.

Kim-Farley, R.J., Lichfield, P.,Orenstein, W.A., Bart, K.J. *et al*. Outbreak of paralytic poliomyelitis, Taiwan. *Lancet* 1984; 2:1322–1324.

Kinnunen, E., Farkkila, M., Hovi, T., Juntunen, J., Weckstrom, P. Incidence of Guillain-Barré syndrome during a nationwide oral poliovirus vaccine campaign. *Neurology* 1989; 39:1034–1036.

Klatzo, I. *et al*. Experimental production of neurofibrillary degeneration. *Journal of Neuropathology and Experimental Neurology* 1965; 24:187.

Kleijnen, J., Knipschild, P., ter Riet, G. Clinical trials of homoeopathy. *British Medical Journal* 1991; 302:316.

Klein, A. *Trial by Fury*. New York: Charles Scribner's Sons, 1972.

Klugman, K.P., Gilbertson, I.T., Koornhof, H.J. et al. Protective activity of Vi capsular polysaccharide vaccine against typhoid fever. *Lancet* 1987; 330:1165–9.

Koch, J., Leet, C., McCarthy, R. *et al.* Adverse events temporally associated with immunizing agents—1987 report. *Canada Diseases Weekly Report* 1989; 15:151–158.

Koff, R.S. Hepatitis vaccines. *Infectious Disease Clinics of North America* 2001; 15(1):83–95.

Kopeloff, L.M. *et al.* Recurrent convulsive seizures in animals produced by immunologic and chemical means. *American Journal of Psychiatry* 1942; 98:881.

Korger, G., Quast, U., Dechert, G. Tetanusimpfung: Vertraglichkeit und Vermeidung von Nebenreaktionen. [Tetanus vaccination: tolerance and avoidance of adverse reactions.] *Klininische Wochenschrift* 1986;64:767–775.

Korn, R.F., Albrecht, R.M., Locke, F.B. The association of parenteral injections with poliomyelitis. *American Journal of Public Health* 1952; 42:153–169.

Kulenkampff, M., Schwartzman, J.S., Wilson, J. Neurological complications of pertussis inoculation. *Archives of Disease in Childhood* 1974; 49:46–49.

Kyle, W.S. Simian retroviruses, poliovaccine, and origin of AIDS. *Lancet* 1992; 339:600–601.

Lambert, H. Epidemiology of a small pertussis outbreak in Kent County, Michigan. *Public Health Rep* 1965; 80:365–369.

Landrigan, P.J., Witte, J.J. Neurologic disorder following live measles-virus vaccination. *Journal of the American Medical Association* 1973; 223:1459–1462.

Lane, J.M. Complications of smallpox vaccination. *New England Journal of Medicine* 1969; 281:1201–1208.

Lane, J.M. Complications of smallpox vaccination, 1968: Results of ten statewide surveys. *Journal of Infectious Disease* 1970; 122:303–309.

Lasky, T., Terracciano, G.J., Magder, L. *et al.* Guillain-Barré syndrome and the 1992–1993 and 1993–1994 influenza vaccines. *New England Journal of Medicine* 1998; 339:1797–802.

Lecatsas, G., Alexander, J.J. Origins of AIDS. *Lancet* 1992; 339:1427.

Leneman, F. The Guillain-Barré syndrome. *Archives of Internal Medicine* 1966; 118:139–144.

Leung, A.K.C. Anaphylaxis due to DPT vaccine (letter). *Journal of the Royal Society of Medicine* 1985; 78:175.

Levine, M.M., Ferreccio, C., Black, R.E., Germanier, R. Chilean Typhoid Committee. Large-scale field trial of Ty21a live oral typhoid vaccine in enteric-coated capsule formulation. *Lancet* 1987; 329:1049–52.

Levine, M.M., Taylor, D.N., Ferreccio, C. Typhoid vaccines come of age. *Pediatric Infectious Disease Journal* 1989; 8:374–81.

Levine, M.M., Ferreccio, C., Cryz, S., Ortiz, E. Comparison of enteric-coated capsules and liquid formulation of Ty21a typhoid vaccine in randomised controlled field trial. *Lancet* 1990; 336:891–4.

Lewis, J.E. Pertussis vaccine encephalopathy (letter) *Journal of the American Medical Association* 1990; 264:2383.

Libman, I. How many people in the US have IDDM? *Washington Post. Health.* April 1, 1997.

License application for pertussis vaccine withdrawn in Sweden. *Lancet* 1989; I:114.

Liebling, T., Rosenman, K.D., Pastides, H. *et al.* Cancer mortality among workers exposed to formaldehyde. *American Journal of Industrial Medicine* 1984; 5(6):423–428.

Lilic, D., Ghosh, S.K. Liver dysfunction and DNA antibodies after hepatitis B vaccination. *Lancet* 1994; 344:1292–1293.

Lin, F.Y., Ho, V.A., Khiem, H.B. *et al.* The efficacy of a Salmonella typhi Vi conjugate vaccine in two-to-five-year-old children. *New England Journal of Medicine* 2001; 344(17):1263–9.

Lo, K-J, Lee, S-D, Tsai, Y-T *et al.* Long-term immunogenicity and efficacy of hepatitis B vaccine in infants born to HBeAg-positive HBsAg carrier mothers. *Hepatology* 1988; 8:1647–1650.

Lockett, D. Internal memo. Advisory Committee on Immunization Practices, Centers for Disease Control. Oct. 19, 1995.

Lorentzen, J.C. Identification of arthritogenic adjuvants of self and foreign origin. *Scandinavian Journal of Immunology* 1999; 49:45–50.

Mack, T.M. Smallpox in Europe, 1950–1971. *J Infectious Disease* 1972; 125:161–169.

Maclaren, N., Atkinson, M. Is insulin-dependent diabetes mellitus environmentally induced? *New England Journal of Medicine* 1992; 327:348–349.

Mahurkar, S.D. *et al.* Dialysis dementia. *Lancet* 1973; 1:1412.

Makela, P.H., Sibakov, M., Herva, E., Henricksen, J. Pneumococcal vaccine and otitis media. *Lancet* 1980; 2:547–551.

Makela, P.H., Leinonen, M., Tukander, J., Karma, P. A study of the pneumococcal vaccine in prevention of clinically acute attacks of recurrent otitis media. *Review of Infectious Disease* 1981; 3:S124–S130.

Mangano, M.F., White, C.J. Varicella vaccine reflux. *Pediatrics* 1992; 89:353–354.

Marchant, D.D., Band, E., Froeschle, J.E., McVerry, P.H. Depression of anticapsular antibody after immunization with *Haemophilus influenzae* type b polysaccharide-diphtheria conjugate vaccine. *Pediatric Infectious Disease Journal* 1989; 8:508–511.

Marcuse, E.K. Why wait for DTP-E-IPV? *American Journal of Diseases of Children* 1989; 143:1006–1007.

Markowitz, L.E., Preblud, S.R., Orenstein, W.A. *et al.* Patterns of transmission in measles outbreaks in the United States, 1985–1986. *New England Journal of Medicine* 1989; 320:75–81.

Marks, J.S., Halpin, T.J. Guillain-Barré syndrome in recipients of A/New Jersey influenza vaccine. *JAMA* 1980; 243(42):2490–4.

Marshall, G.S., Wright, P.F., Fenichel, G.M., Karzon, D.T. Diffuse retinopathy following measles, mumps, and rubella vaccination. *Pediatrics* 1985; 76:989–991.

Martin, W.J. Stealth virus isolated from an autistic child. *Journal of Autism Disorders* 1995; 25:223–224.

Martin, W.J., Ahmed, K.N., Zeng, L.C. *et al.* African green monkey origin of the atypical cytopathic 'stealth virus' isolated from a patient with chronic fatigue syndrome. *Journal of Clinical and Diagnostic Virology* 1995; 4:93–103.

Martin, W.J. Severe stealth virus encephalopathy following chronic fatigue syndrome-like illness: Clinical and histopathological features. *Pathobiology* 1996; 64:1–8.

Martinez, E., Domingo, P. Evans's syndrome triggered by recombinant hepatitis B vaccine. *Clinical Infectious Diseases* 1992; 15:1051.

Martyn, C.N., Osmond, C., Edwardson, J.A. *et al.* Geographical relation between Alzheimer's disease and aluminium in drinking water. *Lancet* 1989; 339:59–62.

Matyszak, M.K. Inflammation in the CNS: balance between immunological privilege and immune responses. *Progress Neurobiology* 1998; 56:19–35.

McCloskey, B.P. The relation of prophylactic inoculations to the onset of poliomyelitis. *Lancet* 1950; 1:659–663.

McCloskey, B.P. Residual paralysis after poliomyelitis following recent inoculation. *Lancet* 1952; 1:1187–1189.

McComb, J.A., Dwyer, R.C. Passive-active immunization with tetanus immune globulin (human). *New England Journal of Medicine* 1963; 268:857–862.

McComb, J.A., Levine, L. Adult immunization: dosage reduction as a solution to increasing reactions to tetanus toxoid. *New England Journal of Medicine* 1961; 265:1152–1153.

McEwen, J. Early-onset reaction after measles vaccination: further Australian reports. *Medical Journal of Australia* 1983; 2:503–505.

McEwen, M. Should there be universal childhood vaccination against hepatitis B? *Pediatric Nursing* 1993; 19:447–452.

Medical Research Council Committee on Inoculation Procedures and Neurological Lesions. Poliomyelitis and prophylactic inoculation. *Lancet* 1956; 2:1223–1231.

Mendelsohn, R. The truth about immunizations. *The People's Doctor,* April 1978, p. 1.

Meselson, M., Guillemin, J., Hugh-Jones, M. *et al.* The Sverdlovsk anthrax outbreak of 1979. *Science.* 1994; 266:1202–1208.

Meyers, J.D. Congenital varicella in term infants: Risk reconsidered. *Journal of Infectious Disease* 1974; 129:215–217.

Michel, P., Commenges, D., Dartigues, J.F. *et al.* Study of the relationship between Alzheimer's disease and aluminum in drinking water [abstr]. *Neurobiology of Aging* 1990; 11:264.

Miller, D., Madge, N., Diamond, J., Wadsworth, J., Ross, E. Pertussis immunisation and serious acute neurological illnesses in children. *British Medical Journal* 1993, 307:1171–1176.

Miller, N.Z. *Vaccines: Are They Really Safe and Effective?* Santa Fe, NM: New Atlantean Press, 1992.

Miller, N.Z. *Immunization, Theory vs. Reality: Exposé on Vaccinations.* Santa Fe, NM: New Atlantean Press, 1996.

Milstien, J.B., Gross, T.P., Kuritsky, J.N. Adverse reactions reported following receipt of *Haemophilus influenzae* type b vaccine: an analysis after 1 year of marketing. *Pediatrics* 1987; 80:270–274.

Mink, C.M., Sirota, N.M., Nugent, S. Outbreak of pertussis in a fully immunized adolescent and adult population. *Archives of Pediatric and Adolescent Medicine* 1994; 148:153–157.

Monath, T.P. Facing up to re-emergence of urban yellow fever. *Lancet* 1999; 353:1541.

Monteyne, P., Andre, F.E. Is there a causal link between hepatitis B vaccination and multiple sclerosis? *Vaccine* 2000; 18(19):1994–2001.

Morgan, C.M., Cherry, J.D., Christenson, P. *et al.* A search for *Bordetella pertussis* infection in university students. *Clinical Infectious Diseases* 1992; 14:464–471.

Morris, J.A., Butler, H. Nature and frequency of adverse reaction following hepatitis B vaccine injection in children in New Zealand, 1985–1988. Submitted to the Vaccine Safety Committee, Institute of Medicine, Washington, DC, May 4, 1992.

Morris, K., Rylance, G. Guillain-Barré syndrome after measles, mumps, and rubella vaccine. *Lancet* 1994; 343:60.

Mortimer, E.A. Immunization against infectious disease. *Science* 1978; 200:902.

Mortimer, E.A., Kimura, M., Cherry, J.D. *et al.* Protective efficacy of the Takeda acellular pertussis vaccine combined with diphtheria and tetanus toxoids following household exposure of Japanese children. *American Journal of Diseases of Children* 1990; 144:899–904.

Moskowitz, R. The case against immunizations. *Journal of the American Institute of Homeopathy* 1983; 76:7–25.

Moskowitz, R. Postscript on immunizations: Directions for future research. *Journal of the American Institute of Homeopathy* 1985; 78:101–104.

Moskowitz, R. Immunizations: The other side. *Mothering* 1984; 31:32–38.

Moskowitz, R. Unvaccinated children. *Mothering* 1987; 34:34–39.

Moskowitz, R. Vaccination: A sacrament of modern medicine. *Journal of the American Institute of Homeopathy* 1991; 84:96–105.

Moxon, E.R. Modern vaccines: The scope of immunisation. *Lancet* 1990; 335(8687):448–451.

Moyer, P. Hepatitis B vaccine linked to onset of diabetes. *WebMD Medical News,* June 13, 2000; http://my.webmd.com/content/article/1728.58430

Mühlebach-Sponer, M., Zbinden, R., da Silva, V.A., Gnehm, H.E. Intrathecal rubella antibodies in an adolescent with Guillain-Barré syndrome after mumps measles rubella vaccination. *European Journal of Pediatrics* 1995; 154:166.

Mukinda, V.B.K. *et al.* Reemergence of human monkeypox in Zaire in 1996. *Lancet* 1997; 349:1449–50.

Munoz, J.J. *et al.* Elicitation of experimental encephalomyelitis in mice with the aid of pertussigen. *Cellular Immunology* 1984; 83(1):92–100.

Murphy, J. *What Every Parent Should Know About Childhood Immunization.* Boston: Earth Healing Products, 1993.

Murphy, T.V., Clements, J.F., Breedlove, J.A., Hansen, E.J. *et al.* Risk of subsequent disease among day-care contacts of patients with systemic *Haemophilus influenzae* type b disease. *New England Journal of Medicine* 1987; 316:5–10.

Murphy, T.V., White, K.E., Pastor, P., Gabriel, L. *et al.* Declining incidence of *Haemophilus influenzae* type b disease since introduction of vaccination. *Journal of the American Medical Association* 1993; 269:246–248.

Myers, M.G., Beckman. C.W., Vosdingh, R.A. *et al.* Primary immunization with tetanus and diphtheria toxoids: reaction rates and immunogenicity in older children and adults. *Journal of American Medical Association* 1982; 248:2478–2480.

Nabe-Nielsen, J., Walter, B. Unilateral deafness as a complication of the mumps, measles, and rubella vaccination. *British Medical Journal* 1988; 297:489.

Nadler, J.P. Multiple sclerosis and hepatitis B vaccination (letter). *Clinical Infectious Disease* 1993; 17:928–29.

Naruse, H., Miwata, H., Ozaki, T., Asano, Y. *et al.* Varicella infection complicated with meningitis after immunization. *Acta Paediatrica Japonica* 1993; 35:345–347.

Nass, M. Anthrax vaccine: Model of a response to the biologic warfare threat. *Infectious Disease Clinics of North America.* 1999; 13:187–208.

Nathanson, N., Langmuir, A.D. The Cutter incident: Poliomyelitis following formaldehyde-inactivated poliovirus vaccination in the United States during the spring of 1955. I. Background; II. Relationship of poliomyelitis to Cutter vaccine. *American Journal of Hygiene* 1963; 78:16–60.

National Institutes of Health. *Acellular pertussis vaccine trials: results and impact on U.S. public health.* June 3–5, 1996. Washington, D.C.

Naylor, G.J., Smith, A.H.W., McHarg, A. *et al.* Raised serum aluminum concentration in Alzheimer's disease. *Trace Elements and Medicine* 1989; 6:93–95.

Nelson, N., Levine, R.J., Albert, R.E. *et al.* Contribution of formaldehyde to respiratory cancer. *Environmental Health Perspectives* 1986; 70:23–35.

Neuzil, K.M., Griffin, M.R., Schaffner, W. Influenza vaccine: Issues and opportunities. *Infectious Disease Clinics of North America* 2001; 15(1):123–141.

Newcomb, E.W., III/DASG-ZH/DSN 223–5820, Possible anthrax vaccine-related reaction. Unclassified Navy document released June 11, 1998.

Nicholson, J.K.A., Holman, R.C., Jones, B.M. *et al.* The effect of measles-rubella vaccination on lymphocyte populations and subpopulations in HIV-infected and healthy individuals. *Journal of Acquired Immune Deficiency Syndromes* 1992; 5:528–537.

Nieminen, U., Peltola, H., Syrjala, M.T. *et al.* Acute thrombocytopenic purpura following measles, mumps and rubella vaccination: A report on 23 patients. *Acta Paediatrica* 1993; 82:267–270.

Nightingale, E.O. Recommendations for a national policy on poliomyelitis vaccination. *New England Journal of Medicine* 1977; 297:249–253.

Niu, M.T. Two-year review of hepatitis A vaccine safety: Data from the Vaccine Adverse Event Reporting System (VAERS). *Clinical Infectious Diseases* 1998; 26:1475–6.

Niu, M.T., Salive, M.E., Ellenberg, S.S. Neonatal deaths after hepatitis B vaccine. *Archives of Pediatric Adolescent Medicine* 1999; 153:1279–82.

Nkowane, B.M., Wassilak, S.G., Orenstein, W.A., Bart, K.J. Vaccine-associated paralytic poliomyelitis, United States: 1973 through 1984. *Journal of the American Medical Association* 1987; 257:1335–1340.

Noble, G.R., Bernier, R.H., Esber, E.C. *et al.* Acellular and whole-cell pertussis vaccines in Japan: Report of a visit by US scientists. *Journal of the American Medical Association* 1987; 257:1351–1356.

Norrby, R. Polyradiculitis in connection with vaccination against morbilli, parotitis and rubella. *Lakartidningen* 1984; 81:1636–1637.

Nowak, R. HIV-2 and SIV may be the same virus. *Journal of National Institute of Health Research* 1992; 4:38–40.

Nuorti, J.P., Butler, J.C., Farley, M.M. *et al.* Cigarette smoking and invasive pneumococcal disease. *New England Journal of Medicine* 2000; 342:681.

Odent, M.R., Culpin, E.F., Kimmel, T. Letter to the editor. Pertussis vaccination and asthma: Is there a link? *JAMA* 1994; 272:592–3.

Ogra, P.L., Ogra, S.S., Chiba, Y. *et al.* Rubella virus infection in juvenile rheumatoid arthritis. *Lancet* 1975; 1.

O'Leary, J. Testimony before Congressional Oversight Committee on Autism and Immunisation. April 6, 2000.

Olsen, J.H., Jensen, S.P., Hink, M. *et al.* Occupational formaldehyde exposure and increased nasal cancer risk in man. *International Journal of Cancer* 1984; 34(5):639–644.

Ortqvisdt, A., Hedlund, J., Burman, L.A. *et al.* Randomized trial of 23-valent pneumococcal capsular polysaccharide vaccine in the prevention of pneumonia in middle-aged and elderly people. *Lancet* 1998; 351:399.

Oski, F.A., Naiman, J.L. Effect of live measles vaccine on the platelet count. *New England Journal of Medicine* 1966; 275:352–356.

Osterholm, M.T., Pierson, L.M., White, K.E., Libby, T.A. *et al.* The risk of subsequent transmission of *Haemophilus influenzae* type b disease among children: Results of a two-year statewide prospective surveillance and contact survey. *New England Journal of Medicine* 1987; 316:1–5.

Osterholm, M.T., Rambeck, J.H., White, K.E. *et al.* Lack of efficacy of Haemophilus b polysaccharide vaccine in Minnesota. *Journal of the American Medical Association* 1988; 260:1423–1428.

Osvath, P., Csorba, S., Endre, L. *et al.* IgE levels of infants with complications after pertussis vaccination. *Allergologia et Immunopathologia* 1979; 7:111–114.

Otten, A., Helmke, K., Stief, T. *et al.* Mumps, mumps vaccination, islet cell antibodies and the first manifestation of diabetes mellitus type I. *Behring Institute Mitteilungen* 1984; 75:83–88.

Ovens, H. Anaphylaxis due to vaccination in the office. *Canadian Medical Association Journal* 1986; 134:369–370.

Papers presented at discussion held at the First International Conference on Live Poliovirus Vaccines. Washington, DC: PAHO, 1959: 324–325.

Pascal, L. What happens when science goes bad. Science and Technology Analysis Working Paper No 9, *Department of Science and Technology Studies,* University of Wollongong, Australia, December 1991.

Pasko, M.T., Beam, T.R. Persistence of anti-HBs among health care personnel immunized with hepatitis B vaccine. *American Journal of Public Health* 1990; 80:590–593.

Pate, J.E. *The School Performance of Post-*Haemophilus influenzae *Meningitic Children: Dallas. Final Report.* Education Resources Information Center, E.D. 067801, U.S. Office of Education, July 1, 1972.

Paterson, J., Boyd, W.E. Potency action: A preliminary study of the alteration of the Schick test by a homeopathic potency, *British Homœopathic Journal* 1941; 301–309.

Peltola, H., Kilpi, T., Anttila, M. Rapid disappearance of *Haemophilus influenzae* type b meningitis after routine childhood immunisation with conjugate vaccines. *Lancet* 1992; 340:592–594.

Pelton, S.I. Acute otitis media in the era of effective pneumococcal conjugate vaccine: will new pathogens emerge? *Vaccine* 2000; 19(Suppl. 1):S96–9.

Perl, D.P., Brody, A.R. Alzheimer's disease: X-ray spectrometric evidence of aluminium accumulation in neurofibrillary tangle-bearing neurones. *Science* 1980; 208:297–299.

Petersen, G.M., Silimperi, D.R., Rotter, J.I. *et al.* Genetic factors in *Haemophilus influenzae* type b disease susceptibility and antibody acquisition. *Journal of Pediatrics* 1987; 110:228–233.

Philip, R.N., Reinhard, K.R., Lackman, D.B. Observations on a mumps epidemic in a "virgin" population. *American Journal of Hygiene* 1959; 69:91–111.

Pichichero, M.E., Francis, A.B., Marsocci, S.M. *et al.* Comparison of a diphtheria and tetanus toxoids and bicomponent acellular pertussis vaccine with diphtheria and tetanus toxoids and whole-cell pertussis vaccine in infants. *American Journal of Diseases of Children* 1992; 147:295–299.

Pierchella, P., Petri, H., Rüping, K.W., Stary, A. [Urticaria after H-B-Vax injection due to hypersensitivity to thiomersal (merthiolate)] Urtikarielle Reaktion nach Injektion von H-B-Vax bei Sensibilisierung auf Thiomersal (Merthiolat). *Allergologie* 1987; 10:97–99.

Plotkin, S. Hell's fire and varicella-vaccine safety. *New England Journal of Medicine* 1988; 318:573–575.

Poliovaccine and AIDS origin link very unlikely. *Lancet* 1992; 340:1090–1091.

Pollard, J.D. Personal communication; University of Sydney, Sydney, Australia, 1993.

Pollard, J.D., Selby, G. Relapsing neuropathy due to tetanus toxoid: report of a case. *Journal of Neurological Science* 1978; 37:113–125.

Pollock, T.M., Morris, J. A 7-year survey of disorders attributed to vaccination in Northwest Thames Region. *Lancet* 1983; 1:753–757.

Popkin, B.M., Adair, L., Akin, J.S., Black, R. *et al. Pediatrics* 1990; 86:874–882.

Poullin, P., Gabriel, B. Thrombocytopenic purpura after recombinant hepatitis B vaccine. *Lancet* 1994; 344:1293.

Preblud, S.R. Varicella: complications and costs. *Pediatrics* 1986; 78 (suppl):728–735.

Rahn, D.W. Lyme vaccine issues and controversies. *Infectious Disease Clinics of North America* 2001; 15(1):171–87.

Read, S.J., Schapel, G.J., Pender, M.P. Acute transverse myelitis after tetanus toxoid vaccination. *Lancet* 1992; 339:1111–1112.

Recker, R.R., Blotcky, A.J., Leffler, J.A., Rack, E.P. Evidence for aluminium absorption from the gastrointestinal tract and bone deposition by aluminium carbonate ingestion with normal renal function. *Journal of Laboratory and Clinical Medicine* 1977; 90:810.

Regamey, R.H. Die Tetanus-Schutzimpfung. [Tetanus immunization in *Handbook of Immunization.*] In Herrlick, A., ed. *Handbuch der Schutzimpfungen.* Berlin: Springer, 1965.

Reilly, D., Taylor, M.A., Beattie, N.G.M. *et al.* Is evidence for homeopathy reproducible? *Lancet* 1994; 344:1601.

Reingold, A.L., Broome, C.V., Hightower, A.W. *et al.* Age-specific differences in duration of clinical protection after vaccination with meningococcal polysaccharide A vaccine. *Lancet* 1985; 2:114–8.

Relihan, M. Reactions to tetanus toxoid. *Journal of the Irish Medical Association* 1969; 62:430–434.

Relyveld, E.H. Current developments in production and testing of tetanus and diphtheria vaccines. In Mizrahi, A., Hertman, I., Klingberg, M., Kohn, A., eds. *New Developments with Human and Veterinary Vaccine*s. New York: Alan R. Liss, 1980.

Rennels, M.B., Edwards, K.M., Keyserling, H.L. *et al*. Safety and immunogenicity of heptavalent pneumococcal vaccine conjugated to CRM197 in United States infants. *Pediatrics* 1998; 101:604–11.

Report of the working group on the possible relationship between hepatitis B vaccination and the chronic fatigue syndrome. *Canadian Medical Journal* 1993; 149:314–319.

Reuman, P.D., Kubilis, P., Hurni, W. *et al*. The effect of age and weight on the response to formalin inactivated alum-adjuvanted hepatitis A vaccine in healthy adults. *Vaccine* 1997; 15:1157.

Ribera, E.F., Dutka, A.J. Polyneuropathy associated with administration of hepatitis B vaccine. *New England Journal of Medicine* 1983; 309:614–615.

Rietschel, R.L., Adams, R.M. Reactions to thimerosal in hepatitis B vaccines. *Dermatologic Clinics* 1990; 8:161–164.

Roberts, S.C. Vaccination and cot deaths in perspective. *Archives of Disease in Childhood* 1987; 62:754–759.

Rosa, F.W., Sever, J.L., Madden, D.L. Absence of antibody response to simian virus 40 after inoculation with killed-poliovirus vaccine of mothers of offspring with neurologic tumors. *New England Journal of Medicine* 1988; 318:1469.

Rosa, F.W., Sever, J.L., Madden, D.L. Response to: Neurologic tumors in offspring after inoculation of mothers with killed poliovirus vaccine. *New England Journal of Medicine* 1988; 319:1226.

Rosenblum, L.S., Villarino, M.E., Nainan, O.V. *et al*. Hepatitis A outbreak in a neonatal intensive care unit: risk factors for transmission and evidence of prolonged viral excretion among preterm infants. *Journal of Infectious Disease* 1991; 164:476–82.

Rosenthal, S.R. Developing new smallpox vaccines. *CDC, Emerging Infectious Diseases* 7,6, Nov-Dec 2001.

Ross, R.T. Varicella and remission of multiple sclerosis. *Lancet* 1991; 337:300.

Russell, S. Critical vaccines, medicine run low: Tetanus shots rationed – Congress probes shortage. *San Francisco Chronicle* Feb. 10, 2002.

Saarinen, U.M. Prolonged breast feeding as prophylaxis for recurrent otitis media. *Acta Paediatrica Scandinavica* 1982; 71:567–571.

Safranek, T.J., Lawrence, D.N., Kurland, L.T. *et al*. Reassessment of the association between Guillain-Barré syndrome and receipt of swine influenza vaccine in 1976–1977: results of a two-state study. Expert Neurology Group. *American Journal of Epidemiology* 1991; 133(9):940–51.

St. Geme, J.W., George, B.L., Bush, B.M. Exaggerated natural measles following attenuated virus immunization. *Pediatrics* 1976; 57:148–150.

Salk, J., Drucker, J. Noninfectious poliovirus vaccine. In Plotkin, S.A., and Mortimer, E.A. *Vaccines.* Philadelphia: W.B. Saunders, 1988.

Sankilampi, U., Honkanen, P.O., Pyhala, R. *et al.* Associations of prevaccination antibody levels with adverse reactions to pneumococcal and influenza vaccines administered simultaneously in the elderly. *Vaccine* 1997; 15:1133.

Santosham, M., Wolff, M., Reid, R., Hohenboken, M. *et al.* The efficacy in Navajo infants of a conjugate vaccine consisting of *Haemophilus influenzae* type b polysaccharide and Neisseria meningitidis outer-membrane protein complex. *New England Journal of Medicine* 1991; 324:1767–1772.

Saroso, J.S., Bahrawi, W., Witjaksono, H. *et al.* A controlled field trial of plain and aluminium hydroxide-adsorbed cholera vaccines in Surabaya, Indonesia, during 1973–75. *Bulletin of the World Health Organization* 1978; 56:619.

Schäfer, T., Enders, F., Przybilla, B. Sensitization to thimerosal and previous vaccination. *Contact Dermatitis* 1995; 32:114–116.

Schaffer, R. A case of oral polio vaccinosis. *Journal of the American Institute of Homeopathy* 1995; 88:33–34.

Schaffner, W., Fleet, W.F., Kilroy, A.W. *et al.* Polyneuropathy following rubella immunization: a follow-up study and review of the problem. *American Journal of Diseases of Children* 1974; 127:684–688.

Scheibner, V. *Vaccination: The Medical Assault on the Immune System.* Santa Fe, NM: New Atlantean Press, distributor, 1993.

Schick, B. Die Diphtherietoxin-Hauktreation des Menschen als Vorprobe der prophylaktischen Diphtherieheilseruminjektion. *Munchen Med. Schnschr.* 1913; 60: 2608–2610.

Schlenska, G.K. Unusual neurological complications following tetanus toxoid administration. *Journal of Neurology* 1977; 215:299–302.

Schneck, S.A. Vaccination with measles and central nervous system disease. *Neurology* 1968; 18 (Part 2):79–82.

Schoenbaum, S.C., Biano, S., Mack, T. Epidemiology of congenital rubella syndrome: The role of maternal parity. *Journal of the American Med Association* 1975; 233:151–155.

Schwartz, M. Monkey virus reportedly found in polio vaccine. *San Jose Mercury News* August 29, 1995.

Schwarz, G., Lanzer, G., List, W.F. Acute midbrain syndrome as an adverse reaction to tetanus immunization. *Intensive Care Medicine* 1988; 15:53–54.

Scott, J. The Treatment of Children by Acupuncture. Sussex, England: *Journal of Chinese Medicine* 1986.

Sell, S.H. *Haemophilus influenzae* type b meningitis: Manifestations and long-term sequelae. *Pediatric Infectious Disease Journal* 1987; 6:775–778.

Sell, S.H., Webb, W.W., Pate, J.E. *et al.* Psychological sequelae to bacterial meningitis: Two controlled studies. *Pediatrics* 1972; 49:212–217.

Shah, K., Nathanson, N. Human exposure to SV40. *American Journal of Epidemiology* 1976; 103:1–12.

Shapiro, E.D., Murphy, T.V., Wald, E.R., Brady, C.A. The protective efficacy of *Haemophilus influenzae* polysaccharide vaccine. *Journal of the American Medical Association* 1988; 260:1419–1422.

Shasby, D.M., Shope, T.C., Downs, H., Herrmann, K.L., Polkowski, J. Epidemic measles in a highly vaccinated population. *New England Journal of Medicine* 1977; 296:585–589.

Shaw, F.E., Graham, D.J., Guess, H.A., Milstien, J.B. *et al.* Postmarketing surveillance for neurologic adverse events reported after hepatitis B vaccination: Experience of the first three years. *American Journal of Epidemiology* 1988; 127:337–352.

Shepherd, D. *Homoeopathy in Epidemic Diseases*. Essex, England: Health Science Press, 1967.

Shimoni, Z., Dobrousin, A., Cohen, J. *et al.* Tetanus in an Immunised Patient. *British Medical Journal Online* (10/16/99); 319(7216):1049.

Shivapurkar, N., Harada, K., Reddy, J., et al. Presence of simian virus 40 DNA sequences in human lymphomas. *Lancet* 2002; 359(9309):851–2.

Shoenfeld, Y., Aron-Maor, A. Vaccination and autoimmunity – 'vaccinosis': a dangerous liaison. *Journal of Autoimmunity* 2000; 14(1):1–10.

Sieber, O.F., Fulginiti, V.A. Is adult immunization more appropriate than immunization of infants? *Pediatrics* 1977; 60:562–563.

Siegel, M., Fuerst, H.T., Peress, N.S. Comparative fetal mortality in maternal virus diseases: A prospective study on rubella, measles, mumps, chickenpox, and hepatitis. *New England Journal of Medicine* 1966; 274:768–771.

Silfverdal, S.A., Bodin, L., Hugosson, S., Garpenholt, O., Werner, B., Esbjorner, E., Lindquist, B., Olcen, P. Protective effect of breastfeeding on invasive Haemophilus influenzae infection: a case-control study in Swedish preschool children. *International Journal of Epidemiology* 1997; 26(2):443–50.

Silfverdal, S.A., Bodin, L., Olcen, P. Protective effect of breastfeeding: an ecologic study of Haemophilus influenzae meningitis and breastfeeding in a Swedish population. *International Journal of Epidemiology* 1999; 28(1):152–6.

Simberkoff, M.S., Cross, A.P., Al-Ibrahim, M. *et al.* Efficacy of pneumococcal vaccine in high-risk patients: Results of a Veterans Administration cooperative study. *New England Journal Med* 1986; 315:1316–1327.

Simpson, N., Simon, L., Randall, R. Parental refusal to have children immunised: extent and reasons. *British Medical Journal* 1995; 310:227.

Singh, V.K. Antibodies to myelin basic protein in children with autistic behavior. *Journal of Neuroimmunology* 1996; 66:143–145.

Singh, V.K., Sheren, X.L., Yang, V.C. Serological association of measles virus and human herpesvirus-6 with brain autoantibodies in autism. *Clinical Immunology and Immunopathology* 1998; 89(1):105–8.

Sirisanthana, T., Nelson, K.E., Ezzell, J.W., Abshire, T.G. Serological studies of patients with cutaneous and oral pharyngeal anthrax from northern Thailand. *Amer Journal Tropical Medicine Hygiene* 1988; 39:575–81.

Skudder, P.A., McCarroll, J.R. Current status of tetanus control: Importance of human tetanus-immune globulin. *Journal of the American Med Association* 1964; 188:625–627.

Slater, D.N., Underwood, J.C.E., Durrant, T.E. *et al.* Aluminium hydroxide granulomas: Light and electron microscopic studies and x-ray microanalysis. *British Journal of Dermatology* 1982; 107:103–108.

Sloyer, J.L., Ploussard, J.H., Howie, V.M. Efficacy of pneumococcal polysaccharide vaccine in preventing acute otitis media in infants in Huntsville, Alabama. *Review of Infectious Disease* 1981; 3:S119–S123.

Smith, H.H., Penna, H.A., Paoliello, A. Yellow fever vaccination with cultured virus (17D) without immune serum. *American Journal of Tropical Medicine* 1938; 18:437–68.

Smith, T. Active immunity produced by so-called balanced or neutral mixtures of diphtheria toxin and antitoxin. *Journal of Experimental Medicine* 1909; 11: 241–256.

Smits, T. The treatment and prevention of post-vaccinal disease. *Journal of the American Institute of Homeopathy* 1995; 88:27–32.

Sood, S.K., Daum, R.S. Disease caused by *Haemophilus influenzae* type b in the immediate period after homologous immunization: immunologic investigation. *Pediatrics* 1990; 85 (4 Pt 2):698–704.

Staak, M., Wirth, E. Zur problematik anaphylaktischer Reaktionen nach aktiver Tetanus-Immunisierung. [Anaphylactic reaction following active tetanus immunization.] *Deutsche Medizinische Wochenschrift* 1973; 98:110–111.

Stayner, L., Smith, A.B., Reeve, G. *et al.* Proportionate mortality study of workers in the garment industry exposed to formaldehyde. *American Journal of Industrial Medicine* 1985; 7(3):229–240.

Stayner, L.T., Elliott, L., Blade, L. *et al.* A retrospective cohort mortality study of workers exposed to formaldehyde in the garment industry. *American Journal of Industrial Medicine* 1988; 13(6):667–681.

Steele, L. Prevalence and patterns of Gulf War illness in Kansas veterans: Association of symptoms with characteristics of person, place, and time of military service. *American Journal of Epidemiology* 2000; 152:992–1002.

Stevens, C.E., Toy, P.T., Taylor, P.E., Lee, T., Yip, H. Prospects for control of hepatitis B virus infection: implications of childhood vaccination and long-term protection. *Pediatrics* 1992; 90:170–173.

Stewart, B.J.A., Prabhu, P.U. Reports of sensorineural deafness after measles, mumps, and rubella immunisation. *Archives of Diseases of Childhood* 1993; 69:153–154.

Stewart, T.A., Hultgren, B., Huang, X. *et al.* Induction of type 1 diabetes by interferon-alpha in transgenic mice. *Science* 1993; 260:1942–6.

Still, C.N. Aluminum neurotoxicity and Alzheimer's disease. *Journal of the South Carolina Medical Association* 1994; November:560–564.

Storsaeter, J., Olin, P., Renemar, B. *et al.* Mortality and morbidity from invasive bacterial infections during a clinical trial of acellular pertussis vaccines in Sweden. *Pediatric Infectious Disease Journal* 1988; 7:637–645.

Strebel, P.M., Aubert-Combiescu, A., Ion-Nedelcu, N. *et al.* Paralytic poliomyelitis in Romania, 1984–1992; evidence for a high risk of vaccine-associated disease and reintroduction of wild-virus infection. *American Journal of Epidemiology* 1994; 140:1111–1124.

Strebel, P.M., Ion-Nedelcu, N., Baughman, A.L. *et al.* Intramuscular injections within 30 days of immunization with oral poliovirus vaccine—a risk factor for vaccine-associated paralytic poliomyelitis. *New England Journal of Medicine* 1995; 332:500–506.

Street, A.C., Weddle, T.Z., Thomann, W.R., Lundbert, E.W. *et al.* Persistence of antibody in healthcare workers vaccinated against hepatitis B. *Infection Control and Hospital Epidemiology* 1990; 11:525–530.

Stuart, G. Reactions following vaccination against yellow fever. In *Yellow Fever.* WHO Monograph Series, No. 30, Geneva, 1956.

Subbarao, K. As good as the real thing. *Journal of Pediatrics* 2000; 136:139–141.

Subcommittee on National Security, Veterans Affairs and International Relations, House Committee on Government Reform. The department of defense anthrax vaccine immunization program: Unproven force protection, Feb. 17, 2000. *http://www.house.gov/reform/ns/reports/anthrax1.pdf.*

Sugiura, A., Yamada, A. Aseptic meningitis as a complication of mumps vaccination. *Pediatric Infectious Disease Journal* 1991; 10:209–213.

Sullivan-Bolyai, J.Z., Yin, E.K., Cox, P. *et al.* Impact of chickenpox on households of healthy children. *Pediatric Infectious Disease Journal* 1987; 6:33–35.

Sultz, H.A., Hart, B.A., Zielezny, M., Schlesinger, E.R. Is mumps virus an etiologic factor in juvenile diabetes mellitus? *Journal of Pediatrics* 1975; 86:654–656.

Sumaya, C.V., Gibbs, R.S. Immunization of pregnant women with influenza A/New Jersey/76 virus vaccine: Reactogenicity and immunogenicity in mother and infant. *Journal of Infectious Disease* 1979; 140:141–6.

Suruda, A., Schulte, P., Boeniger, M. *et al.* Cytogenetic effects of formaldehyde exposure in students of mortuary science. *Cancer Epidemiology, Biomarkers and Prevention* 1993; 2(5):453–460.

Sutter, R.W., Patriarca, P.A., Brogan, S., Malankar, P.G. *et al.* Outbreak of paralytic poliomyelitis in Oman: Evidence for widespread transmission among fully vaccinated children. *Lancet* 1991; 338:715–720.

Sutter, R.W., Patriarca, P.A., Suleiman, A.J.M. *et al.* Attributable risk of DTP (diphtheria and tetanus toxoids and pertussis vaccine) injection in provoking paralytic poliomyelitis during a large outbreak in Oman. *Journal of Infectious Disease* 1992; 165:444–449.

Swartz, T.A., Klingberg, W., Goldwasser, R.A. *et al.* Clinical manifestations, according to age, among females given HPV-77 duck rubella vaccine. *American Journal of Epidemiology* 1971; 94:246–251.

Swenberg, J.A., Kerns, W.D., Mitchell, R.I. *et al.* Induction of squamous cell carcinomas of the rat nasal cavity by inhalation exposure to formaldehyde vapor. *Cancer Research* 1980; 40(9):3398–3402.

Tager, A. Preliminary report on the treatment of recurrent herpes simplex with poliomyelitis vaccine (Sabin's). *Dermatologica* 1974; 149:253–255.

Taylor Reilly, D., Taylor Reilly, M., McSharry, C., Aitchinson, T. Is homoeopathy a placebo response? Controlled trial of homoeopathic potency, with pollen in hayfever as model. *Lancet* 1986; 2:881.

Teele, D.W., Pelton, S.I., Klein, J.O. Bacteriology of acute otitis media unresponsive to initial antimicrobial therapy. *Journal of Pediatrics* 1981; 98:537–539.

Tejani, A., Dobias, B., Sambursky, J. Long-term prognosis after *H. influenzae* meningitis: Prospective evaluation. *Developmental Medicine in Child Neurology* 1982; 24:338–343.

Thompson, G.R., Weiss, J.J., Shillis, J.L., Brackett, R.G. Intermittent arthritis following rubella vaccination: a three-year follow-up. *American Journal of Diseases of Children* 1973; 125:526–530.

Thompson, N.P., Montgomery, S.M., Pounder, R.E., Wakefield, A.J. Is measles vaccination a risk factor for inflammatory bowel disease? *Lancet* 1995; 345:1071–1073.

Thompson, N.P., Montgomery, S.M., Pounder, R.E., Wakefield, A.J. Measles vaccination as a risk factor for inflammatory bowel disease (letter). *Lancet* 1995(a); 345:1364.

Thornton, Russell. *American Indian Holocaust and Survival.* Norman: University of Oklahoma Press, 1987.

Tingle, A.J., Pot, C.H., Chantler, J.K. Prolonged arthritis, viraemia, hypogammaglobulinaemia, and failed seroconversion following rubella immunisation (letter). *Lancet* 1984; 1:1475–1476.

Tingle, A.J., Chantler, J.K., Pot, K.H. *et al.* Postpartum rubella immunization: association with development of prolonged arthritis, neurological sequelae, and chronic rubella viremia. *Journal of Infectious Diseases* 1985; 152:606–612.

Tingle, A.J., Allen, M., Petty, R.E. *et al.* Rubella-associated arthritis. I: Comparative study of joint manifestations associated with natural rubella infection and RA 27/3 rubella immunisation. *Annals of the Rheumatic Diseases* 1986; 45:110–114.

Topaloglu, H., Berker, M., Kansu, T. *et al.* Optic neuritis and myelitis after booster tetanus toxoid vaccination (letter). *Lancet* 1992; 339:178–179.

Toraldo, R., Tolone, C., Catalanotti, P. *et al.* Effect of measles-mumps-rubella vaccination on polymorphonuclear neutrophil functions in children. *Acta Paediatrica* 1992; 81:887–890.

Torch, W. Diphtheria-pertussis-tetanus (DPT) immunization: A potential cause of the sudden infant death syndrome (SIDS). *Neurology* 1982; 32:A169.

Torch, W. Characteristics of diphtheria-pertussis-tetanus (DPT) postvaccinal deaths and DPT-caused sudden infant death syndrome (SIDS): a review (abstract). *Neurology* 1986; 36 (Suppl. 1):148.

Tosti, A., Melino, M., Bardazzi, F. Systemic reactions due to thimerosal. *Contact Dermatitis* 1986; 15:187–188.

Tosti, A., Guerra, L., Bardazzi, F. Hyposensitizing therapy with standard antigenic extracts: An important source of thimerosal sensitization. *Contact Dermatitis* 1989; 20:173–176.

Tourbah, A., Gout, O., Liblau, R. *et al.* Encephalitis after hepatitis B vaccination: recurrent disseminated encephalitis or MS? *Neurology* 1999; 53(2):396–401.

Trevisani, F., Gattinara, G.C., Caraceni, P., Bernardi, M. *et al.* Transverse myelitis following hepatitis B vaccination. *Journal of Hepatology* 1993; 19:317–318.

Troen, P., Kaufman, S.A., Katz, K.H. Mercuric bichloride poisoning. *New England Journal of Medicine* 1951; 244:459–463.

Tsang, S.X., Switzer, W.M., Shanmugam, V., Johnson, J.A. et al. Evidence of Avian Leukosis Virus Subgroup E and Endogenous Avian Virus in Measles and Mumps Vaccines Derived from Chicken Cells: Investigation of Transmission to Vaccine Recipients. *Journal of Virology* 1999; 73(7):5843–5851.

Tucker, Jonathan B. *Scourge: The Once and Future Threat of Smallpox*. New York: Atlantic Monthly Press, 2001.

Tudela, P., Marti, S., Bonal, J. Systemic lupus erythematosus and vaccination against hepatitis B (letter). *Nephron* 1992; 62:236.

Tuomilehto, J., Virtala, E., Karvonen, M. *et al.* Increase in incidence of insulin-dependent diabetes mellitus among children in Finland. *International Journal of Epidemiology* 1995; 24:984–92.

Uhari, M., Rantala, H., Niemala, M. Cluster of childhood Guillain-Barré cases after an oral poliovaccine campaign. *Lancet* 1989; 2:440–441.

Ulhmann, V., Martin, C.M., Sheils, O., Pilkington, L. *et al.* Potential viral pathogenic mechanism for new variant inflammatory bowel disease. *Journal of Clinical Pathology: Molecular Pathology* 2002; 55:0–6.

Unwin, C., Blatchley, N., Coker, W., Ferry, S. *et al.* Health of UK servicemen who served in Persian Gulf War. *Lancet* 1999; 353:169–182.

Vadheim, C.M., Greenberg, D.P., Partridge, S., Jing, J. *et al.* Effectiveness and safety of an *Haemophilus influenzae* type b conjugate vaccine (PRP-T) in young infants. *Pediatrics* 1993; 92:272–279.

Vadheim, C.M., Greenberg, D.P., Eriksen, E., Hemenway, L. *et al.* Eradication of *Haemophilus influenzae* type b disease in Southern California. *Archives Pediatric and Adolescent Medicine* 1994; 148:51–56.

Valensi, J., Carlson, J., Van Nest, G. Systemic cytokin profiles in BALB/c mice immunized with trivalent influenza vaccine containing MF-59 oil emulsion and other advanced adjuvants. *Journal of Immunology* 1994; 153:4029–39.

Vaughan, T.L., Strader, C., Davis, S., Daling, J.R. Formaldehyde and cancers of the pharynx, sinus and nasal cavity: II. Residential exposures. *International Journal of Cancer* 1986; 38:685–688.

Vautier, G., Carty, J.E. Acute sero-positive rheumatoid arthritis occurring after hepatitis vaccination. *British Journal of Rheumatology* 1994; 33:991.

Vilchez, R.A., Madden, C.R., Kozinetz, C.A., et al. Association between simian virus 40 and non-Hodgkin lymphoma. *Lancet* 2002; 359(9309):817–23.

Vogt, T. Water quality and health—a study of a possible relationship between aluminium in drinking water and dementia. Sosiale og okonomiske studier 61:1–99. Oslo: Central Bureau of Statistics of Norway, 1986.

Waisbren, B.A. A commentary regarding personal observations of demyelinizing disease caused by viral vaccines, borrelia infections, and proteolytic enzymes. Paper submitted to the Vaccine Safety Committee, Institute of Medicine, Washington, DC, August 11, 1992.

Waisbren, B.A. Other side of the coin (letter). *Infectious Disease News* 1992; 5:2.

Wakefield, A.J., Ekbom, A., Dhillon, A.P. *et al.* Crohn's disease: pathogenesis and persistent measles virus infection. *Gastroenterology* 1995; 108:911–916.

Wakefield, A.J., Murch, S.H., Anthony, A. *et al.* Ileal-lymphoid-nodular hyperplasia, non-specific colitis, and pervasive developmental disorder in children. *Lancet* 1998; 351:637–41.

Wakefield, A.J. Testimony before Congressional Oversight Committee on Autism and Immunisation. April 6, 2000.

Walker, A.M., Jick, H., Perera, D.R. *et al.* Diphtheria-tetanus-pertussis immunization and sudden infant death syndrome. *Am Journal of Public Health* 1987; 77:945–951.

Walker, A.M. Does pertussis vaccine cause sudden infant death? Presentation for Institute of Medicine Workshop on Possible Adverse Consequences of Pertussis and Rubella Vaccines, Washington, DC, May 14, 1990. Unpublished.

Ward, J. Newer *Haemophilus influenzae* type b vaccines and passive prophylaxis. *Pediatric Infectious Disease Journal* 1987; 6:799–803.

Ward, J., Brenneman, G., Letson, G.W., Heyward, W.L. Alaska *H. Influenzae* Vaccine Study Group. Limited efficacy of a *H. influenzae* type b conjugate vaccine in Alaska Native infants. *New England Journal of Medicine* 1990; 323:1381–1387.

Waters & Krause Law Firm. Press release. October 17, 2001.

Waters *et al.* Yellow fever vaccination, avian leukosis virus, and cancer risk in man. *Science* 1972; 177:76–77.

Watson, B.M., Piercy, S.A., Plotkin, S.A., Starr, S.E. Modified chickenpox in children immunized with the Oka-Merck varicella vaccine. *Pediatrics* 1993; 91:17–22.

Weibel, R.E., Stokes, J., Buynak, E.B., Hilleman, M.R. Influence of age on clinical response to HPV-77 duck rubella vaccine. *Journal of American Medical Association* 1972; 222:805–807.

Weibel, R.E., Caserta, V., Benor, D.E., Evans, G. Acute encephalopathy followed by permanent brain injury or death associated with further attenuated measles vaccines: a review of claims submitted to the National Vaccine Injury Compensation Program. *Pediatrics* 1998; 101 (3 Pt 1): 383–7.

Weiner, L.B., Corwin, R.M., Nieburg, P.I., Feldman, H.A. A Measles outbreak among adolescents. *Journal of Pediatrics* 1977; 90:17–20.

Weiss, K.B., Gergen, P.J., Hodgson, T.A. An economic evaluation of asthma in the United States. *New England Journal of Medicine* 1992; 326:862–866.

Weller, T.H. Varicella and herpes zoster: changing concepts of the natural history, control, and importance of a not-so-benign virus. *New England Journal of Medicine* 1983; 309:1362–1367.

Wentz, K.R., Marcuse, E.K. Diphtheria-tetanus-pertussis vaccine and serious neurologic illness: an updated review of the epidemiologic evidence. *Pediatrics* 1991; 87:287–297.

Werne, J., Garrow, I. Fatal anaphylactic shock: occurrence in identical twins following second injection of diphtheria toxoid and pertussis antigen. *Journal of American Medical Association* 1946; 131:730–735.

Werzberger, A., Mensch, B., Kuter, B. *et al.* A controlled trial of a formalin-inactivated hepatitis A vaccine in healthy children. *New England Journal of Medicine* 1992; 327:453–7.

Wessel, D. Long incubation: A vaccine to prevent chickenpox is near; now, will it be used? *Wall Street Journal* Jan. 16, 1985:1.

White, F. Measles vaccine-associated encephalitis in Canada. *Lancet* 1983, 2:683–684.

White, W.G., Barnes, G.M., Barker, E. *et al.* Reactions to tetanus toxoid. *Journal of Hygiene* 1983; 71:283–297.

WHO. Monkeypox, Zaire. *Widy Epidemiol Aec*, 1996; 71:326.

Williams, R.P. *Bacillus anthracis* and other spore-forming bacilli. In: Braude, A.I., Davis, L.E., Fierer, J., eds. *Infectious Disease and Medical Microbiology*. Philadelphia, PA: WB Saunders Co; 1986:270–78.

Williams, W.W., Hickson, M.A., Kane, M.A. *et al.* Immunization policies and vaccine coverage among adults: the risk for missed opportunities. *Annals of Internal Medicine* 1988; 108:616–625.

Wilson, M.E. Travel-related vaccines. *Infectious Disease Clinics of North America* 2001; 15(1):231–51.

Wise, R.P., Kiminyo, K.P., Salive, M.E. Hair loss after routine immunizations. *JAMA* 1997; 278(14):1176–8.

Wise, R.P., Salive, M.E., Braun, M.M. *et al.* Postlicensure safety surveillance for Varicella vaccine. *JAMA* 2000; 284(10):1271–9.

Wyatt, H.V. Provocation of poliomyelitis by multiple injections. *Transactions of the Royal Society of Tropical Medicine & Hygiene* 1985; 79:355–358.

Yamanishi, K., Matsunaga, Y., Ogino, T., Lopetegui, P. Biochemical transformation of mouse cells by varicella-zoster virus. *Journal Gen Virology* 1981; 56:421–430.

Yazbak, F.E. Autism: Is there a vaccine connection? Part I Vaccination after delivery. 1999
www.garynull.com/documents/autism99b.htm

Yazbak, F.E. Autism: Is there a vaccine connection? Part II Vaccination around pregnancy. 1999(a)
www.garynull.com/documents/autism99b2.htm

Zhen, H.N., Zhang, X., Bu, X.Y. *et al.* Expression of the simian virus 40 large tumor antigen (Tag) and formation of Tag-p53 and Tag-pRb complexes in human brain tumors. *Cancer* 1999; 86(10):2124–32.

Zupanska, B., Lawkowicz, W., Gorska, B. et al. British Journal of Haematology 1976; 34:511–520.

INDEX

SV40 and, 58–60
varicella vaccine and, 154
Centers for Disease Control (CDC),
  19, 20
Central nervous system disorders
  hepatitis B vaccine and, 175–76
  measles vaccine and, 205–6
  mercury and, 76
  rubella vaccine and, 219–20
  tetanus vaccine and, 259–60
CFS. *See* Chronic fatigue syndrome
Chemicals, 69–77
Cherry, James, 21, 22
Chickenpox (varicella), 147–55
  complications of, 148–49
  facts about, 154
  personal strategy for, 155
  symptoms of, 147
  treatment of, 147
  vaccine, 149–50
  vaccine efficacy, 150–52
  vaccine reactions, 152–54
Children. *See also individual*
    vaccines
  breastfeeding and, 109–10, 114
  emotional health of, 118
  nutrition and, 110–12
  supplements for, 112–17
  vaccines for, 3–5
Chinese medicine. *See* Traditional
    Chinese Medicine
Cholera, 266
Chronic fatigue syndrome (CFS),
    65
Colostrum, 114–15, 116
Compulsory vaccinations, 38,
    119–22, 252
Contaminated vaccines, 57–67
Copper, 115, 116
Cowpox, 248
Crohn's disease, 210
Crowe, William, 143
Cytokines, 114, 115

D
Deafness, 208
Deaths
  hepatitis B vaccine and, 173
  measles vaccine and, 40
  meningococcal vaccine and, 196
  pertussis vaccine and, 20,
    229–31, 233
  polio vaccine and, 40
  smallpox vaccine and, 251
  varicella vaccine and, 152–53
DHA, 113, 116
Diabetes, 55–56
  hepatitis B vaccine and, 56,
    176–77
  Hib vaccine and, 55, 193
  mumps/MMR vaccine and,
    214–15
Diphtheria, 100–102, 157–58,
    231–33. *See also* DTP/DTaP
    vaccine
Doctors. *See also* Pediatricians
  changing view of, 14
  vaccine industry's influence on,
    14, 19
DTP/DTaP vaccine, 224–25. *See*
    also Diphtheria; Pertussis;
    Tetanus
  chemicals in, 69–70
  efficacy of, 225–26
  reactions to, 20–23, 51, 226–33

E
Eczema, 251
Elderly
  flu vaccine and, 159–60
  tetanus and, 256
Emotional health, 118
Encephalitis
  pertussis vaccine and, 232–33
  small pox vaccine and, 251
  yellow fever vaccine and, 270
Encephalopathy

finding practitioner of, 91
history of, 87–88
at home, 90
immune system and, 86–87, 89, 92
success of, 86, 87–88
theoretical framework of, 88–89
treating reactions with, 92–94

I

IgA, 109, 114, 115
Immigration, 129–30
Immune system
  breastfeeding and, 109–10, 114
  emotional health and, 118
  homeopathy and, 86–87, 89, 92
  living conditions and, 117–18
  measles vaccine and, 210–11
  nutrition and, 110–17
  strengthening, 13, 93–94, 109–18
  suppression of, by vaccines, 13, 49–54, 89–90, 92, 210–11
Inflammatory bowel disease, 210
Influenza. *See* Flu
Informed choice, making, 5, 15–17, 28–34, 35–36, 275–78
Institute of Medicine Vaccine Safety Committee, 39–44, 53
Interferon gamma, 53
IPV. *See* Polio
IVGG therapy, 94

J

Jenner, Edward, 96

K

Kidneys
  aluminum and, 73
  mercury and, 75

L

Lactoferrin, 114, 115

Lederle Laboratories, 19, 21
Legal requirements, 119–32
  compulsory vaccination and, 38, 119–22, 252
  exemptions from, 120, 121–29
  immigration and, 129–30
  military service and, 130–32
  travel and, 270
Leucocytes, 114, 115
Living conditions, effect of, 117–18
Lyme disease, 181–84
  facts about, 184
  personal strategy for, 184
  vaccine, 182
  vaccine reactions, 182–84
Lysozyme, 114, 115

M

Martin, John, 20, 65
Measles, 201–11. *See also* MMR vaccine; Rubella (German measles)
  atypical, 210
  facts about, 211
  homeopathic prevention of, 97, 99
  incidence of, 202
  living conditions and, 117–18
  personal strategy for, 211
  vaccine efficacy, 202–4
  vaccine reactions, 47–48, 50, 204–11
Medical exemptions, 122–23
Mendelsohn, Robert, 79
Meningitis, 185–99
  Haemophilus influenzae type B (Hib), 51, 52, 55, 110, 185–94
  homeopathic prevention of, 98
  meningococcal vaccine, 195–96
  mumps/MMR vaccine and, 213–14
  pneumococcal vaccine, 197–99

vaccine reactions, 240–43
Pregnancy
  flu vaccine and, 162
  rubella and, 215–17, 221–22
PRP vaccine, 188–90, 192

R

Reactions, 37–56. *See also*
  individual vaccines and
  reactions
  long-term (delayed), 42, 44–56
  short-term (immediate), 38–44
  treating, with natural medicine,
    92–94
  underreporting of, 37–38,
    135–36
  Vaccine Safety Committee's
    findings on, 39–44
Religious exemptions, 123–27
Retroviruses, 60
Rotavirus vaccine, 23–24
Rubella (German measles), 215–22.
  See also MMR vaccine
  facts about, 221
  incidence of, 217
  personal strategy for, 221–22
  vaccine efficacy, 217–18
  vaccine reactions, 47, 218–21

S

Sabin, Albert, 58
Saccharides, 114, 115
Schick test, 100–102
Schools, dealing with, 119,
    120–21, 277. *See also*
    Exemptions
Seizures
  DTP vaccine and, 20–21, 226–27
  Hib vaccine and, 192–93
Shake, recipe for, 116
SIDS, 22, 229–31
SIV, 60–65
Smallpox, 245–54

as biological weapon, 247, 250
facts about, 253
further reading on, 254
history of, 245
homeopathic prevention of,
    98–99
personal strategy for, 253–54
symptoms of, 246–47
vaccine, 248
vaccine efficacy, 248–49
vaccine reactions, 38, 92, 251–53
vaccine strategy, 250
SmithKline Beecham, 19, 54–55,
    182–84
Squalene, 142–43
Stealth virus, 65
Streptococcus pneumonia, 197–99
Stress, 118
Studies, conventional vaccine,
    79–83
Supplements, 112–17
SV40 virus, 58–60, 242–43

T

TCM. *See* Traditional Chinese
    Medicine
Terrorism
  anthrax and, 137, 138–39
  smallpox and, 247, 250
Tetanus, 255–63. *See also*
    DTP/DTaP vaccine
  diphtheria and, 157–58
  facts about, 261
  incidence of, 255–56
  personal strategy for, 261–63
  symptoms of, 255
  treatment of, 90, 255
  vaccine, 256–57
  vaccine efficacy, 257–58
  vaccine reactions, 258–60
Tetanus immune globulin (TIG),
    257, 258, 260, 262, 263
Thimerosal (mercury), 74–76

Thrombocytopenia
  Hib vaccine and, 193
  MMR vaccine and, 40, 209, 221
Thrombocytopenic purpura, 174
Thuja occidentalis, 92, 252
TIG. *See* Tetanus immune globulin
Traditional Chinese Medicine
  (TCM), 86, 90–91
Trans fats, 112–13
Transverse myelitis, 192
Travel, 265–71
  hepatitis A and, 266–67
  typhoid and, 267–68
  yellow fever and, 269–71
Typhoid, 267–68

V

Vaccine Adverse Event Reporting
  System (VAERS), 39, 136
Vaccine-associated paralytic
  poliomyelitis (VAPP), 240–41
Vaccine Compensation
  Amendments, 39
Vaccine manufacturers. *See also*
  individual companies
  governmental protection of, 8,
    38–39
  influence of, on doctors, 14, 19
  influence of, on government,
    19–20, 24
  motivations of, 8–9, 11–12,
    18–19, 24–25, 274
Vaccines. *See also* Reactions;
  individual diseases and
  vaccines
  adult, 6–7
  alternative, 95–107
  checklist of, 281
  chemicals in, 69–77
  childhood, 3–5
  combining, 34
  commonly refused, 30

compulsory, 119–22
contaminated, 57–67
conventional studies of, 79–83
development of new, 273–75
efficacy of, 79–81
history of, 96
making informed choice about, 5,
  15–17, 28–34, 35–36,
  275–78
schedule of, 279, 280
timing, 31–34
Vaccine Safety Committee. *See*
  Institute of Medicine Vaccine
  Safety Committee
Vaccinia immune globulin (VIG),
  252, 254
Vaccinia virus, 248
Vaccinosis, 252
VAERS. *See* Vaccine Adverse Event
  Reporting System
Varicella. *See* Chickenpox
Variola. *See* Smallpox
VIG. *See* Vaccinia immune globulin
Viruses, 57–67. *See also individual*
  viruses
Vitamins
  A, 115
  C, 115
  E, 113, 116

W

Wakefield, Andrew, 20, 45, 46
Whooping cough. *See* Pertussis
Wistar Institute, 63
Wound care, 262–63
Wyeth-Ayerst Laboratories, 24–25

Y

Yellow fever, 67, 87–88, 269–71

Z

Zinc, 115, 116